Modern Statistics for Modern Biology

If you are a biologist and want to get the best out of the powerful methods of modern computational statistics, this is your book. You can visualize and analyze your own data, apply unsupervised and supervised learning, integrate datasets, apply hypothesis testing, and make publication-quality figures using the power of R/Bioconductor and ggplot2.

This book will teach you "cooking from scratch", from raw data to beautiful illuminating output, as you learn to write your own scripts in the R language and to use advanced statistics packages from CRAN and Bioconductor. It covers a broad range of basic and advanced topics important in the analysis of high-throughput biological data, including principal component analysis and multidimensional scaling, clustering, multiple testing, unsupervised and supervised learning, resampling, the pitfalls of experimental design, and power simulations using Monte Carlo, and it even reaches networks, trees, spatial statistics, image data, and microbial ecology. Using a minimum of mathematical notation, it builds understanding from well-chosen examples, simulation, visualization, and above all hands-on interaction with data and code.

- **R package msmb** contains complete code and the example datasets, allowing students to recreate all examples, figures, and results in the book

- **Solutions, slides, and dynamic material** available on the course website

- Introduces **methods on a "need to know" basis**, so students tackle biological questions immediately and understand motivation for the methods

- **Real-life examples** done from scratch, guiding students through realistic complexities and building practical intuition

- Includes a wrap-up chapter that explains the complete workflow from design of experiments to analysis of results, identifying **common pitfalls with big data**

- All figures and results generated by the code in the book, demonstrating how **reproducible research** works

SUSAN HOLMES is Professor of Statistics at Stanford University, California. She specializes in exploring and visualizing multidomain biological data, using computational statistics to draw inferences in microbiology, immunology and cancer biology. She has published over 100 research papers, and has been a key developer of software for the multivariate analyses of complex heterogeneous data. She was the Breiman Lecturer at NIPS 2016, has been named a Fields Institute fellow, and is currently a fellow at the Center for the Advances Study of the Behavioral Sciences.

WOLFGANG HUBER is Research Group Leader and Senior Scientist at the European Molecular Biological Laboratory, where he develops computational methods for new biotechnologies and applies them to biological discovery. He has published over 150 research papers in functional genomics, cancer and statistical methods. He is a founding member of the open-source bioinformatics software collaboration Bioconductor and has co-authored two books on Bioconductor.

Modern Statistics for Modern Biology

Susan Holmes
Stanford University, California

Wolfgang Huber
European Molecular Biology Laboratory

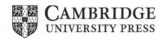

CAMBRIDGE
UNIVERSITY PRESS

CAMBRIDGE
UNIVERSITY PRESS

University Printing House, Cambridge CB2 8BS, United Kingdom

One Liberty Plaza, 20th Floor, New York, NY 10006, USA

477 Williamstown Road, Port Melbourne, VIC 3207, Australia

314–321, 3rd Floor, Plot 3, Splendor Forum, Jasola District Centre, New Delhi – 110025, India

79 Anson Road, #06–04/06, Singapore 079906

Cambridge University Press is part of the University of Cambridge.

It furthers the University's mission by disseminating knowledge in the pursuit of education, learning, and research at the highest international levels of excellence.

www.cambridge.org
Information on this title: www.cambridge.org/9781108705295
DOI: 10.1017/9781108551441

First published 2019

Printed and bound in Great Britain by Clays Ltd, Elcograf S.p.A.

A catalogue record for this publication is available from the British Library.

Library of Congress Cataloging-in-Publication Data

ISBN 978-1-108-70529-5 Paperback

Additional resources for this publication at www.cambridge.org/msmb

Image credits for chapter openers: Chapter 1, Wikicommons;
Chapter 4, xkcd.com/1347; Chapter 5, mikedabell/iStock/Getty Images;
Chapter 6, extract from xkcd.com/882/; Chapter 7, The Matrix: scene 291 Close on Computer Screen © Warner Bros.; Chapter 8, xkcd.com/1725;
Chapter 9, Robert Orchard/Moment/Getty Images;
Chapter 13, University of Adelaide Library: Rare Books and Special Collections, R.A. Fisher Digital Archive,
http://hdl.handle.net/2440/81670.

For Sonia, Sara, Agnès, Johnny, Camille
. . . and the "girls" who make me love the life sciences

For Alexander

Contents

Expanded Contents

13 Design of High-Throughput Experiments and Their Analyses

Introduction

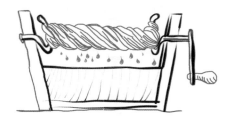

What is happening in biological data analysis?

The two instances of *modern* in the title of this book reflect the two major recent revolutions in biological data analysis:

- Biology, formerly a science with sparse, often only qualitative data, has turned into a field whose production of quantitative data is on par with high energy physics or astronomy and whose data are wildly more heterogeneous and complex.
- Statistics, a field that in the 20th century had become an application ground for probability theory and calculus, often taught loaded with notation and a perceived heavy emphasis on hypothesis testing, has been transformed by the ubiquity of computers and of data in machine-readable form. Exploratory data analysis, visualization, resampling, simulations, pragmatic hybridizations of Bayesian ideas and methods with frequentist data analysis have become parts of the toolset.

The aim of this book is to enable scientists working in biological research to quickly learn many of the important ideas and methods that they need to make the best of their experiments and of other available data. The book takes a hands-on approach. The narrative in each chapter is driven by classes of questions or by certain data types. Methods and theory are introduced on a need-to-know basis. We don't try to systematically deduce from first principles. The book will often throw readers into the water and help them to swim to their destinations despite missing details.

By no means will this book replace systematic training in underlying theory: probability, linear algebra, software engineering, databases, multivariate statistics. Such training takes many semesters of coursework. Perhaps the book will whet your appetite to engage more deeply with one of these fields.

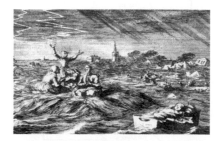

"Watersnood in Groningen, 1686", Jan Luyken, 1698. Rijksmuseum Amsterdam.

The challenge: heterogeneity

Any biological system or organism is composed of tens of thousands of components, which can be in different states and interact in multiple ways. Modern biology aims to understand such systems by acquiring comprehensive – and this means high dimensional – data in their temporal and spatial context, with multiple covariates and interactions. Dealing with this complexity will be our primary challenge. We face real,

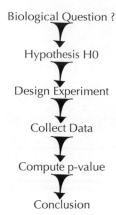

Figure 1: The hypothesis testing paradigm recommended by R.A. Fisher starts with the formulation of a null hypothesis and the design of an experiment before the collection of any data. We could think in a similarly schematic way about model fitting – just replace *Hypothesis H0* by *Parametric Model* and *Compute p-value* by *Fit Parameters*.

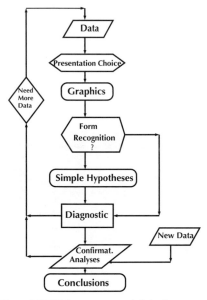

Figure 2: J.W. Tukey recommended starting any analysis with the data and wrote: "No catalogue of techniques can convey a willingness to look for what can be seen, whether or not anticipated" (Holmes Junca, 1985).

---

[1] Called *non-identifiability* or *overfitting*.

biological complexity as well as the complexities and heterogeneities of the data we are able to acquire with our always imperfect instruments.

Biological data come in all sorts of shapes: nucleic acid and protein sequences, rectangular tables of counts, multiple tables, continuous variables, batch factors, phenotypic images, spatial coordinates. Besides data measured in lab experiments, there are clinical data, longitudinal information, environmental measurements, networks, lineage trees, annotation from biological databases in free text or controlled vocabularies, . . .

> "Homogeneous data are all alike;
> all heterogeneous data are heterogeneous in their own way."
> The Anna Karenina principle

It is this heterogeneity that motivates our choice of R and Bioconductor as the computational platform for this book – more on this below.

What's in this book?

Figure 1 outlines a sequential view of statistical data analysis. Motivated by the groundbreaking work on significance and hypothesis testing in the 1930s by Fisher (1935) and Neyman and Pearson (1936), it is well amenable to mathematical formalism, especially the part where we compute the distribution of test statistics under a hypothesis (null or alternative), or where we set up distributional assumptions and search for analytical approximations.

Real scientific discovery rarely works in the caricature manner of Figure 1. Tukey (1977) emphasized two separate approaches. The first he termed **exploratory data analysis (EDA)**. EDA uses the data themselves to decide how to conduct the statistical analysis. EDA is built on simple tools for plotting data. EDA is complemented by **confirmatory data analysis** (CDA): robust inferential methods that do not rely on complex assumptions to reach scientific conclusions. Tukey recommended an iterative approach, schematized in Figure 2, that enables us to see the data at different resolutions and from different perspectives. This enables the refinement of our understanding of the data.

Biology in the late 1990s raised the **large-p small-n problem**: consider a gene expression dataset for $n = 200$ patient samples on $p = 20,000$ genes. If we want to construct a regression or classification model that "predicts" a clinical variable, for instance the disease type or outcome, from the 20,000 genes, or features, we immediately run into problems,[1] since the number of model parameters would have to be orders of magnitudes larger than the number of replicate measurements n. At least, this is the case for common models, say, an ordinary linear model. Statisticians realized that they could remedy the situation by requiring sparsity through the use of regularization techniques (Hastie et al., 2008), i.e., by requiring many of the potential parameters to be either zero or at least close to it.

A generalization of the sparsity principle is attained by invoking one of the most powerful recent ideas in high-dimensional statistics, which goes by the name **empirical Bayes**: we don't try to learn the parameters associated with each feature from scratch, but rather use the fact that some or all of them will be similar, or even the same, across all features, or across groups of related features. There are several important book-long treatments (Efron, 2010) of the subject of large scale inference so essential in modern estimation and hypotheses testing.

This icon signals that we are using a Monte Carlo approximation method, so-called because it harnesses randomness, similar to the randomness of casino games. Ironically, for many casino games the probability of winning is not known analytically, and casinos use their own empirical data to evaluate the odds.

Simulations play an essential role in this book, as *many of the results we need* escape the reach of standard analytic approaches. In other words, simulations liberate us from only considering methods that are analytically tractable, and from worrying about the appropriateness of simplifying assumptions or approximations.

In this book, we try to cover the full range of these developments and their applications to current biological research. We cover many different types of data that modern biologists have to deal with, including RNA-Seq, flow cytometry, taxa abundances, imaging data and single-cell measurements. We assume no prior training in statistics. However, you'll need some familiarity with R and willingness to engage in mathematical and analytical thinking.

Generative models are our basic building blocks. In order to draw conclusions about complicated data *it tends to be useful* to have simple models for the data generated in this or that situation. We do this through the *top-down* use of probability theory and deduction, which we introduce in Chapter 1. We will use examples from immunology and DNA analysis to describe useful generative models for biological data: binomial, multinomial and Poisson random variables.

Once we know how data would look under a certain model, we can start working our way backwards: given some data, what model is most likely able to explain it? This *bottom-up* approach is the core of **statistical inference**, and we explain it in Chapter 2.

We saw the primary role of **graphics** in Tukey's scheme (Figure 2), and so we'll learn how to visualize our data in Chapter 3. We'll use the grammar of graphics and *ggplot2*.

Real biological data often have more complex distributional properties than what we could cover in Chapter 1. We'll use **mixtures** that we explore in Chapter 4; these enable us to build realistic models for heterogeneous biological data and provide solid foundations for choosing appropriate variance-stabilizing transformations.

The large, matrix-like ($n \times p$) datasets in biology lend themselves to **clustering**: once we define a distance measure between matrix rows (the features), we can cluster and group the genes by similarity of their expression patterns, and similarly, for the columns (the patient samples). We'll cover clustering in Chapter 5. Since clustering relies only on distances, we can even apply it to data that are not matrix-shaped, as long as there are objects and distances defined between them.

Further following the path of EDA, we cover the most fundamental unsupervised analysis method for simple matrices – **principal component analysis** – in Chapter 7. We turn to more heterogeneous data that combine multiple data types in Chapter 9. There, we'll see nonlinear unsupervised methods for counts from single-cell data. We'll also address how to use generalizations of the multivariate approaches covered in Chapter 7 to combinations of categorical variables and multiple assays recorded on the same observational units.

The basic **hypothesis testing** workflow outlined in Figure 1 is explained in Chapter 6. We take the opportunity to apply it to one of the most common queries to $n \times p$ datasets: which of the genes (features) are *associated with* a certain property of the samples, say, disease type or outcome? However, conventional significance thresholds would lead to lots of spurious associations: with a false positive rate of $\alpha = 0.05$ we expect $p\alpha = 1000$ false positives if none of the $p = 20,000$ features has a true association. Therefore we also need to deal with multiple testing.

One of the most fruitful ideas in statistics is that of **variance decomposition**, or analysis of variance (ANOVA). We'll explore this, in the framework of linear models and generalized linear models, in Chapter 8. Since we'll draw our example data from an RNA-Seq experiment, this gives us also an opportunity to discuss models for such count data and concepts of *robustness*.

Nothing in biology makes sense except in the light of evolution,[2] and evolutionary relationships are usefully encoded in phylogenetic trees. We'll explore **networks and trees** in Chapter 10.

A rich source of data in biology are **images**, and in Chapter 11 we reinforce our willingness to do EDA on all sorts of heterogeneous data types by exploring feature extraction from images and spatial statistics.

Finally in Chapter 12, we will look at **statistical learning**, i.e., training an algorithm to distinguish between different types of objects depending on their multidimensional feature vector. We'll start simple with low-dimensional feature vectors and linear methods, and then explore classification in high-dimensional settings.

We wrap up in Chapter 13 with considerations on **good practices** in the design of experiments and in data analysis. For this we'll use and reflect on what we have learned in the course of the preceding chapters.

Computational tools for modern biologists

As we'll see over and over again, the analysis approaches, tools and choices to be made are manifold. Our work can only be validated by keeping careful records in a reproducible script format. **R and Bioconductor** provide such a platform.

Although we are tackling many different types of data, questions and statistical methods hands-on, we maintain a consistent computational approach by keeping all the computation under one roof: the R programming language and statistical environment, enhanced by the biological data infrastructure and specialized method packages from the Bioconductor project. The reader will have to start by acquiring some familiarity with R before using the book.

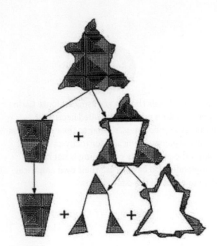

Figure 3: Analyzing data is not a one-step process. Each step involves visualizing and decomposing some of the complexity in the data. Tukey's iterative data structuration can be conceptualized as Total $= V_1 + V_2 + V_3$.

[2] Theodosius Dobzhansky – see *Nothing in Biology Makes Sense Except in the Light of Evolution* on Wikipedia.

R code is a major component of this book. It is how we make the textual explanations explicit. Virtually every data visualization in the book is produced with code that is shown to equip the reader to replicate all of these figures, and any other results shown (as in Figure 4).

Even if you have a basic familiarity with R, don't worry if you don't immediately understand every line of code in the book. Although we have tried to keep the code explicit and give tips and hints at potentially challenging places, there will be instances where

- there is a function invoked that you have not seen before and that does something mysterious, or
- there is a complicated R expression that you don't understand (perhaps involving `apply` functions or data manipulations from the *dplyr* package).

Don't panic. For the mysterious function, have a look at its manual page. Open up RStudio and use the object explorer to look at the variables that go into the expression, and those that come out. Split up the expression to look at intermediate values.

In Chapters 1 and 2, we use *base* R functionality for light doses of plotting and data manipulation. As we successively need more sophisticated operations, we introduce the *ggplot2* way of making graphics in Chapter 3. Besides the powerful grammar of graphics concepts that enable us to produce sophisticated plots using only a limited set of instructions, this implies using the *dplyr* way of data manipulation. Sometimes, we have traded in what would be convoluted loop and `lapply` constructs for elegant *dplyr* expressions, but this requires you to get acquainted with some novelties such as *tibbles*, the `group_by` function and pipes (`%>%`).

Why R and Bioconductor?

There are many reasons why we have chosen to present all analyses on the R (Ihaka and Gentleman, 1996) and Bioconductor (Huber et al., 2015) platforms.

Cutting edge solutions The availability of over 10,000 packages ensures that almost all statistical methods are available, including the most recent developments. Moreover, there are implementations of or interfaces to many methods from computer science, mathematics, machine learning, data management, visualization and internet technologies. This puts thousands of person-years of work by experts at your fingertips.

Open source and community-owned R and Bioconductor have been built collaboratively by a large community of developers. They are constantly tried and tested by thousands of users.

Data input and wrangling Bioconductor packages support the reading of many of the data types and formats produced by measurement instruments used in modern biology, as well as the needed technology-specific "preprocessing" routines. The community is actively keeping these up-to-date with the rapid developments in the instrument market.

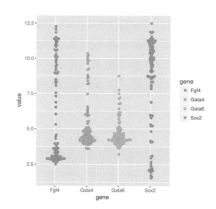

Figure 4: Comparison of the expression levels of four developmentally important genes in the mouse embryo. Each dot represents the measurement from one single cell; the *y*-axis is on a logarithmic scale (arbitrary units). The code that produces this plot is given in Chapter 3.

Download R and Rstudio to follow the code in the book.

Simulation   There are random number generators for every known statistical distribution and powerful numeric routines for linear algebra, optimization, etc.

Visualization and presentation   R can make attractive, publication-quality graphics. We've dedicated Chapter 3 to this, and practice data visualization extensively throughout the book.

Easy-to-use interactive development environment   RStudio is easy and fun to use and helps with all aspects of programming in R. It is an essential tool in following the iterative approach to data analysis schematized in Figure 2.

Reproducibility   As an equivalent to the laboratory notebook that is standard good practice in labwork, we advocate the use of a computational diary written in the R markdown format. We use the *knitr* package to convert R markdown into easy-to-read and shareable HTML or PDF documents. These can even become full-fledged scientific articles or supplements. Together with a version control system, R markdown helps with tracking changes.

Collaborative environment   R markdown enables the creation of websites containing code, text, figures and tables with a minimum of work.

Rich data structures   The Bioconductor project has defined specialized data containers to represent complex biological datasets. These help to keep your data consistent, safe and easy to use.

Interoperability and distributed development   Bioconductor in particular contains packages from diverse authors that cover a wide range of functionalities but still interoperate because of the common data containers.

Documentation   Many R packages come with excellent documentation in their function manual pages and vignettes. The vignettes are usually the best starting point in a package, as they give you a high-level narrative account of what the package does, whereas the manual pages give detailed information on input, output and inner workings of each function. There are online tutorials, forums and mailing lists for many aspects of working with R and Bioconductor.

High-level language   R is an interpreted high-level language. Its roots in LISP and its functional programming features mean that code is data and can be computed on, which enables efficient programming and is fun. These features facilitate constructing powerful domain-specific languages.[3] R is not a fixed language – throughout its history, it has been actively evolving and is constantly improving.

---

[3] Examples include R's formula interface, the grammar of graphics in *ggplot2*, the data manipulation functionality of *dplyr* and R markdown.

How to read this book

The printed version of this book is supplemented by an online version in HTML at `http://bios221.stanford.edu/book/` and `http://www.huber.embl.de/msmb/`.

The online sites:

- provide the `.R` files and all needed input data files;
- are constantly updated to fix typos and make clarifications;

- have up-to-date code that will run with contemporary versions of R, CRAN packages and Bioconductor.

Please do not despair if code in the printed version of the book is not working with your version of R and all the packages. Please do not despair if code on the website is not working with an older version of R or packages. This is fully to be expected and no reason for worries, surprises or even comments. We recommend following the installation instructions – which includes getting the right, matching versions of everything – on the webpage.

The chapters in the book build upon each other, but they are reasonably self-contained, so they can also be studied selectively. Each chapter starts with a section on motivations and goals. Questions in the text help you check whether you are following along. The text contains extensive R code examples throughout. You don't need to scrape R code from the HTML or manually copy it from the book. Use the R files (extension .R) on the book's website. Each chapter concludes with a summary of the main points and a set of exercises. The book ends with an index and a concordance section, which should be useful when looking for specific topics.

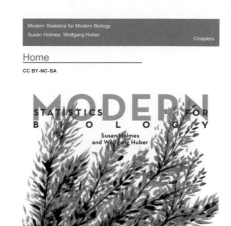

Figure 5: The online version provides the text in HTML, data files and up-to-date code.

Notes and extra information appear under the devil icon: this is the devil who looks after the details.

Chapter 1

Generative Models for Discrete Data

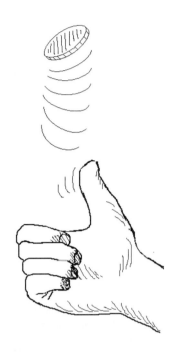

In molecular biology, many situations involve counting events: how many codons use a certain spelling, how many reads of DNA match a reference, how many CG digrams are observed in a DNA sequence. These counts give us *discrete* variables, as opposed to quantities such as mass and intensity that are measured on *continuous* scales.

If we know the rules that the mechanisms under study follow, even if the outcomes are random, we can generate the probabilities of any events we are interested in by computations and standard probability laws. This is a *top-down* approach based upon **deduction** and our knowledge of how to manipulate probabilities. In Chapter 2, you will see how to combine this with data-driven (*bottom-up*) statistical modeling.

1.1   Goals for this chapter

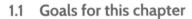

In this chapter we will:

- Learn how to obtain the probabilities of all possible outcomes from a given model and see how we can compare the theoretical frequencies with those observed in real data.
- Explore a complete example of how to use the Poisson distribution to analyze data on epitope detection.
- See how we can experiment with the most useful generative models for discrete data: Poisson, binomial, multinomial.
- Use the R functions for computing probabilities and counting rare events.
- Generate random numbers from specified distributions.

1.2   A real example

Let's dive into a real example, where we know the probability model for the process. We are told that mutations along the genome of HIV (human immunodeficiency virus) occur at random with a rate of 5×10^{-4} per nucleotide per replication cycle. This means

[1] We will give more details later about this type of probability distribution.

that after one cycle, the number of mutations in a genome of about $10^4 = 10,000$ nucleotides will follow a *Poisson distribution*[1] with rate 5. What does that tell us?

This **probability model** predicts that the number of mutations over one replication cycle will be close to 5, and that the variability of this estimate is $\sqrt{5}$ (the standard error). We now have baseline reference values for both the number of mutations we expect to see in a typical HIV strain and its variability.

In fact, we can deduce even more detailed information. If we want to know how often 3 mutations could occur under the Poisson(5) model, we can use an R function to generate the probability of seeing $x = 3$ events, taking the value of the *rate parameter* of the Poisson distribution, called lambda (λ), to be 5.

Greek letters such as λ and μ often denote important parameters that characterize the probability distributions we use.

```
dpois(x = 3, lambda = 5)
## [1] 0.1403739
```

This says the chance of seeing exactly three events is around 0.14, or about 1 in 7.

If we want to generate the probabilities of all values from 0 to 12, we do not need to write a loop. We can simply set the first argument to be the **vector** of these 13 values, using R's sequence operator, the colon " : ". We can see the probabilities by plotting them (Figure 1.1). As with this figure, most figures in the margins of this book are created by the code shown in the text.

Note how the output from R is formatted: the first line begins with the first item in the vector, hence the [1], and the second line begins with the 9th item, hence the [9]. This helps you keep track of elements in long vectors. The term *vector* is R parlance for an ordered list of elements of the same type (in this case, numbers).

```
0:12
##  [1]  0  1  2  3  4  5  6  7  8  9 10 11 12
dpois(x = 0:12, lambda = 5)
##  [1] 0.0067 0.0337 0.0842 0.1404 0.1755 0.1755 0.1462 0.1044
##  [9] 0.0653 0.0363 0.0181 0.0082 0.0034
barplot(dpois(0:12, 5), names.arg = 0:12, col = "red")
```

Mathematical theory tells us that the Poisson probability of seeing the value x is given by the formula $e^{-\lambda}\lambda^x/x!$. In this book, we'll discuss theory from time to time, but give preference to displaying concrete numeric examples and visualizations like Figure 1.1.

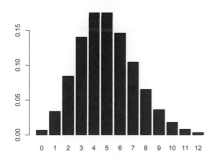

Figure 1.1: Probabilities of seeing 0,1,2,...,12 mutations, as modeled by the Poisson(5) distribution. The plot shows that we will often see four or five mutations but rarely as many as 12. The distribution continues to higher numbers (13, . . .), but the probabilities will be successively smaller, and here we don't visualize them.

The Poisson distribution is a good model for rare events such as mutations. Other useful probability models for **discrete events** are the Bernoulli, binomial and multinomial distributions. We will explore these models in this chapter.

1.3   Using discrete probability models

A point mutation can either occur or not; it is a binary event. The two possible outcomes (yes, no) are called the **levels** of the categorical variable.

Not all events are binary. For example, the genotypes in a diploid organism can take three levels (AA, Aa, aa).

Think of a **categorical variable** as having different alternative values. These are the levels, similar to the different alternatives at a gene locus: alleles.

Sometimes the number of levels in a categorical variable is very large; examples include the number of different types of bacteria in a biological sample (hundreds or thousands) and the number of codons formed of three nucleotides (64 levels).

When we measure a categorical variable on a sample, we often want to tally the frequencies of the different levels in a vector of counts. R has a special encoding for categorical variables and calls them **factors**.[2] Here we capture the different blood genotypes for 19 subjects in a vector that we tabulate.

[2] R makes sure that the factor variable will not accept other, "illegal" values, and this is useful for keeping your calculations safe.

```
genotype = c("AA","AO","BB","AO","OO","AO","AA","BO","BO",
            "AO","BB","AO","BO","AB","OO","AB","BB","AO","AO")
table(genotype)
## genotype
## AA AB AO BB BO OO
##  2  2  7  3  3  2
```

`c()` is a basic function. It collates elements of the same type into a vector. In this code, the elements of `genotype` are character strings.

On creating a factor, R automatically detects the levels. You can access the levels with the `levels` function.

```
genotypeF = factor(genotype)
levels(genotypeF)
## [1] "AA" "AB" "AO" "BB" "BO" "OO"
table(genotypeF)
## genotypeF
## AA AB AO BB BO OO
##  2  2  7  3  3  2
```

▶ **Question 1.1** What if you want to create a factor that has some levels not yet in your data? ◀

▶ **Solution 1.1** Look at the manual page of the `factor` function. □

It is not obvious from the output of the `table` function that the input was a factor; however, if there had been another level with no instances, the table would also have contained that level, with a zero count.

If the order in which the data are observed doesn't matter, we call the random variable **exchangeable**. In that case, all the information available in the factor is summarized by the counts of the factor levels. We then say that the vector of frequencies is **sufficient** to capture all the relevant information in the data, thus providing an effective way of compressing the data.

1.3.1 Bernoulli trials

Tossing a coin has two possible outcomes. This simple experiment, called a Bernoulli trial, is modeled using a so-called Bernoulli random variable. Understanding this building block will take you surprisingly far. We can use it to build more complex models.

Let's try a few experiments to see what some of these random variables look like. We use special R functions tailored to generate outcomes for each type of distribution. They all start with the letter `r`, which stands for random, followed by a specification of the model, here `rbinom`, where `binom` is the abbreviation used for binomial.

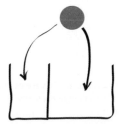

Figure 1.2: Two possible events with unequal probabilities. We model this by a **Bernoulli distribution** with probability parameter $p = \frac{2}{3}$.

Suppose we want to simulate a sequence of 15 fair coin tosses. To get the outcome of 15 Bernoulli trials with a probability of success equal to 0.5 (a fair coin), we write

```
rbinom(15, prob = 0.5, size = 1)
## [1] 1 1 0 0 1 1 0 0 0 1 0 1 0 1 0
```

[3] For R functions, parameters are also called *arguments*.

We use the `rbinom` function with a specific set of **parameters**:[3] the first parameter is the number of trials we want to observe; here we chose 15. We designate by `prob` the probability of success. By `size=1` we declare that each individual trial consists of just one single coin toss.

▶ Question **1.2** Repeat this function call a number of times. Why isn't the answer always the same?   ◀

[4] We call such events **complementary**.

Success and failure can have unequal probabilities in a Bernoulli trial, as long as the probabilities sum to one.[4] To simulate 12 trials of throwing a ball into the two boxes shown in Figure 1.2, with probability of falling in the right-hand box $\frac{2}{3}$ and in the left-hand box $\frac{1}{3}$, we write

```
rbinom(12, prob = 2/3, size = 1)
## [1] 1 1 1 1 0 0 1 1 0 0 1 0
```

The 1 indicates success, meaning that the ball fell in the right-hand box; 0 means the ball fell in the left-hand box.

1.3.2 Binomial success counts

[5] The exchangeability property.

If we only care how many balls go in the right-hand box, then the order of the throws doesn't matter,[5] and we can get this number by just taking the sum of the cells in the output vector. Therefore, instead of the binary vector we saw above, we only need to report a single number. In R, we can do this using one call to the `rbinom` function with the parameter `size` set to 12.

Two outcomes and a size of 1 or more make this experiment a binomial trial. If the size is 1, then this is the special case of the Bernoulli trial.

```
rbinom(1, prob = 2/3, size = 12)
## [1] 5
```

This output tells us how many of the 12 balls fell into the right-hand box (the outcome that has probability $\frac{2}{3}$).

[6] One situation in which trials are exchangeable is if they are independent of each other.

We use a random two-box model when we have only two possible outcomes, such as heads or tails, success or failure, CpG or non-CpG, M or F, Y = pyrimidine or R = purine, diseased or healthy, true or false. We only need to specify the probability, p, of "success" because "failure" (the *complementary* event) will occur with probability $1 - p$. When looking at the results of several such trials, if they are exchangeable,[6] we record only the number of successes. Therefore, SSSSSFSSSSFFFSF is summarized as (#Successes=10, #Failures=5), or as $x = 10$, $n = 15$.

The number of successes in 15 Bernoulli trials with a probability of success of 0.3 is called a **binomial** random variable or a random variable that follows the $B(15, 0.3)$

distribution. To generate samples, we use a call to the `rbinom` function with the number of trials set to 15.

```
set.seed(235569515)
rbinom(1, prob = 0.3, size = 15)
## [1] 5
```

▶ Question 1.3 Repeat this function call 10 times. What seems to be the most common outcome? ◀

What does `set.seed` do here?

▶ Solution 1.3 The most frequent value is 4. In fact, the theoretical proportion of times that we expect 4 to appear is the value of the probability that $X = 4$ if X follows $B(15, 0.3)$. □

The complete **probability mass distribution** is available by typing

```
probabilities = dbinom(0:15, prob = 0.3, size = 15)
round(probabilities, 2)
##  [1] 0.00 0.03 0.09 0.17 0.22 0.21 0.15 0.08 0.03 0.01 0.00 0.00
## [13] 0.00 0.00 0.00 0.00
```

The function `round` keeps the number of printed decimal digits down to two.

We can produce a barplot of this distribution, shown in Figure 1.3.

```
barplot(probabilities, names.arg = 0:15, col = "red")
```

The number of trials is the number we input to R as the `size` parameter and is often written n, while the probability of success is p. Mathematical theory tells us that for X distributed as a binomial distribution with parameters (n, p), written $X \sim B(n, p)$, the probability of seeing $X = k$ successes is

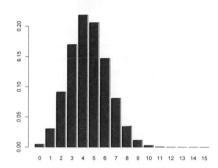

Figure 1.3: Theoretical distribution of $B(15, 0.3)$. The highest bar is at $x = 4$. We have chosen to represent theoretical values in red throughout.

$$P(X = k) = \frac{n \times (n - 1) \ldots (n - k + 1)}{k \times (k - 1) \ldots 1} \, p^k \, (1 - p)^{n-k}$$

$$= \frac{n!}{(n - k)!k!} \, p^k \, (1 - p)^{n-k}$$

$$= \binom{n}{k} \, p^k \, (1 - p)^{n-k}.$$

▶ Question 1.4 What is the output of the formula for $k = 3, p = \frac{2}{3}, n = 4$? ◀

1.3.3 Poisson distributions

The special notation $\binom{n}{k}$, called the binomial coefficient and read "n choose k", is a shortcut for $\frac{n!}{(n-k)!k!}$.

When the probability of success p is small and the number of trials n is large, the binomial distribution $B(n, p)$ can be faithfully approximated by a simpler distribution, the **Poisson distribution** with rate parameter $\lambda = np$. We used this fact, and this distribution, in the HIV example (Figure 1.1).

▶ Question 1.5 What is the probability mass distribution of observing $0:12$ mutations in a genome of $n = 10^4$ nucleotides, when the probability of mutation is $p = 5 \times 10^{-4}$ per nucleotide? Is it similar when modeled by the binomial $B(n, p)$ distribution and by the Poisson($\lambda = np$) distribution? ◀

[7] This formula appeared briefly in Section 1.2.

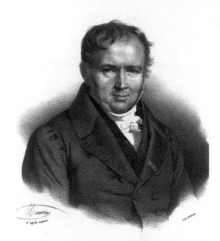

Figure 1.4: Simeon Poisson, after whom the Poisson distribution is named (this is why it always has a capital letter, except in our R code). Image credit: Wikicommons.

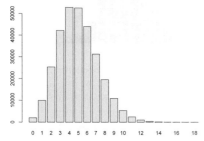

Figure 1.5: Simulated distribution of B(10,000, 10^{-4}) for 300,000 simulations.

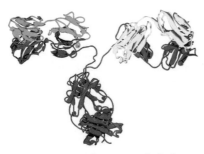

Figure 1.6: Structure of an IgG2 antibody showing several immunoglobulin domains in color. Image credit: Wikicommons.

[8] **Enzyme-linked immunosorbent assay** – see *ELISA* on Wikipedia.

Note that, unlike the binomial distribution, the Poisson does not depend on two separate parameters n and p, but only on their product np. As in the case of the binomial distribution, we also have a mathematical formula for computing Poisson probabilities:[7]

$$P(X = k) = \frac{\lambda^k \, e^{-\lambda}}{k!}.$$

For instance, let's take $\lambda = 5$ and compute $P(X = 3)$.

```
5^3 * exp(-5) / factorial(3)
## [1] 0.1403739
```

which we can compare with what we computed in Section 1.2 using `dpois`.

▶ Task Simulate a mutation process along 10,000 positions with a mutation rate of 5×10^{-4} and count the number of mutations. Repeat this many times and plot the distribution with the `barplot` function (see Figure 1.5). ◀

```
rbinom(1, prob = 5e-4, size = 10000)
## [1] 6
simulations = rbinom(n = 300000, prob = 5e-4, size = 10000)
barplot(table(simulations), col = "lavender")
```

Now we are ready to use probability calculations in a case study.

1.3.4 A generative model for epitope detection

When testing certain pharmaceutical compounds, it is important to detect proteins that provoke an allergic reaction. The molecular sites that are responsible for such reactions are called **epitopes**. The technical definition of an epitope is:

> A specific portion of a macromolecular antigen to which an antibody binds. In the case of a protein antigen recognized by a T cell, the epitope or determinant is the peptide portion or site that binds to a major histocompatibility complex (MHC) molecule for recognition by the T-cell receptor (TCR).

And in case you're not so familar with immunology: an antibody (as schematized in Figure 1.6) is a type of protein made by certain white blood cells in response to a foreign substance in the body, which is called an antigen.

An antibody binds (with more or less specificity) to its antigen. The purpose of the binding is to help destroy the antigen. Antibodies can work in several ways, depending on the nature of the antigen. Some antibodies destroy antigens directly. Others help recruit white blood cells to destroy the antigen. An epitope, also known as antigenic determinant, is the part of an antigen that is recognized by the immune system, specifically by antibodies, B cells or T cells.

ELISA error model with known parameters

ELISA[8] assays are used to detect specific epitopes at different positions along a protein. Suppose the following facts hold for an ELISA assay we are using:

- The baseline noise level per position, or more precisely the false positive rate, is 1%. This is the probability of declaring a hit – we think we have an epitope – when there is none. We write this as $P(\text{declare epitope} \mid \text{no epitope})$.
- The protein is tested at 100 different positions, supposed to be independent.

We are going to examine a collection of 50 patient samples.

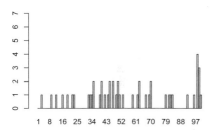

We read the vertical bar in expressions such as $X \mid Y$ as "given" or "conditional on". Thus, "X happens **conditional on** Y being the case".

One patient's data

The data for one patient's assay look like this:

```
##    [1] 0 0 0 0 0 0 0 0 0 0 0 0 0 0 0 0 0 0 0 0 0 0 0 0 0 1 0 0 0 0 0 0 0
##   [30] 0 0 0 0 0 0 0 0 0 0 0 0 0 0 0 0 0 0 0 0 0 0 0 0 0 0 0 0 0
##   [59] 0 0 0 0 0 0 0 0 0 0 0 0 0 0 0 0 0 0 0 0 0 0 0 0 0 0 0 0 0
##   [88] 0 0 0 0 0 0 0 0 0 0 0 0 0
```

where the 1 signifies a hit (and thus the potential for an allergic reaction), and the zeros signify no reaction at that position.

▶ Task Verify by simulation that the sum of 50 independent Bernoulli variables with $p = 0.01$ is – to good enough approximation – the same as a Poisson(0.5) random variable. ◀

Results from the 50 assays

We're going to study the data for all 50 patients tallied at each of the 100 positions. If there are no allergic reactions, the false positive rate of 1% means that for a single patient, each individual position has a probability of 1 in 100 of being a 1. So, after tallying 50 patients, we expect at any given position the sum of the 50 observed 0/1 variables to have a Poisson distribution with parameter 0.5. A typical set of false positives across the 100 positions may look like Figure 1.7.

Now suppose we see actual data as shown in Figure 1.8, loaded as an R object `e100` from the data file `e100.RData`.

```
load("../data/e100.RData")
barplot(e100, ylim = c(0, 7), width = 0.7, xlim = c(-0.5, 100.5),
    names.arg = seq(along = e100), col = "darkolivegreen")
```

The spike in Figure 1.8 is striking. *What are the chances of seeing a value as large as 7, if no epitope is present?*

If we look for the probability of seeing a number as big as 7 (or larger) when considering one Poisson(0.5) random variable, the answer can be calculated in closed form as

$$P(X \geqslant 7) = \sum_{k=7}^{\infty} P(X = k).$$

This is, of course, the same as $1 - P(X \leqslant 6)$. The probability $P(X \leqslant 6)$ is the so-called **cumulative distribution function** at 6, and R has the function `ppois` for computing it, which we can use in either of the following two ways.[9]

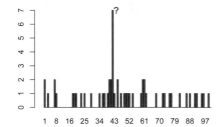

Figure 1.7: Plot of typical data from our generative model for the background, i.e., for the false positive hits: 100 positions along the protein, at each position the count is drawn from a Poisson(0.5) random variable.

Figure 1.8: Output of the ELISA array results for 50 patients at the 100 positions.

[9] Besides the convenience of not having to do the subtraction from 1, the second of these computations also tends to be more accurate when the probability is small. This has to do with limitations of floating point arithmetic.

```
1 - ppois(6, 0.5)
## [1] 1.00238e-06
ppois(6, 0.5, lower.tail = FALSE)
## [1] 1.00238e-06
```

▶ Task Check the manual page of `ppois` for the meaning of `lower.tail`.   ◀

[10] Mathematicians often call small numbers (and children) epsilons.

We denote this number by ϵ, the Greek letter epsilon.[10] We have shown that the probability of seeing a count as large as 7, assuming no epitope reactions, is

$$\epsilon = P(X \geqslant 7) = 1 - P(X \leqslant 6) \simeq 10^{-6}. \tag{1.1}$$

Extreme value analysis for the Poisson distribution

Stop! The above calculation is *not* the correct computation in this case.

▶ Question **1.6** Can you spot the flaw in our reasoning if we want to compute the probability that we observe these data if there is no epitope?   ◀

▶ Solution **1.6** We looked at all 100 positions, looked for the largest value and found that it was 7. Due to this initial selection from all positions, a value as large as 7 is more likely to occur than if we looked at only one position from the start.   □

So instead of asking what the chances are of seeing a Poisson(0.5) as large as 7, we should ask ourselves, what are the chances that the maximum of 100 Poisson(0.5) trials is as large as 7? We will use **extreme value analysis** here.[11] We order the data values $x_1, x_2, \ldots, x_{100}$ and rename them $x_{(1)}, x_{(2)}, x_{(3)}, \ldots, x_{(100)}$, so that $x_{(1)}$ denotes the smallest and $x_{(100)}$ the largest of the counts over the 100 positions. Together, $x_{(1)}, \ldots, x_{(100)}$ are called the **rank statistic** of this sample of 100 values.

[11] Meaning that we're interested in the behavior of the very large or very small values of a random distribution, for instance the maximum or the minimum. This approach allows us to compute the probability of **rare events**.

The maximum value being as large as 7 is the *complementary event* of having all 100 counts be smaller than or equal to 6. Two complementary events have probabilities that sum to 1. Because the positions are supposed to be independent, we can now do the computation:

$$
\begin{aligned}
P(x_{(100)} \geqslant 7) &= 1 - P(x_{(100)} \leqslant 6) \\
&= 1 - P(x_{(1)} \leqslant 6) \times P(x_{(2)} \leqslant 6) \times \cdots \times P(x_{(100)} \leqslant 6) \\
&= 1 - P(x_1 \leqslant 6) \times P(x_2 \leqslant 6) \times \cdots \times P(x_{100} \leqslant 6) \\
&= 1 - \prod_{i=1}^{100} P(x_i \leqslant 6).
\end{aligned}
$$

The notation $\prod$ is just a compact way of writing the product of a series of terms, analogous to $\sum$ for sums.

Because we suppose these 100 events are independent, we can use our result from (1.1) above:

$$\prod_{i=1}^{100} P(x_i \leqslant 6) = (P(x_i \leqslant 6))^{100} = (1 - \epsilon)^{100}.$$

Actually calculating the numbers

We could just let R compute the value of this number, $(1-\epsilon)^{100}$. For those interested in how such calculations can be simplified through approximation, we give some details here. These can be skipped on a first reading.

We recall from above that $\epsilon \simeq 10^{-6}$ is much smaller than 1. To compute the value of $(1-\epsilon)^{100}$ approximately, we can use the binomial theorem and drop all "higher order" terms of ϵ, i.e., all terms with $\epsilon^2, \epsilon^3, \ldots$, because they are negligibly small compared to the remaining ("leading") terms:

$$(1-\epsilon)^n = \sum_{k=0}^{n} \binom{n}{k} 1^{n-k} (-\epsilon)^k = 1 - n\epsilon + \binom{n}{2}\epsilon^2 - \binom{n}{3}\epsilon^3 + \ldots \simeq 1 - n\epsilon \simeq 1 - 10^{-4}.$$

Another, equivalent, route uses the approximation $e^{-\epsilon} \simeq 1 - \epsilon$, which is the same as $\log(1-\epsilon) \simeq -\epsilon$. Hence

$$(1-\epsilon)^{100} = e^{\log\left((1-\epsilon)^{100}\right)} = e^{100\log(1-\epsilon)} \simeq e^{-100\epsilon} \simeq e^{-10^{-4}} \simeq 1 - 10^{-4}.$$

Thus the correct probability of seeing a number of hits as large as or larger than 7 in the 100 positions, if there is no epitope, is about 100 times the probability we wrongly calculated previously.

Both computed probabilities 10^{-6} and 10^{-4} are smaller than standard significance thresholds (say, 0.05, 0.01 or 0.001). The decision to reject the null hypothesis of no epitope would have been the same. However, if one has to stand up in court and defend the p-value to eight significant digits, as in some forensic court cases,[12] that is another matter. The adjusted p-value that takes into account the multiplicity of the test is the one that should be reported, and we will return to this important issue in Chapter 6.

[12] This occurred in the examination of the forensic evidence in the O.J. Simpson case.

Computing probabilities by simulation

In the case we just saw, the theoretical probability calculation was simple and we could figure out the result by an explicit calculation. In practice, things tend to be more complicated, and we do better to compute our probabilities using the **Monte Carlo** method: a computer simulation based on our generative model that finds the probabilities of the events we're interested in. The intuition here is to generate Figure 1.7 again and again, and observe how often the biggest spike is 7 or larger.

We generate 100,000 instances of picking the maximum from 100 Poisson distributed numbers.

We'll often use Monte Carlo simulations such as these instead of analytical calculations.

```
maxes = replicate(100000, {
  max(rpois(100, 0.5))
})
table(maxes)
## maxes
##     1     2     3     4     5     6     7     9
##     7 23028 60840 14364  1604   141    15     1
```

The expression `maxes >= 7` evaluates into a logical vector of the same length as `maxes`, but with values of TRUE and FALSE. Applying the function `mean` to it converts that vector into 0s and 1s, and the result of the computation is the fraction of 1s, which is the same as the fraction of TRUEs.

We postulated the Poisson distribution for the noise, pretending we knew all the parameters, and were able to conclude through mathematical deduction.

In 16 of 100,000 trials, the maximum was 7 or larger. This gives the following approximation for $P(X_{max} \geqslant 7)$.

```
mean( maxes >= 7 )
## [1] 0.00016
```

which more or less agrees with our theoretical calculation. We already see one of the potential limitations of Monte Carlo simulations: the "granularity" of the simulation result is determined by the inverse of the number of simulations (100,000) and so will be around 10^{-5}. Any estimated probability cannot be more precise than this granularity, and indeed the precision of our estimate will be a few multiples of that. Everything we have done up to now is possible only because we know the false positive rate per position, we know the number of patients assayed and the length of the protein, we suppose we have identically distributed independent draws from the model, and there are no unknown parameters. This is an example of **probability or generative modeling**: all the parameters are known and the mathematical theory allows us to work by **deduction** in a *top-down* fashion.

If instead we are in the more realistic situation of knowing the number of patients and the length of the proteins, but don't know the distribution of the data, then we have to use **statistical modeling**. This approach will be developed in Chapter 2. We will see that if we have only the data to start with, we first need to **fit** a reasonable distribution to describe it. However, before we get to this harder problem, let's extend our knowledge of discrete distributions to more than binary success-or-failure outcomes.

1.4   Multinomial distributions: the case of DNA

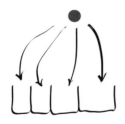

Figure 1.9: The boxes represent four outcomes or levels of a discrete *categorical* variable. The box on the right represents the most likely outcome.

More than two outcomes.   When modeling four possible outcomes, as for instance the boxes in Figure 1.9 or when studying counts of the four nucleotides A, C, G and T, we need to extend the binomial model.

Recall that when using the binomial, we can consider unequal probabilities for the two outcomes by assigning a probability $p = P(1) = p_1$ to the outcome 1 and $1 - p = P(0) = p_0$ to the outcome 0. When there are more than two possible outcomes, say A, C, G and T, we can think of throwing balls into boxes of different sizes corresponding to different probabilities, and we can label these probabilities p_A, p_C, p_G, p_T. Just as in the binomial case, the sum of the probabilities of all possible outcomes is 1, that is, $p_A + p_C + p_G + p_T = 1$.

You are secretly meeting a continuous distribution here, the *uniform distribution*: `runif`.

▶ Task   Experiment with the random number generator that generates all possible numbers between 0 and 1 through the function called `runif`. Use it to generate a random variable with four levels (A, C, G, T) where $p_A = \frac{1}{8}, p_C = \frac{3}{8}, p_G = \frac{3}{8}, p_T = \frac{1}{8}$.   ◀

Mathematical formulation. Multinomial distributions are the most important models for tallying counts, and R uses a general formula to compute the probability of a

multinomial vector of counts $(x_1, \ldots, x_m)$ for outcomes that have m boxes with probabilities $p_1, \ldots, p_m$:

$$P(x_1, x_2, \ldots, x_m \mid p_1, \ldots, p_m) = \frac{n!}{\prod x_i!} \prod p_i^{x_i}$$

$$= \binom{n}{x_1, x_2, \ldots, x_m} p_1^{x_1} p_2^{x_2} \cdots p_m^{x_m}.$$

The first term reads: the joint probability of observing count x_1 in box 1 and x_2 in 2 and … x_m in box m, given that box 1 has probability p_1, box 2 has probability p_2, … and box m has probability p_m.

▶ Question **1.7** Suppose we have four boxes that are equally likely. Using the formula, what is the probability of observing four in the first box, two in the second box and none in the two other boxes? ◀

The term in brackets is a shortcut called the multinomial coefficient:

$$\binom{n}{x_1, x_2, \ldots, x_m} = \frac{n!}{x_1! x_2! \cdots x_m!}.$$

It generalizes the binomial coefficient – for $m = 2$ they are the same.

▶ Solution **1.7**

$$P(4, 2, 0, 0) = \frac{6 \times 5 \times 4 \times 3 \times 2}{4 \times 3 \times 2 \times 2} \frac{1}{4^6} = \frac{15}{4^6} \simeq 0.0037.$$

```
dmultinom(c(4, 2, 0, 0), prob = rep(1/4, 4))
## [1] 0.003662109
```

We often run simulation experiments to check whether the data we see are consistent with the simplest possible four-box model where each box has the same probability $\frac{1}{4}$. We'll see more examples of this in Chapter 2. Here we use a few R commands to generate such vectors of counts.

First, suppose we have eight characters of four different, equally likely types.

```
pvec = rep(1/4, 4)
t(rmultinom(1, prob = pvec, size = 8))
##      [,1] [,2] [,3] [,4]
## [1,]    1    3    1    3
```

▶ Question **1.8** Try the code without the `t()` function; what does t stand for? ◀

▶ Question **1.9** How do you interpret the difference between `rmultinom(n = 8, prob = pvec, size = 1)` and `rmultinom(n = 1, prob = pvec, size = 8)`? Hint: remember what we did in Sections 1.3.1 and 1.3.2. ◀

1.4.1 Simulating for power

Let's see an example of using Monte Carlo for the multinomial in a way that is related to a problem scientists often have to solve when planning their experiments: how big a sample size do I need?

The term **power** has a special meaning in statistics. It is the probability of detecting something if it *is* there, also called the **true positive rate**.

Conventionally, experimentalists aim for a power of 80% (or more) when planning experiments. This means that if the same experiment is run many times, about 20% of the time it will fail to yield significant results even though it should.

$\mathfrak{n}?$

sample size

Ask a statistician about sample size and they will always tell you they need more data. The larger the sample size, the more sensitive the results. However, lab work is expensive, so there is a tricky cost–benefit trade-off to be considered. This is such an important problem that we have dedicated a whole chapter to it at the end of the book (Chapter 13).

We compute the probability of rejecting by simulation. We generate 1000 simulated instances from an alternative process, parameterized by pvecA.

```
pvecA = c(3/8, 1/4, 3/12, 1/8)
observed = rmultinom(1000, prob = pvecA, size = 20)
dim(observed)
## [1]    4 1000
observed[, 1:7]
##      [,1] [,2] [,3] [,4] [,5] [,6] [,7]
## [1,]   10    4    8    8    4    7    7
## [2,]    3   10    5    6    6    7    2
## [3,]    5    3    5    6    4    2    6
## [4,]    2    3    2    0    6    4    5
apply(observed, 1, mean)
## [1] 7.469 4.974 5.085 2.472
expectedA = pvecA * 20
expectedA
## [1] 7.5 5.0 5.0 2.5
```

As with the simulation from the null hypothesis, the observed values vary considerably. The question is: how often (out of 1000 instances) will our test detect that the data depart from the null?

The test doesn't reject the first observation, $(10, 3, 5, 2)$, because the value of the statistic is within the 95th percentile.

```
stat(observed[, 1])
## [1] 7.6
S1 = apply(observed, 2, stat)
q95
## 95%
## 7.6
sum(S1 > q95)
## [1] 199
power = mean(S1 > q95)
power
## [1] 0.199
```

Run across 1000 simulations, the test identified 199 as coming from an alternative distribution. We've thus computed that the probability $P(\text{reject } H_0 \mid H_A)$ is 0.199.

With a sequence length of $n = 20$ we have a power of about 20% to detect the difference between the fair generating process and our **alternative**.

▶ Task   In practice, as we mentioned, an acceptable value of power is 0.8 or more. Repeat the simulation experiments and suggest a new sequence length n that will ensure that the power is acceptable.   ◀

Classical statistics for classical data

We didn't need to simulate the data using Monte Carlo to compute the 95th percentiles; there is an adequate theory to help us with the computation.

Our statistic `stat` actually has a well-known distribution, called the **chi-squared distribution** (with three degrees of freedom) and written χ_3^2.

We will see in Chapter 2 how to compare distributions using QQ-plots (see Figure 2.8). We could have used a more standard test instead of running a handmade simulation. However, the procedure we've learned extends to many situations in which the chi-squared distribution doesn't apply, for instance, when some of the boxes have extremely low probabilities and their counts are mostly zero.

1.5   Summary of this chapter

We have used mathematical formulas and R to compute probabilities of various discrete events that can be modeled with a few basic distributions:

The *Bernoulli* distribution is our most basic building block – it is used to represent a single binary trial such as a coin flip. We can code the outcomes as 0 and 1. We call p the probability of success (the 1 outcome).

The *binomial* distribution is used for the number of 1s in n binary trial, and we generate the probabilities of seeing k successes using the R function `dbinom`. We also saw that we could simulate an n-trial binomial using the function `rbinom`.

The *Poisson* distribution is most appropriate for cases when p is small (the 1s are rare). It has only one parameter, λ, and the Poisson distribution for $\lambda = np$ is approximately the same as the binomial distribution for (n, p) if p is small. We used the Poisson distribution to model the number of randomly occurring false positives in an assay that tests for epitopes along a sequence, presuming that the per-position false positive rate p is small. We saw how such a parametric model enables us to compute the probabilities of extreme events, as long as we know all the parameters.

The *multinomial* distribution is used for discrete events that have more than two possible outcomes, or levels. The power example showed us how to use Monte Carlo simulation to decide how much data we need to collect if we want to test whether a multinomial model with equal probabilities is consistent with the data.

We used probability distributions and probabilistic models to evaluate hypotheses about how our data were generated, by making assumptions about the generative models. We term the probability of seeing the data, given a hypothesis, a **p-value**. This is not the same as the probability that the hypothesis is true!

1.6   Further reading

- The elementary book by Freedman et al. (1997) provides the best introduction to probability through the type of box models we mention here.

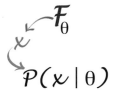

Figure 1.11: We have studied how a probability model has a distribution; we call this F. F often depends on parameters, which are denoted by Greek letters such as θ. The observed data are generated via the brown arrow and are represented by Roman letters such as x. The vertical bar in the probability computation stands for *supposing that* or *conditional on*.

$P(H_0 \mid \text{data})$ is not the same as a p-value $P(\text{data} \mid H_0)$.

- The book by Durbin et al. (1998) covers many useful probability distributions and provides in its appendices a more complete view of the theoretical background in probability and its application to sequences in biology.
- Monte Carlo methods are used extensively in modern statistics. Robert and Casella (2009) provides an introduction to these methods using R.
- Chapter 6 will cover the subject of hypothesis testing. We also suggest Rice (2006) for more advanced material useful on the type of probability distributions – beta, gamma, exponential – that we often use in data analyses.

1.7   Exercises

▶ Exercise **1.1** R can generate numbers from all known distributions. We now know how to generate random discrete data using the specialized R functions tailored for each type of distribution. We use the functions that start with an `r`, as in `rXXXX`, where `XXXX` could be `pois`, `binom`, `multinom`. If we need a theoretical computation of a probability under one of these models, we use the functions `dXXXX`, such as `dbinom`, which computes the probabilities of events in the discrete binomial distribution, and `dnorm`, which computes the **probability density function** for the continuous normal distribution. When computing tail probabilities such as $P(X > a)$, it is convenient to use the cumulative distribution functions, which are called `pXXXX`. Find two other discrete distributions that could replace the `XXXX` above.   ◀

▶ Exercise **1.2** In this chapter we concentrated on *discrete* random variables, where the probabilities are concentrated on a countable set of values. How would you calculate the *probability mass* at the value $X = 2$ for a binomial $B(10, 0.3)$ with `dbinom`? Use `dbinom` to compute the *cumulative* distribution at the value 2, corresponding to $P(X \leqslant 2)$, and check your answer with another R function.   ◀

▶ Exercise **1.3** Whenever we keep needing a certain sequence of commands, it's good to put them into a function. The function body contains the instructions that we want to do over and over again, and the function arguments take those things that we may want to vary. Write a function to compute the probability of having a maximum as big as `m` when looking across `n` Poisson variables with rate `lambda`.   ◀

▶ Exercise **1.4** Rewrite the function in Exercise 1.3 to have **default** values for its arguments (i.e., values it uses if the argument is not specified in a call to the function).

◀

▶ Exercise **1.5** In the epitope example, use a simulation to find the probability of having a maximum of 9 or larger in 100 trials. How many simulations do you need if you would like to prove that "the probability is smaller than 0.000001"?   ◀

▶ Exercise **1.6** Use `?Distributions` in R to get a list of available distributions.[14] Make plots of the probability mass or density functions for various distributions (using the functions named `dXXXX`), and list five distributions that are not discrete.   ◀

[14] These are just the distributions that come with a basic R installation. More are available in additional packages; see the *CRAN task view on probability distributions*.

▶ Exercise **1.7** Generate 100 instances of a Poisson(3) random variable. What is the mean? What is the variance as computed by the R function `var`?   ◀

▶ Exercise **1.8 C. elegans genome nucleotide frequency**. Is the mitochondrial sequence of *C. elegans* consistent with a model of equally likely nucleotides?

a. Explore the nucleotide frequencies of chromosome M by using a dedicated function in the *Biostrings* package from Bioconductor.
b. Test whether the *C. elegans* data is consistent with the uniform model (all nucleotide frequencies the same) using a simulation.

This is our opportunity to use **Bioconductor** for the first time. You will need to source the biocLite function and install the Bioconductor packages in a special way.

```
source("http://bioconductor.org/biocLite.R")
biocLite(c("Biostrings", "BSgenome.Celegans.UCSC.ce2"))
```

After that, we can load the genome sequence package *BSgenome.Celegans.UCSC.ce2* as we load any other R packages.   ◀

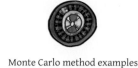

Monte Carlo method examples

CHAPTER 2

Statistical Modeling

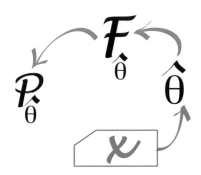

In Chapter 1, knowing both the generative model and the values of the parameters allowed us to deduce probabilities we could use for decision making – for instance, whether we had really found an epitope. In many real situations, neither the generative model nor the parameters are known, and we need to estimate them using data we have collected. Statistical modeling works from the data *upwards* to a model that *might* plausibly explain the data.[1] This upward-reasoning step is called statistical **inference**. This chapter will show us some of the distributions and estimation mechanisms that serve as building blocks for inference. Although the examples in this chapter are all parametric (i.e., the statistical models only have a small number of unknown parameters), the principles we discuss will generalize.

[1] Even if we have found a model that perfectly explains all our current data, it could always be that reality is more complex. A new set of data lets us conclude that another model is needed, and may include the current model as a special case or approximation.

2.1 Goals for this chapter

In this chapter we will:

- See that there is a difference between two subjects that are often confused: "Probability" and "Statistics".
- Fit data to probability distributions using histograms and other visualization tricks.
- Have a first encounter with an estimating procedure known as maximum likelihood through a simulation experiment.
- Make inferences from data for which we have prior information. For this we will use the Bayesian paradigm, which will involve new distributions with specially tailored properties. We will use simulations and see how Bayesian estimation differs from simple application of maximum likelihood.
- Use statistical models and estimation to evaluate dependencies in binomial and multinomial distributions.
- Analyze some historically interesting genomic data assembled into tables.
- Make Markov chain models for dependent data.
- Do a few concrete applications counting motifs in whole genomes and manipulate special Bioconductor classes dedicated to genomic data.

In a statistical setting, we start with the data X and use them to *estimate* the parameters of a distribution. These estimates are denoted by Greek letters with what we call hats on them, as in $\widehat{\theta}$.

$$\lambda,\ \mu,\ \theta$$

Examples of parameters. The single parameter λ defines a Poisson distribution. The letter μ is often used for the mean of the normal. More generally, we use the Greek letter θ to designate a generic tuple of parameters necessary to specify a probability model. For the binomial distribution, $\theta = (n, p)$ comprises two numbers, a positive integer and a real number between 0 and 1.

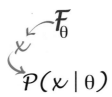

Figure 2.1: The probabilistic model we obtained in Chapter 1. The data are represented as x in green. We can use the observed data to compute the probability of observing x when we know the true value of θ.

Parameters are the key. We saw in Chapter 1 that knowing all the parameter values in the epitope example enabled us to use our probability model and test a null hypothesis based on the data we had at hand. We will see different approaches to statistical modeling through some real examples and computer simulations, but let's start by making a distinction between two situations depending on how much information is available.

2.2   The difference between statistical and probabilistic models

A probabilistic analysis is possible when we know a good generative model for the randomness in the data *and* we are provided with the parameters' actual values.

In the epitope example, knowing that false positives occurred as Bernoulli(0.01) per position, the number of patients assayed and the length of the protein ensured that there were *no unknown parameters*.

In such a case, we can use mathematical **deduction** to compute the probability of an event, as schematized in Figure 2.1. In the epitope example, we used the Poisson probability as our **null model** with the given parameter $\lambda = 0.5$. We were able to conclude through mathematical deduction that the chance of seeing a maximum value of 7 or larger was around 10^{-4} and thus that in fact the observed data were highly unlikely under that model (or "null hypothesis").

Now suppose that we know the number of patients and the length of the proteins (these are given by the experimental design) but not the distribution itself and the false positive rate. Once we observe data, we need to go **up** from the data to estimate both a probability model F (Poisson, normal, binomial) and eventually the missing parameter(s) for that model. This is the type of statistical **inference** we will explain in this chapter.

2.3   A simple example of statistical modeling

Start with the data

There are two parts to the modeling procedure. First we need a reasonable probability distribution to model the data-generating process. As we saw in Chapter 1, discrete count data may be modeled by simple probability distributions such as binomial, multinomial or Poisson distributions. The normal distribution, or bell-shaped curve, is often a good model for continuous measurements. Distributions can also be more complicated mixtures of these elementary ones (more on this in Chapter 4).

Let's revisit the epitope data from Chapter 1, starting without the tricky outlier.

```
load("../data/e100.RData")
e99 = e100[-which.max(e100)]
```

Goodness of fit: visual evaluation

Our first step is to find a fit from candidate distributions; this requires consulting graphical and quantitative goodness-of-fit plots.

For discrete data,[2] we can plot a barplot of frequencies as in Figure 2.2.

```
barplot(table(e99), space = 0.8, col = "chartreuse4")
```

However, it is hard to decide which theoretical distribution fits the data best without using a comparison. One visual **goodness-of-fit** diagram is known as the **rootogram** (Cleveland, 1988); it hangs the bars with the observed counts from the theoretical red points. If the counts correspond exactly to their theoretical values, the bottoms of the boxes will align exactly with the horizontal axis.

```
library("vcd")
gf1 = goodfit( e99, "poisson")
rootogram(gf1, xlab = "", rect_gp = gpar(fill = "chartreuse4"))
```

▶ **Question 2.1** To calibrate what such a plot looks like with a known Poisson variable, use `rpois` with $\lambda = 0.05$ to generate 100 Poisson distributed numbers and draw their rootogram. ◀

▶ **Solution 2.1**

```
simp = rpois(100, lambda = 0.05)
gf2 = goodfit(simp, "poisson")
rootogram(gf2, xlab = "")
```
□

We see from the rootogram in Figure 2.3 that the Poisson model seems to fit the `e99` data reasonably well. But remember, to make this happen we removed the outlier. The Poisson is completely determined by one parameter, often called the Poisson mean λ. In most cases where we can guess that the data follow a Poisson distribution, we will need to estimate the Poisson parameter from the data.

The most common way of estimating λ is to choose the value $\hat{\lambda}$ that makes the observed data the most likely. This is called the **maximum likelihood estimator** (Rice, 2006, Chapter 8, Section 5), often abbreviated **MLE**. We will illustrate this rather paradoxical idea in the next section.

Although above we took out the extreme observation before taking a guess at the probability distribution, we are going to return to the data *with* that observation for the rest of our analysis. In practice we would not know whether there are any outliers, and which data points they are. The effect of leaving it in is to make our estimate of the mean for the null model higher. In turn, this would make it more likely that we'd observe a value of 7 or larger under the null model, resulting in a larger p-value. So, if the p-value we obtain is small even with the outlier included, we are assured that our analysis is on to something real. We call such an approach **conservative**: we err on the side of caution, of not (over)detecting something.

[2] For continuous data, we would look at the histogram.

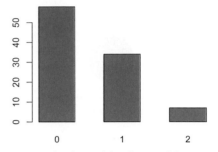

Figure 2.2: The observed distribution of the epitope data without the outlier.

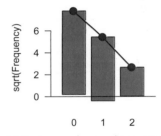

Figure 2.3: Rootogram showing the square roots of the theoretical Poisson values as red dots and the square roots of the observed frequencies as drop-down rectangles. (We'll see later how the `goodfit` function decides which λ to use.)

The parameter is called the Poisson mean because it is the mean of the theoretical distribution *and*, as it turns out, is estimated by the sample mean. This overloading of the word is confusing to everyone.

We explore the values taken by the distribution by randomly sampling from it.

Estimating the parameter of the Poisson distribution

What value for the Poisson mean makes the data the most probable? In a first step, we tally the outcomes.

```
table(e100)
## e100
##  0  1  2  7
## 58 34  7  1
```

Then we try out different values for the Poisson mean to see which gives the best fit to our data. If the mean λ of the Poisson distribution were 3, the counts would look something like this:

```
table(rpois(100, 3))
##
##  0  1  2  3  4  5  6  7  8
##  3 10 23 23 18 18  2  2  1
```

which has many more 2s and 3s than we see in our data. So we see that $\lambda = 3$ is unlikely to have produced our data, as the counts do not match up so well.

▶ **Question 2.2** Repeat this simulation with different values of λ. Can you find one that gives counts close to the observed counts just by trial and error?   ◀

So we can try out many possible values and proceed by brute force. However, we'll do something more elegant and use a little mathematics to see which value maximizes the probability of observing our data. Let's calculate the probability of seeing the data if the value of the Poisson mean is m. Since we suppose the data derive from independent draws, this probability is simply the product of individual probabilities:

$$P(58 \text{ zeroes}, 34 \text{ ones}, 7 \text{ twos}, 1 \text{ seven} \mid \text{data are Poisson}(m))$$
$$= P(0)^{58} \times P(1)^{34} \times P(2)^7 \times P(7)^1.$$

We use R's **vectorization** here: the call to `dpois` returns four values, corresponding to the four different numbers. We then take these to the powers of 58, 34, 7 and 1, respectively, using the ^ operator, resulting again in four values. Finally, we collapse them into one number, the product, with the `prod` function.

For $m = 3$ we can compute this:

```
prod(dpois(c(0, 1, 2, 7), lambda = 3) ^ (c(58, 34, 7, 1)))
## [1] 1.392143e-110
```

▶ **Question 2.3** Compute the probability as above for $m = 0, 1, 2$. Does m have to be an integer? Try computing the probability for $m = 0.4$, for example.   ◀

▶ **Solution 2.3**

```
prod(dpois(c(0, 1, 2, 7), lambda = 0.4) ^ (c(58, 34, 7, 1)))
## [1] 8.5483e-46
```
    □

Here L stands for likelihood and $f(k) = e^{-\lambda} \lambda^k / k!$, the Poisson probability we saw in Chapter 1.

This probability is the **likelihood function** of λ, given the data, and we write it

$$L(\lambda, \ x = (k_1, k_2, k_3, \ldots)) = \prod_{i=1}^{100} f(k_i).$$

Instead of working with multiplications of a hundred small numbers, it is convenient to take the logarithm.[3] Since the logarithm is strictly increasing, if there is a point where the logarithm achieves its maximum within an interval, it will also be the maximum for the probability.

[3] That's usually true both for pencil and paper and for computer calculations.

Let's start with a computational illustration. We compute the likelihood for many different values of the Poisson parameter. To do this, we need to write a small function that computes the probability of the data for different values.[4]

```
loglikelihood  = function(lambda, data = e100) {
  sum(log(dpois(data, lambda)))
}
```

[4] Again, we use R's vector syntax to write the computation without an explicit loop over the data points. Compared to the code above, here we call dpois on each of the 100 data points, rather than tabulating data with the table function before calling dpois only on the distinct values. This is a simple example of alternative solutions whose results are equivalent but that may differ in how easy it is to read the code or how long it takes to execute.

Now we can compute the likelihood for a whole series of `lambda` values from 0.05 to 0.95 (Figure 2.4).

```
lambdas = seq(0.05, 0.95, length = 100)
loglik = vapply(lambdas, loglikelihood, numeric(1))
plot(lambdas, loglik, type = "l", col = "red", ylab = "", lwd = 2,
     xlab = expression(lambda))
m0 = mean(e100)
abline(v = m0, col = "blue", lwd = 2)
abline(h = loglikelihood(m0), col = "purple", lwd = 2)
m0

## [1] 0.55
```

▶ **Question 2.4** What does the `vapply` function do in the above code? Hint: check its manual page. ◀

▶ **Solution 2.4** `vapply` takes its first argument, the vector `lambdas` in this case, and iteratively applies the function `loglikelihood` (its second argument) to each of the vector elements. As a result, it returns a vector of the results. The function also needs a third argument, `numeric(1)` in this case, that specifies what type of value each individual call to `loglikelihood` is supposed to return: a single number. (In general, it could happen that the function sometimes returns something else, say, a character string or two numbers; in that case it would not be possible to assemble the overall results into a coherent vector, and `vapply` would complain.) □

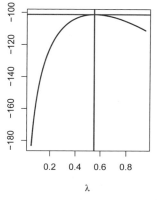

Figure 2.4: The red curve is the log-likelihood function. The vertical line shows the value of m (the mean) and the purple horizontal line the log-likelihood of m. It looks like m maximizes the likelihood.

In fact, there is a shortcut: the function `goodfit`.

```
gf  = goodfit(e100, "poisson")
names(gf)

## [1] "observed" "count"    "fitted"   "type"     "method"
## [6] "df"       "par"

gf$par

## $lambda
## [1] 0.55
```

The output of `goodfit` is a composite object called a list. One of its components is called `par` and contains the value(s) of the fitted parameter(s) for the distribution studied. In this case it's only one number, the estimate of λ.

▶ Question **2.5** What are the other components of the output from the `goodfit` function? ◀

▶ Task Compare the value of m to the value that we used previously for λ, 0.5. Redo the modeling that we did in Chapter 1 with m instead of 0.5. ◀

2.3.1 Classical statistics for classical data

Here is a formal proof of our computational finding that the mean maximizes the (log-)likelihood:

$$
\log L(\lambda, x) = \sum_{i=1}^{100} -\lambda + k_i \log \lambda - \log(k_i!)
$$

$$
= -100\lambda + \log \lambda \left(\sum_{i=1}^{100} k_i \right) + \text{const.} \tag{2.1}
$$

We use the catch-all "const." for terms that do not depend on λ (although they do depend on x, i.e., on the k_i). To find the λ that maximizes this, we compute the derivative in λ and set it to zero:

$$
\frac{d}{d\lambda} \log L = -100 + \frac{1}{\lambda} \sum_{i=1}^{100} k_i \overset{?}{=} 0, \tag{2.2}
$$

$$
\lambda = \frac{1}{100} \sum_{i=1}^{100} k_i = \bar{k}. \tag{2.3}
$$

You have just seen the first steps of a **statistical approach**, starting "from the ground up" (from the data) to infer the model parameter(s): this is statistical **estimation** of a parameter from data. Another important component is choosing which family of distributions our data come from; that part is done by evaluating the **goodness of fit**. We will encounter more of this later in Sections 2.6 and 2.7.

In the classical **statistical testing** framework, we consider one single model, which we call the **null model**, for the data. The null model formulates an "uninteresting" baseline, such as that all observations come from the same random distribution regardless of which group or treatment they are from. We then test whether there is something more interesting going on by computing the probability that the data are compatible with that model. Often, this is the best we can do, since we do not know in sufficient detail what the "interesting", non-null or alternative model should be. In other situations, we have two competing models that we can compare, as we will see later in Section 2.10.1.

▶ Question **2.6** What is the value of modeling with a known distribution? For instance, why is it interesting to know that a variable has a Poisson distribution? ◀

▶ **Solution 2.6**   Models are concise but expressive representations of the data-generating process. For the Poisson for instance, knowing one number allows us to know everything about the distribution, including, as we saw earlier, the probabilities of extreme or rare events.   □

Another useful direction is **regression**. We may be interested in knowing how our count-based response variable (e.g., the result of counting sequencing reads) depends on a continuous covariate, say, temperature or nutrient concentration. You may already have encountered linear regression, where our model is that the response variable y depends on the covariate x via the equation $y = ax + b + e$, with parameters a and b (that we need to estimate), and with **residual** e, whose probability model is a normal distribution (whose variance we usually also need to estimate). For count data, the same type of regression model is possible, although the probability distribution for the residuals then needs to be non-normal. In that case we use the **generalized linear model** framework. We will see examples when studying RNA-Seq in Chapter 8 and another type of next-generation sequencing data, 16S rRNA data, in Chapter 9.

Knowing that our probability model involves a Poisson, binomial or multinomial distribution or another parametric family enables us to have quick answers to questions about the parameters of the model and compute quantities such as p-values and confidence intervals.

2.4   Binomial distributions and maximum likelihood

In a binomial distribution, there are two parameters: the number of trials n, which is typically known, and the probability p of seeing a 1 in a trial. This probability is often unknown.

2.4.1   An example

Suppose we take a sample of $n = 120$ males and test them for red–green color blindness. We can code the data as 0 if the subject is not color blind and 1 if he is. We summarize the data by the table:

```
table(cb)
## cb
##   0    1
## 110   10
```

▶ Question 2.7   Which value of p is the most likely given these data?   ◀

▶ **Solution 2.7** $\hat{p} = \frac{1}{12}$.   □

In this special case, your intuition may give you the estimate $\hat{p} = \frac{1}{12}$, which turns out to be the maximum likelihood estimate. We put a hat over the letter to remind us

Be careful: sometimes ML estimates are not intuitive, and are hard to guess and to compute (see Exercise 2.2).

that this is not (necessarily) the underlying true value, but an estimate we make from the data.

As before in the case of the Poisson, if we compute the likelihood for many possible p, we can plot it and see where its maximum falls.

```
probs    =  seq(0, 0.3, by = 0.005)
likelihood = dbinom(sum(cb), prob = probs, size = length(cb))
plot(probs, likelihood, pch = 16, xlab = "probability of success",
        ylab = "likelihood", cex=0.6)
probs[which.max(likelihood)]
## [1] 0.085
```

Note. 0.085 is not exactly the value we expected ($\frac{1}{12}$), and that is because the set of values that we tried (in `probs`) did not include the exact value of $\frac{1}{12} \simeq 0.0833$, so we obtained the next best one. We could use numerical optimization methods to overcome that.

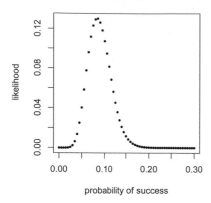

Figure 2.5: Plot of the likelihood as a function of the probabilities. The likelihood is a function on $[0, 1]$; here we zoom into the range $[0, 0.3]$, as the likelihood is practically zero for larger values of p.

Likelihood for the binomial distribution

One can come up with different criteria than ML that lead to other estimators: they all wear hats. We'll see other examples in Chapter 4.

The likelihood and the probability are the same mathematical function, only interpreted in different ways – in one case, it tells us how probable it is to see a particular set of values of the data given the parameters; in the other case, we consider the data as fixed and ask for the particular parameter value that makes the data more likely. Suppose $n = 300$ and we observe $y = 40$ successes. Then, for the binomial distribution,

$$f(\theta \mid n, y) = f(y \mid n, \theta) = \binom{n}{y} \theta^y (1 - \theta)^{(n-y)}. \tag{2.4}$$

[5] It's around e^{115}, and this can be seen from Stirling's formula. We can also use R: `choose(300, 40)` = `9.8e+49`.

As $\binom{n}{y}$ is very large,[5] we use the logarithm of the likelihood to give

$$\log f(\theta|y) = 115 + 40 \log(\theta) + (300 - 40) \log(1 - \theta).$$

Here's a function we use to calculate it:

```
loglikelihood = function(theta, n = 300, k = 40) {
    115 + k * log(theta) + (n - k) * log(1 - theta)
}
```

which we plot for the range of θ from 0 to 1 (Figure 2.6).

```
thetas = seq(0, 1, by = 0.001)
plot(thetas, loglikelihood(thetas), xlab = expression(theta),
     ylab = expression(paste("log f(", theta, " | y)")),type = "l")
```

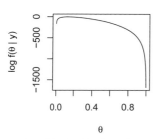

Figure 2.6: Plot of the log-likelihood function for $n = 300$ and $y = 40$.

The maximum lies at $40/300 = 0.1333\ldots$, consistent with intuition, but we see that other values of θ are almost equally likely, as the function is quite flat around the maximum. We will see in Section 2.9 how Bayesian methods allow us to use a range of values for θ.

2.5   More boxes: multinomial data

2.5.1   DNA count modeling: base pairs

There are four basic molecules of DNA: A – adenine, C – cytosine, G – guanine, T – thymine. The nucleotides are classified into two groups: purines (A and G) and pyrimidines (C and T). The binomial would work as a model for the purine/pyrimidine groupings but not if we want to use A, C, G, T; for that we need the multinomial model from Section 1.4. Let's look at noticeable patterns that occur in these frequencies.

2.5.2   Nucleotide bias

This section combines estimation and testing by simulation in a real example. Data from one strand of DNA for the genes of *Staphylococcus aureus* bacterium are available in a `fasta` file, `staphsequence.ffn.txt`, which we can read with a function from the Bioconductor package *Biostrings*.

```
library("Biostrings")
staph = readDNAStringSet("../data/staphsequence.ffn.txt", "fasta")
```

Let's look at the first gene.

```
staph[1]
```

```
##   A DNAStringSet instance of length 1
##     width seq                                    names
## [1]  1362 ATGTCGGAAAAAGAA...ATAAGAAATGTATAA lcl|NC_002952.2_c...
```

```
letterFrequency(staph[[1]], letters = "ACGT", OR = 0)
```

```
##   A   C   G   T
## 522 219 229 392
```

▶ Question **2.8** Why did we use double square brackets in the second line?   ◀

▶ Solution **2.8** The double square brackets `[[i]]` extract the sequence of the `i`th gene as a *DNAString*, as opposed to the pair of single brackets `[i]`, which return a *DNAStringSet* with just a single *DNAString* in it. If you look at the length of `staph[1]`, it is 1, whereas `staph[[1]]` has length 1362.   □

▶ Question **2.9** Following a similar procedure to Exercise 1.8, test whether the nucleotides are equally distributed across the four possibilities for this first gene.   ◀

Due to differences between physical properties of nucleotides, evolutionary selection can act on the nucleotide frequencies. So we can ask whether, say, the first 10 genes from these data come from the same multinomial. We do not have a prior reference; we just want to decide whether the nucleotides occur in the same proportions in the first 10 genes. If not, this would provide us with evidence of varying selective pressure on these genes.

```
letterFrq = vapply(staph, letterFrequency, FUN.VALUE = numeric(4),
            letters = "ACGT", OR = 0)
colnames(letterFrq) = paste0("gene", seq(along = staph))
tab10 = letterFrq[, 1:10]
computeProportions = function(x) { x/sum(x) }
prop10 = apply(tab10, 2, computeProportions)
round(prop10, digits = 2)

##    gene1 gene2 gene3 gene4 gene5 gene6 gene7 gene8 gene9 gene10
## A  0.38  0.36  0.35  0.37  0.35  0.33  0.33  0.34  0.38   0.27
## C  0.16  0.16  0.13  0.15  0.15  0.15  0.16  0.16  0.14   0.16
## G  0.17  0.17  0.23  0.19  0.22  0.22  0.20  0.21  0.20   0.20
## T  0.29  0.31  0.30  0.29  0.27  0.30  0.30  0.29  0.28   0.36

p0 = rowMeans(prop10)
p0

##         A         C         G         T
## 0.3470531 0.1518313 0.2011442 0.2999714
```

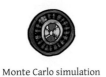

Monte Carlo simulation

So let's suppose p0 is the vector of multinomial probabilities for all 10 genes and use a Monte Carlo simulation to test whether the departures between the observed letter frequencies and expected values under this supposition are within a plausible range.

We compute the expected counts by taking the "outer" product of the vector of probabilities p0 with the sums of nucleotide counts from each of the 10 columns, cs.

```
cs = colSums(tab10)
cs

##  gene1  gene2  gene3  gene4  gene5  gene6  gene7  gene8  gene9
##   1362   1134    246   1113   1932   2661    831   1515   1287
## gene10
##    696

expectedtab10 = outer(p0, cs, FUN = "*")
round(expectedtab10)

##   gene1 gene2 gene3 gene4 gene5 gene6 gene7 gene8 gene9 gene10
## A   473   394    85   386   671   924   288   526   447    242
## C   207   172    37   169   293   404   126   230   195    106
## G   274   228    49   224   389   535   167   305   259    140
## T   409   340    74   334   580   798   249   454   386    209
```

We can now create a random table with the correct column sums using the rmultinom function. This table is generated according to the null hypothesis that the true proportions are given by p0.

```
randomtab10 = sapply(cs, function(s) { rmultinom(1, s, p0) } )
all(colSums(randomtab10) == cs)

## [1] TRUE
```

Now we repeat this $B = 1000$ times. For each table, we compute our test statistic from Section 1.4.1 in Chapter 1 (the function stat) and store the results in the vector simulstat. Together, these values constitute our null distribution, as they were generated under the null hypothesis that p0 is the vector of multinomial proportions for each of the 10 genes.

```
stat = function(obsvd, exptd = 20 * pvec) {
  sum((obsvd - exptd)^2 / exptd)
}
B = 1000
simulstat = replicate(B, {
  randomtab10 = sapply(cs, function(s) { rmultinom(1, s, p0) })
  stat(randomtab10, expectedtab10)
})
S1 = stat(tab10, expectedtab10)
sum(simulstat >= S1)

## [1] 0

hist(simulstat, col = "lavender", breaks = seq(0, 75, length.out=50))
abline(v = S1, col = "red")
abline(v = quantile(simulstat, probs = c(0.95, 0.99)),
       col = c("darkgreen", "blue"), lty = 2)
```

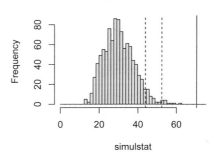

Figure 2.7: Histogram of `simulstat`. The value of S1 is marked by the vertical red line and those of the 0.95 and 0.99 quantiles (see next section) by the dotted lines.

The histogram is shown in Figure 2.7. We see that the probability of seeing a value as large as S1= 70.1 is very small under the *null model*. It happened zero times in our 1000 simulations that a value as big as S1 occurred. Thus the 10 genes do not seem to come from the same multinomial model.

2.6 The χ^2 distribution

In fact, we could have used statistical theory to come to the same conclusion without running these simulations. The theoretical distribution of the `simulstat` statistic is called the **chi-squared (χ^2) distribution**[6] with parameter 30 ($= 10 \times (4 - 1)$). We can use this for computing the probability of having a value as large as S1 = 70.1. As we just saw above, small probabilities are difficult to compute by Monte Carlo: the granularity of the computation is $1/B$, so we cannot estimate any probabilities smaller than that, and in fact the uncertainty of the estimate is larger. So if any theory is applicable, that tends to be useful. We can check how well theory and simulation match in our case using another visual goodness-of-fit tool: the **quantile–quantile (QQ) plot**. When comparing two distributions, whether from two different samples or from one sample versus a theoretical model, just looking at histograms is not informative enough. We use a method based on the quantiles of the distributions.

[6] Strictly speaking, the distribution of `simulstat` is *approximately* described by a χ^2 distribution; the approximation is particularly good if the counts in the table are large.

2.6.1 Intermezzo: quantiles and the quantile–quantile plot

In Chapter 1, we ordered the 100 sample values from smallest to largest: $x_{(1)}, x_{(2)}, \ldots, x_{(100)}$. Say we want the 22nd percentile. We can take any value between the 22nd and 23rd values; that is, any value that fulfills $x_{(22)} \leqslant c_{0.22} < x_{(23)}$ is acceptable as a 0.22 **quantile** ($c_{0.22}$). In other words, $c_{0.22}$ is defined by

$$\frac{\#x_i \leqslant c_{0.22}}{n} = 0.22.$$

In Section 3.6.6, we'll introduce the **empirical cumulative distribution function (ECDF)** $\widehat{F}$, and we'll see that our definition of $c_{0.22}$ can also be written as $\widehat{F}_n(c_{0.22}) = 0.22$. In Figure 2.7, our histogram of the distribution of `simulstat`, the quantiles $c_{0.95}$ and $c_{0.99}$ are also shown.

▶ Question **2.10** (a) Compare the `simulstat` values and 1000 randomly generated χ^2_{30} random numbers by displaying them in histograms with 50 bins each.
(b) Compute the quantiles of the `simulstat` values and compare them to those of the χ^2_{30} distribution. Hint:

```
qs = ppoints(100)
quantile(simulstat, qs)
quantile(qchisq(qs, df = 30), qs)                    ◀
```

▶ Question **2.11** Do you know another name for the 0.5 quantile?   ◀

▶ Solution **2.11** The median.   □

A name collision occurs here. Statisticians call the summary statistic we just computed as `simulstat` (sum of squares of weighted differences) the **chi-squared** or χ^2 **statistic**. The theoretical distribution χ^2_ν is a distribution in its own right, with a parameter ν called the degrees of freedom. When reading about the chi-squared or χ^2, you will need to pay attention to the context to see which meaning is intended.

▶ Question **2.12** In the above definition, we were a little vague on how the quantile is defined in general, i.e., not just for 0.22. How is the quantile computed for any number between 0 and 1, including numbers that are not multiples of $1/n$?   ◀

▶ Solution **2.12** Check the manual page of the `quantile` function and its argument named `type`.   □

Now that we have an idea what quantiles are, we can make a quantile-quantile plot. We plot the quantiles of the `simulstat` values, which we simulated under the null hypothesis, against the theoretical null distribution χ^2_{30} (Figure 2.8).

```
qqplot(qchisq(ppoints(B), df = 30), simulstat, main = "",
    xlab = expression(chi[nu==30]^2), asp = 1, cex = 0.5, pch = 16)
abline(a = 0, b = 1, col = "red")
```

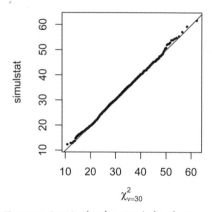

Figure 2.8: Our simulated statistic's distribution compared to χ^2_{30} using a QQ-plot, which shows the theoretical quantiles for the χ^2_{30} distribution on the horizontal axis and the sampled ones on the vertical axis.

Having convinced ourselves that `simulstat` is well described by a χ^2_{30} distribution, we can use that to compute our p-value, i.e., the probability that under the null hypothesis (counts are distributed as multinomial with probabilities $p_A = 0.35$, $p_C = 0.15$, $p_G = 0.2$, $p_T = 0.3$) we observe a value as high as $S1 = 70.1$.

```
1 - pchisq(S1, df = 30)
## [1] 4.74342e-05
```

With such a small p-value, the null hypothesis seems improbable. Note that this computation did not require the 1000 simulations and was faster.

2.7 Chargaff's Rule

The most important pattern in nucleotide frequencies was discovered by Erwin Chargaff (Elson and Chargaff, 1952).

Long before DNA sequencing was available, using the weight of the molecules, he asked whether the nucleotides occurred at equal frequencies. He called this the tetranucleotide hypothesis. We would translate that into asking whether $p_A = p_C = p_G = p_T$.

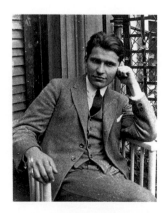

Erwin Chargaff

Unfortunately, Chargaff only published the *percentages* of the mass present in different organisms for each of the nucleotides, not the measurements themselves.

```
load("../data/ChargaffTable.RData")
ChargaffTable
```

```
##                    A     T     C     G
## Human-Thymus    30.9  29.4  19.9  19.8
## Mycobac.Tuber   15.1  14.6  34.9  35.4
## Chicken-Eryth.  28.8  29.2  20.5  21.5
## Sheep-liver     29.3  29.3  20.5  20.7
## Sea Urchin      32.8  32.1  17.7  17.3
## Wheat           27.3  27.1  22.7  22.8
## Yeast           31.3  32.9  18.7  17.1
## E.coli          24.7  23.6  26.0  25.7
```

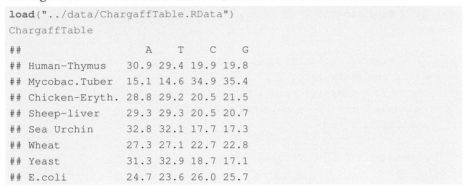

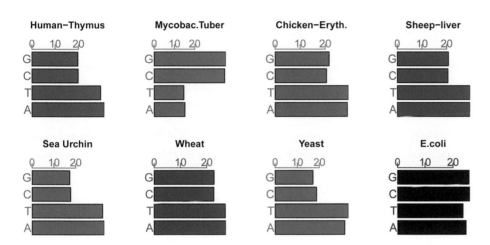

Figure 2.9: Barplots for the different rows in `ChargaffTable`. Can you spot the pattern?

▶ Question 2.13 (a) Do these data seem to come from equally likely multinomial categories?

(b) Can you suggest an alternative pattern?

(c) Can you do a quantitative analysis of the pattern, perhaps inspired by the simulations above?   ◀

▶ Solution 2.13 Chargaff *saw* the answer to this question and postulated a pattern called **base pairing**, which ensured a perfect match of the amount of adenine (A) in the DNA of an organism to the amount of thymine (T). Similarly, whatever the amount of guanine (G), the amount of cytosine (C) would be the same. This is now called Chargaff's rule. On the other hand, the amount of C/G in an organism could be quite different from the amount of A/T, with no obvious pattern across organisms.

Based on Chargaff's rule, we might define a statistic

$$(p_C - p_G)^2 + (p_A - p_T)^2,$$

summed over all rows of the table. We are going to look at a comparison between the data and what would occur if the nucleotides were "exchangeable", in the sense that the probabilities observed in each row were in no particular order, so that there were

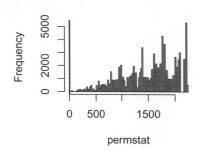

Figure 2.10: Histogram of our statistic `statChf` computed from simulations using per-row permutations of the columns. The value it yields for the observed data is shown by the red line.

no special relationships between the proportions of As and Ts or between those of Cs and Gs.

```
statChf = function(x) {
  sum((x[, "C"] - x[, "G"])^2 + (x[, "A"] - x[, "T"])^2)
}
chfstat = statChf(ChargaffTable)
permstat = replicate(100000, {
    permuted = t(apply(ChargaffTable, 1, sample))
    colnames(permuted) = colnames(ChargaffTable)
    statChf(permuted)
})
pChf = mean(permstat <= chfstat)
pChf

## [1] 0.00012

hist(permstat, breaks = 100, main = "", col = "lavender")
abline(v = chfstat, lwd = 2, col = "red")
```

The histogram in Figure 2.10 shows that it is quite rare to have a value as small as the observed 11.1, where the red line is drawn. The probability of observing a value as small or smaller is `pChf`=1.2×10^{-4}. Thus the data strongly support Chargaff's insight.   □

▶ Question **2.14** When computing `pChf`, we only looked at the values in the null distribution smaller than the observed value. Why did we do this in a one-sided way here?

◀

2.7.1 Two categorical variables

Up to now, we have visited cases where the data are taken from a sample that can be classified into different boxes: the binomial for yes/no binary boxes and the multinomial distribution for categorical variables such as A, C, G, T or different genotypes such as aa, aA, AA. However, it might be that we measure two (or more) categorical variables on a set of subjects, for instance eye color and hair color. We can then cross-tabulate the counts for every combination of eye and hair color. We obtain a table of counts called a **contingency table**. This concept is useful for many types of biological data.

```
HairEyeColor[,, "Female"]

##        Eye
## Hair    Brown Blue Hazel Green
##    Black    36    9     5     2
##    Brown    66   34    29    14
##    Red      16    7     7     7
##    Blond     4   64     5     8
```

▶ Question **2.15** Explore the `HairEyeColor` object in R. What data type, shape and dimensions does it have?

◀

▶ Solution **2.15** It is a numeric array with three dimensions.

```
str(HairEyeColor)
##  table [1:4, 1:4, 1:2] 32 53 10 3 11 50 10 30 10 25 ...
##  - attr(*, "dimnames")=List of 3
##   ..$ Hair: chr [1:4] "Black" "Brown" "Red" "Blond"
##   ..$ Eye : chr [1:4] "Brown" "Blue" "Hazel" "Green"
##   ..$ Sex : chr [1:2] "Male" "Female"
? HairEyeColor                                            □
```

Color blindness and sex

Deuteranopia is a form of red–green color blindness reflecting the absence of medium-wavelength-sensitive cones (green). A deuteranope can distinguish only two to three different hues, whereas somebody with normal vision sees seven different hues. A survey for this type of color blindness in human subjects produced a two-way table crossing color blindness and sex.

```
load("../data/Deuteranopia.RData")
Deuteranopia

##          Men Women
## Deute      19     2
## NonDeute 1981  1998
```

How do we test whether there is a relationship between sex and the occurrence of color blindness? We postulate the null model – of no relationship – with two independent binomials: one for sex and one for color blindness. Under this model we can estimate all the cells' multinomial probabilities, and we can compare the observed counts to the expected counts. This is done using the `chisq.test` function in R.

```
chisq.test(Deuteranopia)
##
##  Pearson's Chi-squared test with Yates' continuity
##  correction
##
## data:  Deuteranopia
## X-squared = 12.255, df = 1, p-value = 0.0004641
```

The small p-value tells us that we should expect to see our observed table with only a very small probability under the null model – i.e., the model that assumes the fractions of deuteranopic color blind among women and men are the same.

We'll see another test for this type of data called Fisher's exact test (also known as the hypergeometric test) in Section 10.3.2. This test is widely used for testing the over-representation of certain types of genes in a list of significantly expressed ones.

2.7.2 A special multinomial: Hardy–Weinberg equilibrium

Here we highlight the use of a multinomial with three possible levels created by combining two alleles, M and N. Suppose that the overall frequency of allele M in the population is p, so that of N is $q = 1 - p$. The Hardy–Weinberg model looks at the relationship between p and q if there is independence of the frequency of both alleles in a genotype, the so-called **Hardy–Weinberg equilibrium** (HWE). This would be the case if there is random mating in a large population with equal distribution of the alleles among sexes. The probabilities of the three genotypes are then as follows:

$$p_{MM} = p^2, \quad p_{NN} = q^2, \quad p_{MN} = 2pq. \tag{2.5}$$

We only observe the frequencies (n_{MM}, n_{MN}, n_{NN}) for the genotypes MM, MN, NN and the total number $S = n_{MM} + n_{MN} + n_{NN}$. We can write the likelihood, i.e., the probability of the observed data when the probabilities of the categories are given by (2.5), using the multinomial formula

$$P(n_{MM}, n_{MN}, n_{NN} \mid p) = \binom{S}{n_{MM}, n_{MN}, n_{NN}}(p^2)^{n_{MM}} \times (2pq)^{n_{MN}} \times (q^2)^{n_{NN}},$$

and the log-likelihood under HWE

$$L(p) = n_{MM} \log(p^2) + n_{MN} \log(2pq) + n_{NN} \log(q^2).$$

The value of p that maximizes the log-likelihood is

$$p = \frac{n_{MM} + n_{MN}/2}{S}.$$

See Rice (2006, chapter 8, section 5) for the proof. Given the data (n_{MM}, n_{MN}, n_{NN}), the log-likelihood L is a function of only one parameter, p. Figure 2.11 shows this log-likelihood function for different values of p for the 216th row of the Mourant data,[7] computed in the following code.

[7] This is genotype frequency data of blood group alleles from Mourant et al. (1976), available through the R package *HardyWeinberg*.

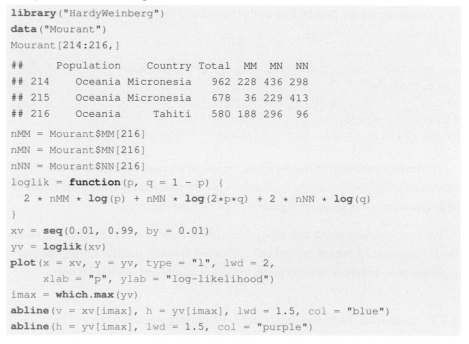

```
library("HardyWeinberg")
data("Mourant")
Mourant[214:216,]

##         Population    Country Total  MM  MN  NN
## 214      Oceania Micronesia   962 228 436 298
## 215      Oceania Micronesia   678  36 229 413
## 216      Oceania     Tahiti   580 188 296  96

nMM = Mourant$MM[216]
nMN = Mourant$MN[216]
nNN = Mourant$NN[216]
loglik = function(p, q = 1 - p) {
  2 * nMM * log(p) + nMN * log(2*p*q) + 2 * nNN * log(q)
}
xv = seq(0.01, 0.99, by = 0.01)
yv = loglik(xv)
plot(x = xv, y = yv, type = "l", lwd = 2,
    xlab = "p", ylab = "log-likelihood")
imax = which.max(yv)
abline(v = xv[imax], h = yv[imax], lwd = 1.5, col = "blue")
abline(h = yv[imax], lwd = 1.5, col = "purple")
```

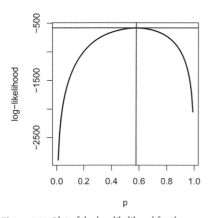

Figure 2.11: Plot of the log-likelihood for the Tahiti data.

The maximum likelihood estimate for the probabilities in the multinomial is also obtained by using the observed frequencies as in the binomial case; however, the estimates have to account for the relationships between the three probabilities. We can compute $\hat{p}_{MM}$, $\hat{p}_{MN}$ and $\hat{p}_{NN}$ using the `af` function from the *HardyWeinberg* package.

```
phat    =   af(c(nMM, nMN, nNN))
phat

## [1] 0.5793103

pMM    =   phat^2
qhat   =   1 - phat
```

The expected values under Hardy–Weinberg equilibrium are then

```
pHW = c(MM = phat^2, MN = 2*phat*qhat, NN = qhat^2)
sum(c(nMM, nMN, nNN)) * pHW

##       MM        MN        NN
## 194.6483 282.7034 102.6483
```

which we can compare to the observed values above. We can see that they are quite close to the observed values. We could further test whether the observed values allow us to reject the Hardy–Weinberg model, by doing either a simulation or a χ^2 test as above. A visual evaluation of the goodness of fit of Hardy–Weinberg was designed by de Finetti (de Finetti, 1926; Cannings and Edwards, 1968). It places every sample at a point whose coordinates are given by the proportions of each of the different alleles.

Visual comparison to the Hardy–Weinberg equilibrium

There are graphical tests for Hardy–Weinberg equilibrium based on a ternary plot (also known as a de Finetti diagram). We can use the `HWTernaryPlot` function for this.

```
pops = c(1, 69, 128, 148, 192)
genotypeFrequencies = as.matrix(Mourant[, c("MM", "MN", "NN")])
HWTernaryPlot(genotypeFrequencies[pops, ],
       markerlab = Mourant$Country[pops],
       alpha = 0.0001, curvecols = c("red", rep("purple", 4)),
       mcex = 0.75, vertex.cex = 1)
```

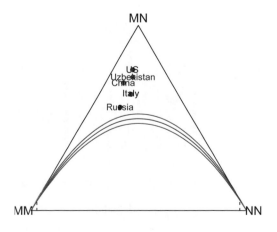

Figure 2.12: This *de Finetti plot* shows the points as barycenters of the three genotypes using the frequencies as weights on each corner of the triangle. The Hardy–Weinberg model is the red curve, and the region where we cannot reject the model is between the two purple lines. We see that the US is the farthest from being in HW equilibrium.

▶ Question **2.16** Make the ternary plot as in the code above, then add the other data points to it. What do you notice? You can back up your discussion using the `HWChisq` function.   ◀

▶ Solution **2.16**

```
HWTernaryPlot(genotypeFrequencies[-pops, ], alpha = 0.0001,
    newframe = FALSE, cex = 0.5)
```

▶ Question **2.17** Divide all total frequencies by 50, keeping the same proportions for each of the genotypes, and recreate the ternary plot.
(a) What happens to the points?
(b) What happens to the confidence regions and why?   ◀

▶ Solution **2.17**

```
newgf = round(genotypeFrequencies / 50)
HWTernaryPlot(newgf[pops, ],
    markerlab = Mourant$Country[pops],
    alpha = 0.0001, curvecols = c("red", rep("purple", 4)),
    mcex = 0.75, vertex.cex = 1)
```

2.7.3   Concatenating several multinomials: sequence motifs and logos

The *Kozak motif* is a sequence that occurs close to the start codon ATG of a coding region. The start codon itself always has a fixed spelling, but in position 5 to the left of it, there is a nucleotide pattern in which the letters are quite far from being equally likely. We summarize this by giving the **position weight matrix** (PWM) or **position-specific scoring matrix** (PSSM), which provides the multinomial probabilities at every position. This is encoded graphically by the **sequence logo** (Figure 2.13).

```
library("seqLogo")
load("../data/kozak.RData")
kozak
```

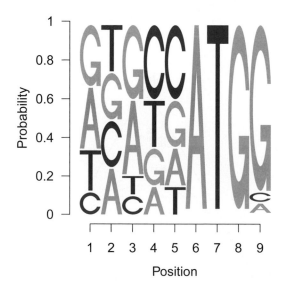

Figure 2.13: This diagram is called a sequence logo for the position-dependent multinomial used to model the Kozak motif. It codifies the amount of variation in each of the positions on a log scale. The large letters represent positions where there is no uncertainty about which nucleotide occurs.

```
##   [,1] [,2] [,3] [,4] [,5] [,6] [,7] [,8] [,9]
## A 0.33 0.25  0.4 0.15 0.20    1    0    0 0.05
## C 0.12 0.25  0.1 0.40 0.40    0    0    0 0.05
## G 0.33 0.25  0.4 0.20 0.25    0    0    1 0.90
## T 0.22 0.25  0.1 0.25 0.15    0    1    0 0.00
pwm = makePWM(kozak)
seqLogo(pwm, ic.scale = FALSE)
```

Over the past few sections, we've seen how the different "boxes" in the multinomial distributions we have encountered very rarely have equal probabilities. In other words, the parameters $p_1, p_2, \dots$ are often different, depending on what is being modeled. Examples of multinomials with unequal frequencies include the 20 different amino acids, blood types and hair color.

If we have multiple categorical variables, we have seen that they are rarely independent (sex and color blindness, hair and eye color, etc.). We will see in Chapter 9 that we can explore the patterns in these dependencies by using multivariate decompositions of the contingency tables. Here, we'll look at an important special case of dependencies between categorical variables: those that occur along a sequence (or "chain") of categorical variables, e.g., over time or along a biopolymer.

2.8 Modeling sequential dependencies: Markov chains

If we want to predict tomorrow's weather, a reasonably good guess is that it will be the same as today's weather. In addition, we may state probabilities for various kinds of possible changes.[8] This method of weather forecasting is an application of the Markov assumption: the prediction for tomorrow depends only on the state of things today, but not on yesterday or three weeks ago (all information we could potentially use is already contained in today's weather). The weather example also highlights that such an assumption need not be exactly true, but it should be a good enough assumption. It is fairly straightforward to extend this assumption to dependencies on the previous k days, where k is a finite and hopefully not too large number. The essence of the Markov assumption is that the process has a finite "memory", so that predictions need to look back for only a finite amount of time.

Instead of temporal sequences, we can also apply this to biological sequences. In DNA, we may see specific successions of patterns so that pairs of nucleotides, called digrams, say, CG, CA, CC and CT, are not equally frequent. For instance, in parts of the genome we see more frequent instances of CA than we would expect under independence:

$$P(CA) \neq P(C)\,P(A).$$

We model this dependency in the sequence as a **Markov chain**:

$$P(CA) = P(NCA) = P(NNCA) = P(\dots CA) = P(C)\,P(A|C),$$

where N stands for any nucleotide and $P(A|C)$ stands for "the probability of A, given that the preceding base is a C". Figure 2.14 shows a schematic representation of such transitions on a graph.

[8] The same reasoning applies in reverse: we can "predict" yesterday's weather from today's.

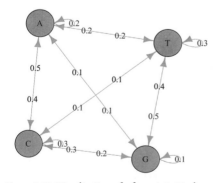

Figure 2.14: Visualization of a four-state Markov chain. The probability of each possible digram (e.g., CA) is given by the weight of the edge between the corresponding nodes. So, for instance, the probability of CA is given by the edge C→A. We'll see in Chapter 10 how to use R packages to draw these types of network graphs.

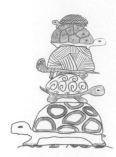

Figure 2.15: Turtles all the way down. Bayesian modeling of the uncertainty of a parameter of a distribution uses a random variable whose own distribution may depend on parameters whose uncertainty can be modeled as random variables; these are called *hierarchical models*.

[9] For so-called frequentists, such a probability does not exist. Their viewpoint is that, although the truth is unknown, in reality the hypothesis is either true or false; there is no meaning in calling it, say, "0.7-true".

2.9 Bayesian thinking

Up to now we have followed a classical approach where the parameters of our distributions, i.e., the probabilities of the possible different outcomes, represent long-term frequencies. The parameters are – at least conceptually – definite, knowable, fixed numbers. We may not know them, so we estimate them from the data at hand. However, such an approach does not take into account any information that we might already know, and that might constrain our parameters or make certain parameters more likely than others even *before* we have seen any of the current set of data. For that we need a different approach, in which we use probability distributions to express our knowledge about the parameters and use data to *update* this knowledge, for instance by shifting those distributions or making them more narrow; this is provided by the Bayesian paradigm (Figure 2.15).

The **Bayesian paradigm** is a practical approach in which **prior** and **posterior** distributions are used as models of our knowledge *before* and *after* collecting some data and making an observation. It is particularly useful for integrating or combining information from different sources.

Suppose we have a certain hypothesis, call it H, and we want to use data to decide whether the hypothesis is true. We can formalize our prior knowledge about H in the form of a prior probability, written $P(H)$.[9] After we see the data, D, we have the posterior probability. We write it as $P(H \mid D)$, the probability of H given that we saw D. This may be higher or lower than $P(H)$, depending on what the data D were.

Haplotypes

To keep the mathematical formalism to a minimum, we will start with an example. We study a forensics example using combined signatures from the Y chromosome called haplotypes.

A **haplotype** is a collection of alleles (DNA sequence variants) that are spatially adjacent on a chromosome, are usually inherited together (recombination tends not to disconnect them), and thus are genetically linked. In this case we are looking at linked variants on the Y chromosome.

First we'll look at the motivation behind haplotype frequency analysis, then we'll revisit a little the idea of likelihood. After this, we'll explain how we can think of unknown parameters as being random numbers themselves, modeling their uncertainty with a prior distribution. Then we will see how to incorporate new data observed into the probability distributions and compute posterior confidence statements about the parameters.

2.9.1 Example: haplotype frequencies

We want to estimate the proportion of a particular Y-haplotype that consists of a set of different short tandem repeats (STRs). The combinations of STR numbers at the specific

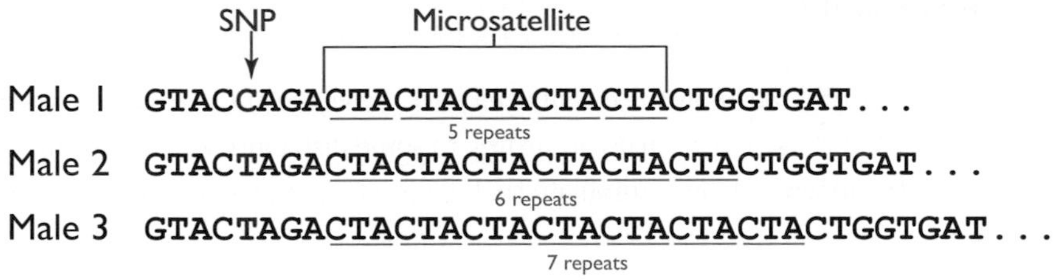

SNP   Microsatellite

Male 1 GTACCAGA<u>CTACTACTACTACTAC</u>TGGTGAT . . .
5 repeats

Male 2 GTACTAGA<u>CTACTACTACTACTACTAC</u>TGGTGAT . . .
6 repeats

Male 3 GTACTAGA<u>CTACTACTACTACTACTACTAC</u>TGGTGAT . . .
7 repeats

Figure 2.16: A short tandem repeat (STR) in DNA occurs when a pattern of two or more nucleotides is repeated and the repeated sequences are directly adjacent to each other. An STR is also known as a microsatellite. The pattern can range in length from 2 to 13 nucleotides, and the number of repeats is highly variable across individuals. STR numbers can be used as genetic signatures.

STR locations used for DNA forensics are labeled by the number of repeats at the specific positions. Here is a short excerpt of an STR haplotype table.

	Individual	DYS19	DXYS156Y	DYS389m	DYS389n	DYS389p
1	H1	14	12	4	12	3
2	H3	15	13	4	13	3
3	H4	15	11	5	11	3
4	H5	17	13	4	11	3
5	H7	13	12	5	12	3
6	H8	16	11	5	12	3

The US Y-STR database can be accessed at http://www.usystrdatabase.org.

This says that haplotype H1 has 14 repeats at position DYS19, 12 repeats at position DXYS156Y, ... We need to find the underlying proportion θ of the haplotype of interest in the population of interest. We are going to consider the occurrence of a haplotype as a "success" in a binomial distribution using collected observations.

The haplotypes created through the use of these Y-STR profiles are shared by men in the same patriarchal lineages. For this reasons it is possible that two different men share the same profile.

2.9.2 Simulation study of the Bayesian paradigm for the binomial

Instead of assuming that our parameter θ has one single value, the Bayesian world view allows us to see it as a draw from a statistical distribution. The distribution expresses our belief about the possible values of the parameter θ. In principle, we can use any distribution that we like whose possible values are permissible for θ. When we are looking at a parameter that expresses a proportion or a probability, and that takes its values between 0 and 1, it is convenient to use the **beta distribution**.

Its density formula is written

$$f_{\alpha,\beta}(x) = \frac{x^{\alpha-1}(1-x)^{\beta-1}}{B(\alpha,\beta)}, \quad \text{where} \quad B(\alpha,\beta) = \frac{\Gamma(\alpha)\Gamma(\beta)}{\Gamma(\alpha+\beta)}.$$

Dividing by $B(\alpha,\beta)$, called the beta function, is necessary to make the total probability integrate to one; $\Gamma(\cdot)$ is the function defined on page 98. We can see in Figure 2.17 how this function depends on the two parameters α and β, making it a very flexible family of distributions (so it can "fit" a lot of different situations). It has a nice mathematical property: if we start with a prior belief on θ that is beta-shaped, observe a dataset of n binomial trials, then update our belief, the posterior distribution on θ will also have a beta distribution, albeit with updated parameters. This is a mathematical fact. We will not prove it; however, we will demonstrate it by simulation.

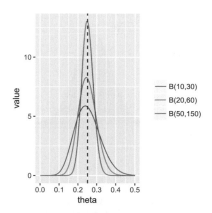

Figure 2.17: Beta distributions with $\alpha = 10, 20, 50$ and $\beta = 30, 60, 150$ used as priors for the probability of success. These three distributions have the same mean ($\frac{\alpha}{\alpha+\beta}$), but different concentrations around the mean.

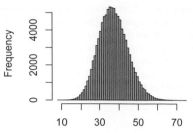

Figure 2.18: Marginal distribution of Y.

The distribution of Y

For a given choice of θ, we know the distribution of Y, by virtue of (2.4). But what is the distribution of Y if θ itself also varies according to some distribution? We call this the **marginal distribution** of Y. Let's simulate that. First we generate a random sample of 10,000 θs.

In the code chunk, we again use `vapply` to apply a function, the unnamed (or "anonymous") function of `th`, across all elements of `rtheta` to obtain as a result another vector `y` of the same length. For each of these θs, we then generate a random sample of Y (Figure 2.18).

```
rtheta = rbeta(100000, 50, 350)
y = vapply(rtheta, function(th) {
  rbinom(1, prob = th, size = 300)
}, numeric(1))
hist(y, breaks = 50, col = "orange", main = "", xlab = "")
```

▶ **Question 2.18** Verify that we can get the same result as in the above code chunk by using R's vectorization capabilities and writing `rbinom(length(rtheta), rtheta, size = 300)`. ◀

Histogram of all the thetas such that $Y = 40$: the posterior distribution

So let's now compute the posterior distribution of θ by conditioning on outcomes where Y is 40. We compare it to the theoretical posterior, `densPostTheory`,[10] of which more below. The results are shown in Figure 2.19.

[10] We use `thetas`, defined in Section 2.4.

```
thetaPostEmp = rtheta[ y == 40 ]
hist(thetaPostEmp, breaks = 40, col = "chartreuse4", main = "",
  probability = TRUE, xlab = expression("posterior"~theta))
densPostTheory  = dbeta(thetas, 90, 610)
lines(thetas, densPostTheory, type="l", lwd = 3)
```

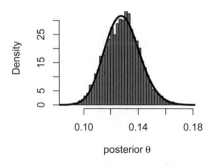

Figure 2.19: Choosing only the values of the distribution with $Y = 40$ gives the posterior distribution of θ. The histogram (green) shows the simulated values for the posterior distribution; the line is the theoretical density of a beta distribution with the theoretical posterior parameters.

We can also check the means of both distributions computed above and see that they are close to four significant digits.

```
mean(thetaPostEmp)
## [1] 0.1285074
dtheta = thetas[2]-thetas[1]
sum(thetas * densPostTheory * dtheta)
## [1] 0.1285714
```

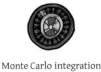

Monte Carlo integration

To approximate the mean of the theoretical density `densPostTheory`, we literally computed the integral $\int_0^1 \theta f(\theta)\, d\theta$ using numerical integration, i.e., the `sum` over the integrand. Direct calculation is not always convenient (or feasible), in particular if our parameters are high dimensional, i.e., if our model parameter θ is not a single scalar but rather a high-dimensional object, as is for instance common in the case of image analysis, and if the integral cannot be computed analytically. So, let's see how we can use **Monte Carlo integration** instead. The method is similar to the code above, where we used numerical integration to compute the posterior mean from `thetaPostEmp` by calling R's `mean` function.

```
thetaPostMC = rbeta(n = 1e6, 90, 610)
mean(thetaPostMC)

## [1] 0.1285704
```

We can check the concordance between our Monte Carlo sample `thetaPostMC` and our sample `thetaPostEmp` using a QQ-plot (Figure 2.20).

```
qqplot(thetaPostMC, thetaPostEmp, type = "l", asp = 1)
abline(a = 0, b = 1, col = "blue")
```

▶ Question **2.19** What is the difference between the simulation that results in `thetaPostEmp` and the Monte Carlo simulation that leads to `thetaPostMC`? ◀

Posterior distribution is also a beta

Now we have seen that the posterior distribution is also a beta. In our case, its parameters $\alpha = 90$ and $\beta = 610$ were obtained by summing the prior parameters $\alpha = 50$ and $\beta = 350$ with the observed successes $y = 40$ and the observed failures $n - y = 260$, thus obtaining the posterior

$$\text{beta}(90, 610) = \text{beta}(\alpha + y, \beta + (n - y)).$$

We can use it to give the best[11] estimate we can for θ with its uncertainty given by the posterior distribution.

Suppose we have a second series of data.   After seeing our previous data, we now have a new prior, $\text{beta}(90, 610)$.

- Now we collect a new set of data with $n = 150$ observations and $y = 25$ successes, thus 125 failures.
- Now what do we take to be our best guess at θ?

Using the same reasoning as before, the new posterior will be: $\text{beta}(90 + 25 = 115, 610 + 125 = 735)$. The mean of this distribution is $\frac{115}{115+735} = \frac{115}{850} \simeq 0.135$, thus one estimate of θ is 0.135.

The theoretical **maximum a posteriori (MAP) estimate** would be the mode of $\text{beta}(115, 735)$, i.e., $\frac{114}{848} \simeq 0.134$. Let's check this numerically.

```
densPost2 = dbeta(thetas, 115, 735)
mcPost2   = rbeta(1e6, 115, 735)

sum(thetas * densPost2 * dtheta)   # mean, by numeric integration
## [1] 0.1352941

mean(mcPost2)                       # mean, by MC
## [1] 0.1352946

thetas[which.max(densPost2)]        # MAP estimate
## [1] 0.134
```

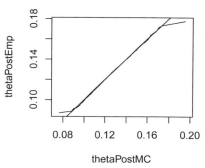

Figure 2.20: QQ-plot of our Monte Carlo sample `thetaPostMC` from the theoretical distribution and our simulation sample `thetaPostEmp`. The curve lies on the line $y = x$, which indicates good agreement, with some random differences at the tails. We could similarly compare either of these two distributions to the theoretical distribution function `pbeta(., 90, 610)`.

[11] We could take the value that maximizes the posterior distribution as our best estimate. This is called the MAP estimate, and in this case it would be $\frac{\alpha-1}{\alpha+\beta-2} = \frac{89}{698} \doteq 0.1275$.

The last line of this code uses a Monte Carlo method for finding the MAP estimate from a sample from `rbeta(., 115, 735)`.

▶ **Question 2.20** Redo all the computations replacing our original prior with a softer prior (less peaked), meaning that we use less prior information. How much does this change the final result?   ◀

As a general rule, the prior rarely changes the posterior distribution substantially except if it is very peaked. This would be the case if, at the outset, we were already rather sure of what to expect. Another case when the prior has an influence is if there is very little data.

The best situation to be in is to have enough data to swamp the prior so that its choice doesn't have much impact on the final result.

Confidence statements for the proportion parameter

Now it is time to reach a conclusion about where the proportion actually lies given the data. One summary is a posterior credibility interval, which is a Bayesian analog of the confidence interval. We can take the 2.5th and 97.5th percentiles of the posterior distribution $P(L \leqslant \theta \leqslant U) = 0.95$ using R.

```
quantile(mcPost2, c(0.025, 0.975))
```

```
##      2.5%      97.5%
## 0.1131418 0.1590589
```

2.10   Example: occurrence of a nucleotide pattern in a genome

The examples we have seen up to now have concentrated on distributions of discrete counts and categorical data. Let's look at an example of distributions of distances, which are quasi-continuous. This case study of the distributions of the distances between instances of a specific motif in genome sequences will also allow us to explore specific genomic sequence manipulations in Bioconductor.

The *Biostrings* package provides tools for working with sequence data. The essential data structures, or *classes* as they are known in R, are *DNAString* and *DNAStringSet*. These enable us to work with one or multiple DNA sequences efficiently.

```
library("Biostrings")
```

▶ **Question 2.21** Explore some of the useful data and functions provided in the *Biostrings* package by exploring the tutorial vignette.   ◀

▶ **Solution 2.21** The first line prints genetic code information, the second one returns IUPAC nucleotide ambiguity codes. The third line lists all the vignettes available in the *Biostrings* package, the fourth displays one particular vignette.

```
GENETIC_CODE
IUPAC_CODE_MAP
vignette(package = "Biostrings")
vignette("BiostringsQuickOverview", package = "Biostrings")                  □
```

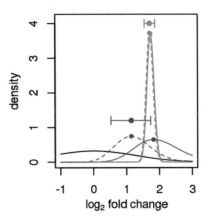

Figure 2.21: An example from Love et al. (2014) shows plots of the likelihoods (solid lines, scaled to integrate to 1) and the posteriors (dashed lines) for the green and purple genes and of the prior (solid black line): due to the higher dispersion of the purple gene, its likelihood is wider and less peaked (indicating less information), and the prior has more influence on its posterior than it does for the green gene. The stronger curvature of the green posterior at its maximum translates to a smaller reported standard error for the MAP logarithmic fold change (LFC) estimate (horizontal error bar).

The *Biostrings* package contains additional classes for representing amino acid and general biological strings.

The `vignette` command will open a list in your browser window from which you can access the documentation.

The *BSgenome* package provides access to many genomes, and you can access the names of the data packages that contain the whole genome sequences by typing

Vignettes are manuals for R packages, complete with examples and case studies.

```
library("BSgenome")
ag = available.genomes()
length(ag)
## [1] 87
ag[1:2]
## [1] "BSgenome.Alyrata.JGI.v1"
## [2] "BSgenome.Amellifera.BeeBase.assembly4"
```

We are going to explore the occurrence of the `AGGAGGT` motif[12] in the genome of *E. coli*. We use the genome sequence of one particular strain, **Escherichia coli** str. K12 substr. DH10B,[13] whose NCBI accession number is NC_010473.

[12] This is the *Shine–Dalgarno motif*, which helps initiate protein synthesis in bacteria.

[13] It is known as the laboratory workhorse, often used in experiments.

```
library("BSgenome.Ecoli.NCBI.20080805")
Ecoli
shineDalgarno = "AGGAGGT"
ecoli = Ecoli$NC_010473
```

We can count the pattern's occurrence in windows of width 50,000 using the `countPattern` function.

```
window = 50000
starts = seq(1, length(ecoli) - window, by = window)
ends   = starts + window - 1
numMatches = vapply(seq_along(starts), function(i) {
  countPattern(shineDalgarno, ecoli[starts[i]:ends[i]],
            max.mismatch = 0)
  }, numeric(1))
table(numMatches)
## numMatches
##  0  1  2  3  4
## 48 32  8  3  2
```

▶ Question **2.22** What distribution might this table fit?   ◀

▶ Solution **2.22** The Poisson is a good candidate, as a quantitative and graphical evaluation (see Figure 2.22) of these data shows.

```
library("vcd")
gf = goodfit(numMatches, "poisson")
summary(gf)
##
##   Goodness-of-fit test for poisson distribution
##
##                       X^2 df  P(> X^2)
## Likelihood Ratio 4.134932  3 0.2472577
distplot(numMatches, type = "poisson")
```

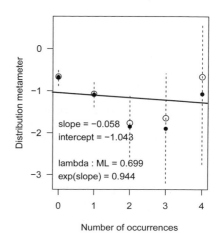

Figure 2.22: Evaluation of a Poisson model for motif counts along the sequence `Ecoli$NC_010473`.

We can inspect the matches using the `matchPattern` function.

```
sdMatches = matchPattern(shineDalgarno, ecoli, max.mismatch = 0)
```

You can type `sdMatches` in the R command line to obtain a summary of this object. It contains the locations of all 65 pattern matches, represented as a set of so-called **views** on the original sequence. Now what are the distances between them?

```
betweenmotifs = gaps(sdMatches)
```

So these are in fact the 66 complementary regions. Now let's find a model for the distribution of the gap sizes between motifs. If the motifs occur at random locations, we expect the gap lengths to follow an **exponential distribution**.[14] The code below (whose output is shown in Figure 2.23) assesses this assumption. If the exponential distribution is a good fit, the points should lie roughly on a straight line. The exponential distribution has one parameter, the rate, and the line with slope corresponding to an estimate from the data is also shown.

```
library("Renext")
expplot(width(betweenmotifs), rate = 1/mean(width(betweenmotifs)),
          labels = "fitted exponential")
```

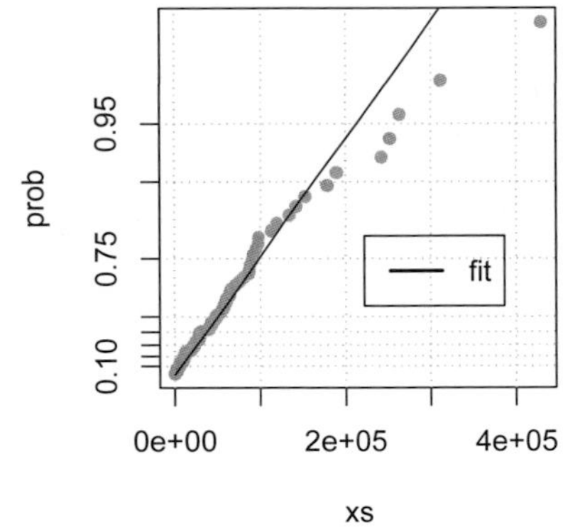

▶ **Question 2.23** There appears to be a slight deviation from the fitted line in Figure 2.23 at the right tail of the distibution, i.e., for the largest values. What could be the reason?

◀

[14] How could we guess that the exponential is the right fit here? Whenever we have independent, random Bernoulli occurrences along a sequence, the gap lengths are exponential. You may be familiar with radioactive decay, where the waiting times between emissions are also exponentially distributed. It is a good idea if you are not familiar with this distribution to look up more details on Wikipedia.

Figure 2.23: Evaluation of fit to the exponential distribution of the gaps between the motifs.

2.10.1 Modeling in the case of dependencies

As we saw in Section 2.8, nucleotide sequences are often dependent: the probability of seeing a certain nucleotide at a given position tends to depend on the surrounding sequence. Here we are going to put into practice dependency modeling using a *Markov chain*. We are going to look at regions of chromosome 8 of the human genome to try to discover differences between regions called CpG islands and the rest.[15]

We use data (generated by Irizarry et al. (2009)) that tell us where the start and end points of the islands are in the genome and look at the frequencies of nucleotides and of the digrams CG, CT, CA, CC. So we can ask whether there are dependencies between the nucleotide occurrences and, if so, how to model them.

[15] CpG stands for 5'-C-phosphate-G-3'; this means that a C is connected to a G through a phosphate along the strand (this is unrelated to C–G base-pairing of Section 2.7). The cytosines in the CpG dinucleotide can be methylated, changing the levels of gene expression. This type of gene regulation is part of **epigenetics**. More information is on Wikipedia: see *CpG site* and *epigenetics*.

```
library("BSgenome.Hsapiens.UCSC.hg19")
chr8   = Hsapiens$chr8
CpGtab = read.table("../data/model-based-cpg-islands-hg19.txt",
                    header = TRUE)
nrow(CpGtab)
## [1] 65699
head(CpGtab)
##      chr  start    end length CpGcount GCcontent pctGC obsExp
## 1 chr10  93098  93818    721       32       403 0.559  0.572
## 2 chr10  94002  94165    164       12        97 0.591  0.841
## 3 chr10  94527  95302    776       65       538 0.693  0.702
```

```
## 4 chr10 119652 120193    542        53       369 0.681   0.866
## 5 chr10 122133 122621    489        51       339 0.693   0.880
## 6 chr10 180265 180720    456        32       256 0.561   0.893
irCpG = with(dplyr::filter(CpGtab, chr == "chr8"),
       IRanges(start = start, end = end))
```

In the last line of code, we subset (`filter`) the data frame `CpGtab` to only chromosome 8, and then we create an *IRanges* object whose start and end positions are defined by the equally named columns of the data frame. In the `IRanges` function call (which constructs the object from its arguments), the first `start` is the argument name of the function, the second `start` refers to the column in the data frame obtained as an output from `filter`, and similarly for `end`.

IRanges is a general container for mathematical intervals. We create the biological context with the next line.[16]

```
grCpG = GRanges(ranges = irCpG, seqnames = "chr8", strand = "+")
genome(grCpG) = "hg19"
```

Now let's visualize; see the output in Figure 2.24.

```
library("Gviz")
ideo = IdeogramTrack(genome = "hg19", chromosome = "chr8")
plotTracks(
  list(GenomeAxisTrack(),
    AnnotationTrack(grCpG, name = "CpG"), ideo),
    from = 2200000, to = 5800000,
    shape = "box", fill = "#006400", stacking = "dense")
```

We now define so-called views on the chromosome sequence that correspond to the CpG islands, `irCpG`, and to the regions in between, `gaps(irCpG)`. The resulting objects, `CGIview` and `NonCGIview`, contain only the coordinates, not the sequences themselves (these stay in the big object `Hsapiens$chr8`), so they are fairly lightweight in terms of storage.

```
CGIview    = Views(unmasked(Hsapiens$chr8), irCpG)
NonCGIview = Views(unmasked(Hsapiens$chr8), gaps(irCpG))
```

We compute transition counts in CpG islands and non-islands using the data.

```
seqCGI      = as(CGIview, "DNAStringSet")
seqNonCGI   = as(NonCGIview, "DNAStringSet")
dinucCpG    = sapply(seqCGI, dinucleotideFrequency)
dinucNonCpG = sapply(seqNonCGI, dinucleotideFrequency)
dinucNonCpG[, 1]

## AA  AC  AG  AT  CA  CC  CG  CT  GA  GC  GG  GT  TA  TC  TG  TT
## 389 351 400 436 498 560 112 603 359 336 403 336 330 527 519 485

NonICounts = rowSums(dinucNonCpG)
IslCounts  = rowSums(dinucCpG)
```

For a four-state Markov chain as we have, we define the transition matrix as a matrix where the rows are the "from" state and the columns are the "to" state.

We use the `::` operator to call the `filter` function specifically from the `dplyr` package – and not from any other packages that may happen to be loaded and defining functions of the same name. This precaution is particularly advisable in the case of the `filter` function, since this name is used by many other packages. You can think of the normal (without `::`) way of calling R functions as calling people by their first (given) names, whereas the fully qualified version with `::` corresponds to calling people by their full names. At least within the reach of the CRAN and Bioconductor repositories, such fully qualified names are guaranteed to be unique.

[16]The "I" in *IRanges* stands for "interval", the "G" in *GRanges* for "genomic".

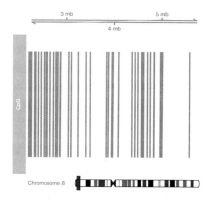

Figure 2.24: *Gviz* plot of CpG locations in a selected region of chromosome 8.

```
TI  = matrix( IslCounts, ncol = 4, byrow = TRUE)
TnI = matrix(NonICounts, ncol = 4, byrow = TRUE)
dimnames(TI) = dimnames(TnI) =
  list(c("A", "C", "G", "T"), c("A", "C", "G", "T"))
```

The transition probabilities are *probabilities*, so the rows need to sum to 1.

We use the counts of numbers of transitions of each type to compute frequencies and put them into two matrices.

```
MI = TI /rowSums(TI)
MI

##            A         C         G         T
## A 0.20457773 0.2652333 0.3897678 0.1404212
## C 0.20128250 0.3442381 0.2371595 0.2173200
## G 0.18657245 0.3145299 0.3450223 0.1538754
## T 0.09802105 0.3352314 0.3598984 0.2068492

MN = TnI / rowSums(TnI)
MN

##            A         C          G         T
## A 0.3351380 0.1680007 0.23080886 0.2660524
## C 0.3641054 0.2464366 0.04177094 0.3476871
## G 0.2976696 0.2029017 0.24655406 0.2528746
## T 0.2265813 0.1972407 0.24117528 0.3350027
```

▶ Question **2.24** Are the transitions different in the different rows? This would mean that, for instance, $P(A \mid C) \neq P(A \mid T)$. ◀

▶ Solution **2.24** The transitions are different. For instance, the transitions from C to A and T to A in the islands (MI) transition matrix seem very different (0.201 versus 0.098). □

▶ Question **2.25** Are the relative frequencies of the different nucleotides different in CpG islands compared to elsewhere? ◀

▶ Solution **2.25**

```
freqIsl=alphabetFrequency(seqCGI,baseOnly=TRUE,collapse=TRUE)[1:4]
freqIsl / sum(freqIsl)
##         A         C         G         T
## 0.1781693 0.3201109 0.3206298 0.1810901

freqNon=alphabetFrequency(seqNonCGI,baseOnly=TRUE,collapse=TRUE)[1:4]
freqNon / sum(freqNon)
##         A         C         G         T
## 0.3008292 0.1993832 0.1993737 0.3004139
```

This output shows an inverse pattern: in the CpG islands, C and G have frequencies around 0.32, whereas in the non-CpG islands, it is A and T that have frequencies around 0.30. □

▶ Question **2.26** How can we use these differences to decide whether a given sequence comes from a CpG island? ◀

▶ Solution **2.26** Use a χ^2 statistic to compare the frequencies between the observed and `freqIsl` and `freqNon` frequencies. For shorter sequences, this test may not be sensitive enough, and a more sensitive approach is given below.   □

Given a sequence for which it's unknown whether it is in a CpG island or not, we can ask what is the probability that it belongs to a CpG island compared to somewhere else. We compute a score based on what is called the odds ratio. Let's do an example: suppose our sequence x is ACGTTATACTACG and we want to decide whether it comes from a CpG island or not.

If we model the sequence as a first-order Markov chain we can write, supposing that the sequence comes from a CpG island:

$$P_i(x = \text{ACGTTATACTACG}) = P_i(\text{A})\, P_i(\text{AC})\, P_i(\text{CG})\, P_i(\text{GT})\, P_i(\text{TT})$$
$$\times P_i(\text{TA})\, P_i(\text{AT})\, P_i(\text{TA})\, P_i(\text{AC})\, P_i(\text{CG}). \qquad (2.6)$$

We are going to compare this probability to the probability for non-islands. As we saw above, these probabilities tend to be quite different. We will take their ratio and see if it is larger or smaller than 1. These probabilties are going to be products of many small terms and become very small. We can work around this by taking logarithms:

$$\log \frac{P(x \mid \text{island})}{P(x \mid \text{non island})} =$$
$$\log \left(\frac{P_i(\text{A})\, P_i(\text{A} \to \text{C})\, P_i(\text{C} \to \text{G})\, P_i(\text{G} \to \text{T})\, P_i(\text{T} \to \text{T})\, P_i(\text{T} \to \text{A})}{P_n(\text{A})\, P_n(\text{A} \to \text{C})\, P_n(\text{C} \to \text{G})\, P_n(\text{G} \to \text{T})\, P_n(\text{T} \to \text{T})\, P_n(\text{T} \to \text{A})} \right.$$
$$\left. \times \frac{P_i(\text{A} \to \text{T})\, P_i(\text{T} \to \text{A})\, P_i(\text{A} \to \text{C})\, P_i(\text{C} \to \text{G})}{P_n(\text{A} \to \text{T})\, P_n(\text{T} \to \text{A})\, P_n(\text{A} \to \text{C})\, P_n(\text{C} \to \text{G})} \right). \qquad (2.7)$$

This is the **log-likelihood ratio** score. To speed up the calculation, we compute the log-ratios $\log(P_i(\text{A})/P_n(\text{A})), \ldots, \log(P_i(\text{T} \to \text{A})/P_n(\text{T} \to \text{A}))$ once and for all and then sum up the relevant ratios to obtain our score.

```
alpha = log((freqIsl/sum(freqIsl)) / (freqNon/sum(freqNon)))
beta  = log(MI / MN)
```

```
x = "ACGTTATACTACG"
scorefun = function(x) {
  s = unlist(strsplit(x, ""))
  score = alpha[s[1]]
  if (length(s) >= 2)
    for (j in 2:length(s))
      score = score + beta[s[j-1], s[j]]
  score
}
scorefun(x)

##          A
## -0.2824623
```

In the code below, we pick sequences of length `len = 100` out of the 2855 sequences in the `seqCGI` object, and then out of the 2854 sequences in the `seqNonCGI` object (each of them is a *DNAStringSet*). In the first three lines of the `generateRandomScores` function, we drop sequences that contain any letters other than A, C, T, G, for example "." (a character used for undefined nucleotides). Among the remaining sequences,

Worked-out examples and many useful details can be found in Durbin et al. (1998).

we sample with probabilities proportional to their length minus `len` and then pick subsequences of length `len` out of them. The start points of the subsequences are sampled uniformly, with the constraint that the subsequences have to fit in.

```r
generateRandomScores = function(s, len = 100, B = 1000) {
  alphFreq = alphabetFrequency(s)
  isGoodSeq = rowSums(alphFreq[, 5:ncol(alphFreq)]) == 0
  s = s[isGoodSeq]
  slen = sapply(s, length)
  prob = pmax(slen - len, 0)
  prob = prob / sum(prob)
  idx  = sample(length(s), B, replace = TRUE, prob = prob)
  ssmp = s[idx]
  start = sapply(ssmp, function(x) sample(length(x) - len, 1))
  scores = sapply(seq_len(B), function(i)
    scorefun(as.character(ssmp[[i]][start[i]+(1:len)]))
  )
  scores / len
}
scoresCGI    = generateRandomScores(seqCGI)
scoresNonCGI = generateRandomScores(seqNonCGI)
```

```r
br = seq(-0.6, 0.7, length.out = 50)
h1 = hist(scoresCGI,    breaks = br, plot = FALSE)
h2 = hist(scoresNonCGI, breaks = br, plot = FALSE)
plot(h1, col = rgb(0, 0, 1, 1/4), xlim = c(-0.5, 0.5), ylim=c(0,120))
plot(h2, col = rgb(1, 0, 0, 1/4), add = TRUE)
```

We can consider these our *training data*: from data for which we know the types, we can see whether our score is useful for discriminating – see Figure 2.25.

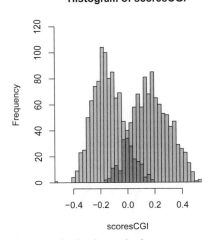

Histogram of scoresCGI

Figure 2.25: Island and non-island scores as generated by the function `generateRandomScores`. This is the first instance of a *mixture* we have encountered. We will revisit mixtures in Chapter 4.

2.11 Summary of this chapter

In this chapter we experienced the basic yoga of statistics: how to go from the data back to the possible generating distributions and how to estimate the parameters that define these distributions.

Statistical models We showed some specific statistical models for experiments with categorical outcomes (binomial and multinomial).

Goodness of fit We used different visualizations and showed how to run simulation experiments to test whether our data could be fit by a fair four-box multinomial model. We encountered the chi-square statistic and saw how to compare simulation and theory using a QQ-plot.

Estimation We explained maximum likelihood and Bayesian estimation procedures. These approaches were illustrated on examples involving nucleotide pattern discovery and haplotype estimation.

Prior and posterior distributions When assessing data of a type that has been been previously studied, such as haplotypes, it can be beneficial to compute the posterior distribution of the data. This enables us to incorporate uncertainty in the decision making, by way of a simple computation. The choice of the prior has little effect on the result as long as there is sufficient data.

CpG islands and Markov chains We saw how dependencies along DNA sequences can be modeled by Markov chain transitions. We used this to build scores based on likelihood ratios that enable us to see whether long DNA sequences come from CpG islands or not. When we made the histogram of scores, we saw in Figure 2.25 a noticeable feature: it seemed to be made of two pieces. This **bimodality** was our first encounter with mixtures; they are the subject of Chapter 4.

This was also our first attempt to build a model on some training data: sequences that we knew were in CpG islands and could use later to classify new data. We will develop a much more complete way of learning from data in Chapter 12.

2.12 Further reading

One of the best introductory statistics books available is Freedman et al. (1997). It uses box models to explain the important concepts. If you have never taken a statistics class, or you feel you need a refresher, we highly recommend it. Many introductory statistics classes do not cover statistics for discrete data in any depth. The subject is an important part of what we need for biological applications. A book-long introduction to these types of analyses can be found in Agresti (2007).

Here we gave examples of simple unstructured multinomials. However, sometimes the categories (or boxes) of a multinomial have specific structure. For instance, the 64 possible codons code for 20 amino acids and the stop codons (61+3). So we can see the amino acids themselves as a multinomial with 20 degrees of freedom. Within each amino acid there are multinomials with differing numbers of categories (proline has four: CCA, CCG, CCC, CCT; see Exercise 2.3). Some multivariate methods have been specifically designed to decompose the variability between codon usage within the differently abundant amino acids (Grantham et al., 1981; Perrière and Thioulouse, 2002), and this enables discovery of latent gene transfer and translational selection. We will cover the specific methods used in those papers when we delve into the multivariate exploration of categorical data in Chapter 9.

There are many examples of successful uses of the Bayesian paradigm to quantify uncertainties. In recent years the computation of the posterior distribution has been revolutionized by special types of Monte Carlo that use either a Markov chain or random walk or Hamiltonian dynamics. These methods provide approximations that converge to the correct posterior distribution after quite a few iterations. For examples and much more, see Robert and Casella (2009), Marin and Robert (2007) and McElreath (2015).

2.13 Exercises

▶ **Exercise 2.1** Generate 1000 random 0/1 variables that model mutations occurring along a 1000-long gene sequence. These occur independently at a rate of 10^{-4} each. Sum the 1000 positions to count how many mutations occur in sequences of length 1000.

Find the correct distribution for these mutation sums using a goodness-of-fit test and make a plot to visualize the quality of the fit.   ◄

▶ **Exercise 2.2** Make a function that generates *n* random uniform numbers between 0 and 7 and returns their maximum. Execute the function for *n* = 25. Repeat this procedure *B* = 100 times. Plot the distribution of these maxima.

What is the maximum likelihood estimate of the maximum of a sample of size 25 (call it $\hat{\theta}$)?

Can you find a theoretical justification and the true maximum θ?   ◄

▶ **Exercise 2.3** A sequence of three nucleotides (a **codon**) taken in a coding region of a gene can be transcribed into one of 20 possible amino acids. There are $4^3 = 64$ possible codon sequences, but only 20 amino acids. We say the **genetic code** is redundant: there are several ways to *spell* each amino acid.

The multiplicity (the number of codons that code for the same amino acid) varies from two to six. The different codon spellings of each amino acid do not occur with equal probabilities. Let's look at the data for the standard laboratory strain of tuberculosis (H37Rv).

```
mtb = read.table("../data/M_tuberculosis.txt", header = TRUE)
head(mtb, n = 4)

##   AmAcid Codon Number PerThous
## 1    Gly   GGG  25874    19.25
## 2    Gly   GGA  13306     9.90
## 3    Gly   GGT  25320    18.84
## 4    Gly   GGC  68310    50.82
```

The codons for the amino acid proline are of the form $CC*$, and they occur with the following frequencies in Mycobacterium tuberculosis.

```
pro  =  mtb[ mtb$AmAcid == "Pro", "Number"]
pro/sum(pro)

## [1] 0.54302025 0.10532985 0.05859765 0.29305225
```

a. Explore the data `mtb` using `table` to tabulate the `AmAcid` and `Codon` variables.
b. How was the `PerThous` variable created?
c. Write an R function that you can apply to the table to find which of the amino acids shows the strongest **codon bias**, i.e., the strongest departure from uniform distribution among its possible spellings.   ◄

▶ **Exercise 2.4** Display GC content in a running window along the sequence of *Staphylococcus aureus*. Read in a `fasta` file sequence from a file.

```
staph = readDNAStringSet("../data/staphsequence.ffn.txt", "fasta")
```

a. Look at the complete `staph` object and then display the first three sequences in the set.
b. Find the GC content in sequence windows of width 100.

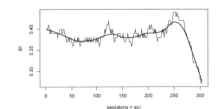

Figure 2.26: Smoothed GC content along sequence 364 of the *Staphylococcus aureus* genome.

c. Display the GC content in a sliding window as a fraction.

d. How could we visualize the overall trends of these proportions along the sequence?

◀

▶ Exercise **2.5** Redo a figure similar to Figure 2.17, but include two other distributions: the uniform (which is beta(1, 1)) and the beta($\frac{1}{2}, \frac{1}{2}$). What do you notice?   ◀

▶ Exercise **2.6** Choose your own prior for the parameters of the beta distribution. You can do this by sketching it here: `https://jhubiostatistics.shinyapps.io/ drawyourprior`. Once you have set up a prior, reanalyze the data from Section 2.9.2, where we saw $Y = 40$ successes out of $n = 300$ trials. Compare your posterior distribution to the one we obtained in that section using a QQ-plot.   ◀

CHAPTER 3

High-Quality Graphics in R

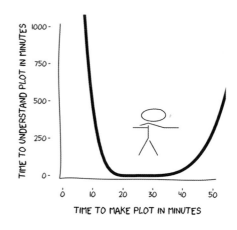

There are (at least) two types of data visualization. The first enables a scientist to explore data and make discoveries about the complex processes at work. The other type of visualization provides informative, clear and visually attractive illustrations of her results that she can show to others and eventually include in a publication.

Both of these types of visualizations can be made with R. In fact, R offers multiple graphics systems. This is because R is extensible, and because progress in R graphics over the years has proceeded largely not by replacing the old functions, but by adding packages. Each of the different graphics systems has its advantages and limitations. In this chapter we will get to know two of them. First we have a cursory look at the base R plotting functions.[1] Subsequently we will switch to *ggplot2*.

Base R graphics came historically first: simple, procedural, conceptually motivated by drawing on a canvas. There are specialized functions for different types of plots. These are easy to call – but when you want to combine them to build up more complex plots or exchange one for another, this quickly gets messy, or even impossible. The user plots (the word harks back to some of the first graphics devices – see Figure 3.1) directly onto a (conceptual) canvas. She explicitly needs to deal with decisions such as how much space to allocate to margins, axis labels, titles, legends, subpanels; once something is "plotted", it cannot be moved or erased.

There is a more high-level approach: in the *grammar of graphics*, graphics are built up from modular logical pieces, so that we can easily try different visualization types for our data in an intuitive and easily deciphered way, just as we can switch in and out parts of a sentence in human language. There is no concept of a canvas or a plotter; rather, the user gives *ggplot2* a high-level description of the plot she wants, in the form of an R object, and the rendering engine takes a holistic view of the scene to lay out the graphics and render them on the output device.

[1] They live in the *graphics* package, which ships with every basic R installation.

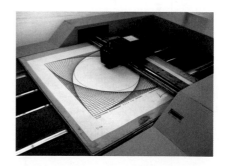

Figure 3.1: The ZUSE Plotter Z64 (presented in 1961). Image credit: Wikicommons.

3.1 Goals for this chapter

In this chapter we will:

- Learn how to rapidly and flexibly explore datasets by visualization.
- Create beautiful and intuitive plots for scientific presentations and publications.

- Review the basics of base R plotting.
- Understand the logic behind the *grammar of graphics* concept.
- Introduce *ggplot2*'s `ggplot` function.
- See how to plot data in one, two, and even three to five dimensions, and explore faceting.
- Create "along-genome" plots for molecular biology data (or along other sequences, e.g., peptides).
- Discuss some of our options for interactive graphics.

3.2   Base R plotting

The most basic function is `plot`. In the code below, the output of which is shown in Figure 3.2, it is used to plot data from an enzyme-linked immunosorbent assay (ELISA). The assay was used to quantify the activity of the enzyme deoxyribonuclease (DNase), which degrades DNA. The data are assembled in the R object `DNase`, which conveniently comes with base R. The object `DNase` is a dataframe whose columns are `Run`, the assay run; `conc`, the protein concentration that was used; and `density`, the measured optical density.

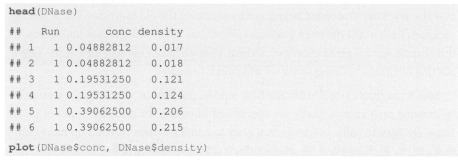

```
head(DNase)

##   Run        conc density
## 1   1 0.04882812   0.017
## 2   1 0.04882812   0.018
## 3   1 0.19531250   0.121
## 4   1 0.19531250   0.124
## 5   1 0.39062500   0.206
## 6   1 0.39062500   0.215

plot(DNase$conc, DNase$density)
```

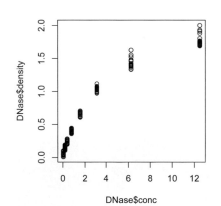

Figure 3.2: Plot of concentration vs. density for an ELISA assay of DNase.

This basic plot can be customized, for example by changing the plot symbol and axis labels using the parameters `xlab`, `ylab` and `pch` (plot character), as shown in Figure 3.3. Information about the variables is stored in the object `DNase`, and we can access it with the `attr` function.

```
plot(DNase$conc, DNase$density,
  ylab = attr(DNase, "labels")$y,
  xlab = paste(attr(DNase, "labels")$x, attr(DNase, "units")$x),
  pch = 3,
  col = "blue")
```

▶ Question **3.1** Annotating dataframe columns with "metadata" such as longer descriptions, physical units, provenance information, etc., seems like a useful feature. Is this way of storing such information, as in the `DNase` object, standardized across the R ecosystem? Are there other standardized or common ways of doing this?   ◀

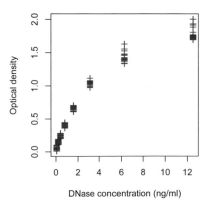

Figure 3.3: Same data as in Figure 3.2 but with better axis labels and a different plot symbol.

▶ Solution **3.1** There is no good or widely used infrastructure in regular R *data.frame*s for this, nor in the tidyverse (*data_frame*, *tibble*). But have a look at the *DataFrame* class in the Bioconductor package *S4Vectors*. Among other things, it is used to annotate the rows and columns of a *SummarizedExperiment*.   □

Besides scatterplots, we can also use built-in functions to create histograms and boxplots (Figure 3.4).

```
hist(DNase$density, breaks=25, main = "")
```

```
boxplot(density ~ Run, data = DNase)
```

Boxplots are convenient for showing multiple distributions next to each other in a compact space. We will see more about plotting multiple univariate distributions in Section 3.6.

The base R plotting functions are great for quick interactive exploration of data, but we soon run into their limitations if we want to create more sophisticated displays. We are going to use a visualization framework called the grammar of graphics, implemented in the package *ggplot2*, that enables step-by-step construction of high-quality graphics in a logical and elegant manner. First let us introduce and load an example dataset.

3.3   An example dataset

To properly test-drive the *ggplot2* functionality, we need a dataset that is big enough and has some complexity so that it can be sliced and viewed from many different angles. We'll use a gene expression microarray dataset that reports the transcriptomes of around 100 individual cells from mouse embryos at different time points in early development. The mammalian embryo starts out as a single cell, the fertilized egg. Through synchronized waves of cell division, the egg multiplies into a clump of cells that at first show no discernible differences between them. At some point, though, cells choose different lineages. By further and further specification, the different cell types and tissues arise that are needed for a full organism. The aim of the experiment, explained by Ohnishi et al. (2014), was to investigate the gene expression changes associated with the first symmetry-breaking event in the embryo. We'll further explain the data as we go. More details can be found in the paper and in the documentation of the Bioconductor data package *Hiiragi2013*. We first load the data.

```
library("Hiiragi2013")
data("x")
dim(exprs(x))
## [1] 45101   101
```

You can print out a more detailed summary of the *ExpressionSet* object x by typing x at the R prompt. The 101 columns of the data matrix (accessed above through the `exprs` function) correspond to the samples (and each of these to a single cell), and the 45,101 rows correspond to the genes probed by the array, an Affymetrix mouse4302 array. The data were normalized using the RMA method (Irizarry et al., 2003). The raw data are also available in the package (in the data object a) and at EMBL–EBI's ArrayExpress database under accession code E-MTAB-1681.

Figure 3.4: Histogram of the density from the ELISA, and boxplots of these values stratified by assay run. The boxes are ordered along the axis in lexicographical order because the runs were stored as text strings. We could use R's type conversion functions to achieve numerical ordering.

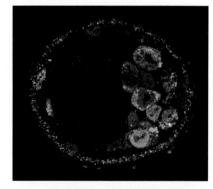

Figure 3.5: Single-section immunofluorescence image of the E3.5 mouse blastocyst stained for Serpinh1, a marker of primitive endoderm (blue), Gata6 (red) and Nanog (green).

It is unfortunate that the data object has the rather generic name x, rather than a more descriptive name. To avoid name collisions, a pragmatic solution is to run code such as `esHiiragi = x; rm(list="x")`.

[2] The notation #CAB2D6 is a hexadecimal representation of the RGB coordinates of a color; more on this in Section 3.10.2.

Let's have a look at what information is available about the samples.[2]

```
head(pData(x), n = 2)

##          File.name Embryonic.day Total.number.of.cells lineage
## 1 E3.25   1_C32_IN         E3.25                    32
## 2 E3.25   2_C32_IN         E3.25                    32
##          genotype   ScanDate sampleGroup sampleColour
## 1 E3.25        WT 2011-03-16       E3.25      #CAB2D6
## 2 E3.25        WT 2011-03-16       E3.25      #CAB2D6
```

The information provided is a mix of information about the cells (i.e., age, size and genotype of the embryo from which they were obtained) and technical information (scan date, raw data file name). By convention, time in the development of the mouse embryo is measured in days and reported as, for instance, E3.5. Moreover, in the paper the authors divided the cells into eight biological groups (sampleGroup), based on age, genotype and lineage, and they defined a color scheme to represent these groups (sampleColour[3]). Using the following code – see below for explanations – we define a small dataframe groups that contains summary information for each group: the number of cells and the preferred color.

[3] This identifier in the dataset uses the British spelling. Everywhere else in this book, we use the US spelling (color). The *ggplot2* package generally accepts both spellings.

```
library("dplyr")
groups = group_by(pData(x), sampleGroup) %>%
  summarise(n = n(), color = unique(sampleColour))
groups

## # A tibble: 8 x 3
##   sampleGroup         n color
##   <chr>           <int> <chr>
## 1 E3.25              36 #CAB2D6
## 2 E3.25 (FGF4-KO)    17 #FDBF6F
## 3 E3.5 (EPI)         11 #A6CEE3
## 4 E3.5 (FGF4-KO)      8 #FF7F00
## 5 E3.5 (PE)          11 #B2DF8A
## 6 E4.5 (EPI)          4 #1F78B4
## 7 E4.5 (FGF4-KO)     10 #E31A1C
## 8 E4.5 (PE)           4 #33A02C
```

The cells in the groups whose names contain FGF4-KO are from embryos in which the FGF4 gene, an important regulator of cell differentiation, was knocked out. Starting from E3.5, the wild-type cells (without the FGF4 knockout) undergo the first symmetry-breaking event and differentiate into different cell lineages, called pluripotent epiblast (EPI) and primitive endoderm (PE).

Since the code chunk above is the first instance where we encounter the pipe operator %>% and the functions group_by and summarise from the package *dplyr*, let's unpack the code. First, look at the pipe %>%. Generally, the pipe is useful for making nested function calls easier to read for humans. The following two lines of code are equivalent to R.[4]

[4] This is not quite true; there are some subtle differences in how variable names are resolved, as described in the manual function for %>%. For our uses, these differences are not important.

```
f(x) %>% g(y) %>% h
h(g(f(x), y))
```

They say: "Evaluate f(x), then pass the result to function g as the first argument, while y is passed to g as the second argument. Then pass the output of g to the function h." You could repeat this ad infinitum. Especially if the arguments x and y are complex expressions themselves, or if there is quite a chain of functions involved, the first version tends to be easier to read.

The `group_by` function simply "marks" the dataframe with a note that all subsequent operations should not be applied to the whole dataframe at once, but to blocks defined by the `sampleGroup` factor. Finally, `summarise` computes summary statistics; this could be, e.g., the `mean`, `sum`, for which we just compute the number of rows in each block, `n()`, and the prevalent color.

3.4   ggplot2

ggplot2 is a package by Hadley Wickham (Wickham, 2016) that implements the idea of the **grammar of graphics** – a concept created by Leland Wilkinson in his book of that title (Wilkinson, 2005). We will explore some of its functionality in this chapter, and you will see many examples of how it can be used in the rest of this book. Comprehensive documentation for the package can be found *on its website*. The online documentation includes example use cases for each graphic type introduced in this chapter (and many more) and is an invaluable resource when creating figures.

Let's start by loading the package and redoing the simple plot of Figure 3.2.

```
library("ggplot2")
ggplot(DNase, aes(x = conc, y = density)) + geom_point()
```

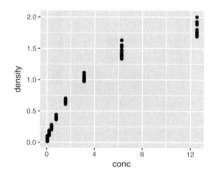

Figure 3.6: Our first *ggplot2* figure, similar to the base graphics in Figure 3.2.

We just wrote our first "sentence" using the grammar of graphics. Let's deconstruct this sentence. First, we specified the dataframe that contains the data, `DNase`. The `aes` (this stands for *aesthetic*) argument states which variables we want to see mapped to the *x*- and *y*-axes, respectively. Finally, we stated that we want the plot to use points (as opposed to, say, lines or bars), by adding the result of calling the function `geom_point`.

Now let's turn to the mouse single-cell data and plot the number of samples for each of the eight groups using the `ggplot` function. The result is shown in Figure 3.7.

```
ggplot(groups, aes(x = sampleGroup, y = n)) +
  geom_bar(stat = "identity")
```

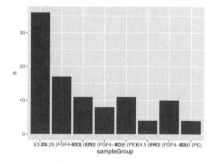

Figure 3.7: A barplot produced with the `ggplot` function from the table of group sizes in the mouse single-cell data.

With `geom_bar` we told `ggplot` that we wanted each data item (each row of `groups`) to be represented by a bar. Bars are one example of geometric objects (`geom` in the *ggplot2* package's parlance) that `ggplot` knows about. We have already seen another such object in Figure 3.6: points, indicated by the `geom_point` function. We will encounter many other geoms later. We used `aes` to indicate that we wanted the groups shown along the *x*-axis and the sizes along the *y*-axis. Finally, we provided the argument `stat = "identity"` (in other words, do nothing) to the `geom_bar` function, since otherwise it would try to compute a histogram of the data (the default value of `stat` is `"count"`). `stat` is short for *statistic*, which is what we call any function of data. Besides the identity and count statistics, there are others, such as smoothing, averaging, binning or other operations that reduce the data in some way.

These concepts – data, geometric objects, statistics – are some of the ingredients of the grammar of graphics, just as nouns, verbs and adverbs are ingredients of an English sentence.

▶ **Task**   Flip the *x*- and *y*-aesthetics to produce a horizontal barplot.   ◀

The plot in Figure 3.7 is not bad, but several improvements are needed to make it a good plot. We can use color for the bars to help us quickly see which bar corresponds to which group. This is particularly useful if we use the same color scheme in several plots. To this end, let's define a named vector `groupColor` that contains our desired colors for each possible value of `sampleGroup`.[5]

```
groupColor = setNames(groups$color, groups$sampleGroup)
```

Another thing that we need to fix in Figure 3.7 is the readability of the bar labels. Right now they are running into each other – a common problem when you have descriptive names.

```
ggplot(groups, aes(x = sampleGroup, y = n, fill = sampleGroup)) +
  geom_bar(stat = "identity") +
  scale_fill_manual(values = groupColor, name = "Groups") +
  theme(axis.text.x = element_text(angle = 90, hjust = 1))
```

This is now already a longer and more complex sentence. Let's dissect it. We added an argument, `fill`, to the `aes` function that states that we want the bars to be colored (filled) based on `sampleGroup` (which in this case coincidentally is also the value of the `x` argument, but that need not always be so). Furthermore, we added a call to the `scale_fill_manual` function, which takes as its input a color map – i.e., the mapping from the possible values of a variable to the associated colors – as a named vector. We also gave this color map a title (note that in more complex plots, there can be several different color maps involved). Had we omitted the call to `scale_fill_manual`, *ggplot2* would have used its choice of default colors. We also added a call to `theme` stating that we want the *x*-axis labels rotated by 90 degrees and right-aligned (`hjust`: the default would be to center).

3.4.1   Data flow

The function `ggplot` expects your data in a dataframe. If they are in a matrix, in separate vectors or in other types of objects, you will have to convert them. The packages *dplyr* and *broom*, among others, offer facilities to this end. We will discuss this more in Section 13.10, and you will see examples of such conversions throughout the book.

The result of a call to the `ggplot` is a *ggplot* object. Let's recall a piece of code from earlier.

```
gg = ggplot(DNase, aes(x = conc, y = density)) + geom_point()
```

We have now assigned the output of `ggplot` to the object `gg` instead of sending it directly to the console, where it was "printed" and produced Figure 3.6. The situation is completely analogous to what you're used to from working with the R console: when

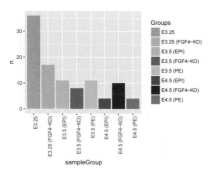

Figure 3.8: Similar to Figure 3.7, but with colored bars and better bar labels.

The expected data format could be the base R *data.frame* as well as the *tibble* (and synonymous *data_frame*) classes from the *tibble* package in the tidyverse.

you enter an expression such as `1+1` and hit "Enter", the result is printed. When the expression is an assignment, such as `s = 1+1`, the side effect takes place (the name `"s"` is bound to an object in memory that represents the value of `1+1`), but nothing is printed. Similarly, when an expression is evaluated as part of a script called with `source`, it is not printed. Thus, the above code also does not create any graphic output, since no `print` method is invoked. To print `gg`, type its name (in an interactive session) or call `print` on it.

```
gg
print(gg)
```

3.4.2 Saving figures

ggplot2 has a built-in plot-saving function called `ggsave`.

```
ggsave("DNAse-histogram-demo.pdf", plot = gg)
```

There are two major ways of storing plots: vector graphics and raster (pixel) graphics. In vector graphics, the plot is stored as a series of geometrical primitives such as points, lines, curves, shapes and typographic characters. The preferred format in R for saving plots in a vector graphics format is PDF. In raster graphics, the plot is stored in a dot matrix data structure. The main limitation of raster formats is their limited resolution, which depends on the number of pixels available. In R, the most commonly used device for raster graphics output is `png`. Generally, it's preferable to save your plots in a vector graphics format, since it is always possible later to convert a vector graphics file into a raster format of any desired resolution, while the reverse is fundamentally limited by the resolution of the original file. And you don't want the figures in your talks or papers to look poor because of pixelization artifacts!

3.5 The grammar of graphics

The components of *ggplot2*'s grammar of graphics are

1. one or more datasets;
2. one or more geometric objects that serve as the visual representations of the data, for instance, points, lines, rectangles, contours;
3. descriptions of how the variables in the data are mapped to visual properties (aesthetics) of the geometric objects, and an associated scale (e.g., linear, logarithmic, rank);
4. one or more coordinate systems;
5. statistical summarization rules;
6. a facet specification, i.e. the use of multiple similar subplots to look at subsets of the same data; and
7. optional parameters that affect the layout and rendering, such as text size, font and alignment, legend positions.

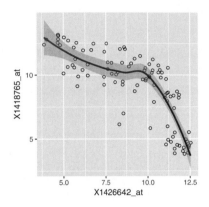

Figure 3.9: A scatterplot with three layers that show different statistics of the same data: points (`geom_point`), a smooth regression line and a confidence band (the latter two from `geom_smooth`).

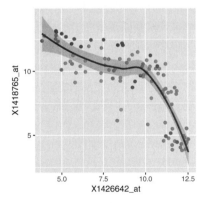

Figure 3.10: As Figure 3.9, but with points colored by time point and cell lineage (as defined in Figure 3.8). We can now see that the expression values of the gene Timd2 (targeted by the probe 1418765_at) are consistently high at the early time points, whereas they go down in the EPI samples at days 3.5 and 4.5. In the FGF4-KO, this decrease is delayed – at E3.5, its expression is still high. Conversely, the gene Fn1 (1426642_at) is off in the early time points and then goes up at days 3.5 and 4.5. The PE samples (green) show a high degree of cell-to-cell variability.

Note the use of the `::` operator to call the `select` function by its fully qualified name, including the package. We encountered this in Chapter 2.

In the examples above, Figures 3.7 and 3.8, the dataset was `groupsize`; the variables were the numeric values and the names of `groupsize`, which we mapped to the aesthetics y-axis and x-axis, respectively; the scale was linear on the y-axis and rank-based on the x-axis (the bars are ordered alphanumerically and each has the same width); and the geometric object was the rectangular bar.

Items 4–7 in the above list are optional. If you don't specify them, then the Cartesian is used as the coordinate system, the statistical summary is the trivial one (i.e., the identity) and no facets or subplots are made (we'll see examples later on, in Section 3.8). The first three items are required: a valid *ggplot2* "sentence" needs to contain at least one of each of them.

In fact, *ggplot2*'s implementation of the grammar of graphics allows you to use the same type of component multiple times, in what are called **layers** (Wickham, 2010). For example, the code below uses three types of geometric objects in the same plot, for the same data: points, a line and a confidence band.

```
dftx = data.frame(t(exprs(x)), pData(x))
ggplot( dftx, aes( x = X1426642_at, y = X1418765_at)) +
  geom_point( shape = 1 ) +
  geom_smooth( method = "loess" )
```

Here we had to assemble a copy of the expression data (`exprs(x)`) and the sample **annotation data** (`pData(x)`) all together into the dataframe `dftx` – since this is the data format that *ggplot2* functions most easily take as input (more on this in Section 13.10).

We can further enhance the plot by using colors – since each of the points in Figure 3.9 corresponds to one sample, it makes sense to use the `sampleColour` information in the object `x`.

```
ggplot( dftx, aes( x = X1426642_at, y = X1418765_at ))  +
  geom_point( aes( color = sampleColour), shape = 19 ) +
  geom_smooth( method = "loess" ) +
  scale_color_discrete( guide = FALSE )
```

▶ Question **3.2** In the code above, we defined the `color` aesthetics (`aes`) only for the `geom_point` layer, while we defined the `x` and `y` aesthetics for all layers. What happens if we set the `color` aesthetics for all layers, i.e., move it into the argument list of `ggplot`? What happens if we omit the call to `scale_color_discrete`? ◀

▶ Question **3.3** Is it always meaningful to visualize scatterplot data together with a regression line as in Figures 3.9 and 3.10? ◀

As an aside, if we want to find out which genes are targeted by these probe identifiers and what they might do, we can call:

```
library("mouse4302.db")
```

```
AnnotationDbi::select(mouse4302.db,
    keys = c("1426642_at", "1418765_at"), keytype = "PROBEID",
    columns = c("SYMBOL", "GENENAME"))
```

```
##       PROBEID SYMBOL
## 1 1426642_at    Fn1
## 2 1418765_at  Timd2
##
##                                        GENENAME
## 1                                   fibronectin 1
## 2 T cell immunoglobulin and mucin domain containing 2
```

Often when using `ggplot` you will only need to specify the data, aesthetics and a geometric object. Most geometric objects implicitly call a suitable default statistical summary of the data. For example, if you are using `geom_smooth`, then *ggplot2* uses `stat = "smooth"` by default and displays a line; if you use `geom_histogram`, the data are binned and the result is displayed in barplot format. Here's an example.

```
dfx = as.data.frame(exprs(x))
ggplot(dfx, aes(x = `20 E3.25`)) + geom_histogram(binwidth = 0.2)
```

▶ **Question 3.4** What is the difference between the objects `dfx` and `dftx`? Why did we need to create them both?   ◀

Let's come back to the barplot example from above.

```
pb = ggplot(groups, aes(x = sampleGroup, y = n))
```

This creates a plot object `pb`. If we try to display it, it creates an empty plot, because we haven't specified what geometric object we want to use. All we have in our `pb` object so far are the data and the aesthetics (Figure 3.12).

```
class(pb)
## [1] "gg"      "ggplot"
pb
```

Now we can simply add on the other components of our plot through using the + operator (Figure 3.13).

```
pb = pb + geom_bar(stat = "identity")
pb = pb + aes(fill = sampleGroup)
pb = pb + theme(axis.text.x = element_text(angle = 90, hjust = 1))
pb = pb + scale_fill_manual(values = groupColor, name = "Groups")
pb
```

This stepwise buildup – taking a graphics object already produced in some way and then further refining it – can be more convenient and easier to manage than, say, providing all the instructions up front to the single function call that creates the graphic.

We can quickly try different visualization ideas without having to rebuild our plots each time from scratch. Instead, we store the partially finished object and then modify it in different ways. For example, we can switch our plot to polar coordinates to create an alternative visualization of the barplot.

```
pb.polar = pb + coord_polar() +
  theme(axis.text.x = element_text(angle = 0, hjust = 1),
        axis.text.y = element_blank(),
        axis.ticks = element_blank()) +
  xlab("") + ylab("")
pb.polar
```

Here we need to use the original feature identifiers (e.g., "1426642_at", without the leading "X"). This is the notation used by the microarray manufacturer, by the Bioconductor annotation packages, and also inside the object `x`. The leading "X" that we used above when working with `dftx` was inserted during the creation of `dftx` by the constructor function `data.frame`, since its argument `check.names` is set to `TRUE` by default. Alternatively, we could have kept the original identifier notation by setting `check.names=FALSE`, but then we would need to work with the backticks, such as `aes(x = `1426642_at`, ...)`, to make sure R understands the identifiers correctly.

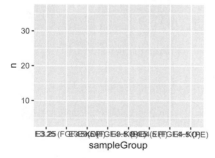

Figure 3.11: Histogram of probe intensities for one particular sample, cell number 20, which was from day E3.25.

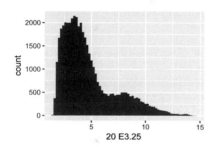

Figure 3.12: `pb`: without a geometric object, the plot remains empty.

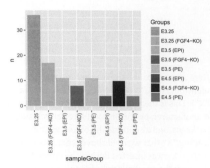

Figure 3.13: The graphics object bp in its full glory.

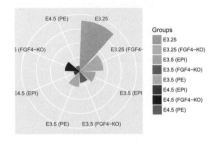

Figure 3.14: A barplot in a polar coordinate system.

[6] You can read more about these genes in Ohnishi et al. (2014).

[7] We'll talk more about the concepts and mechanics of different data representations in Section 13.10.

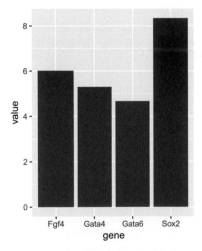

Figure 3.15: Barplot showing the means of the distributions of expression measurements from four probes.

[8] In fact, if the mean is not an appropriate summary, such as for highly skewed or multimodal distributions or for datasets with large outliers, this kind of visualization can be outright misleading.

Note above that we can override previously set `theme` parameters by simply setting them to new values – no need to go back to recreating pb, where we originally set them.

3.6   Visualizing data in 1D

A common task in biological data analysis is comparison between several samples of univariate measurements. In this section we'll explore some possibilities for visualizing and comparing such samples. As an example, we'll use the intensities of a set of four genes, Fgf4, Gata4, Gata6 and Sox2.[6] On the array, they are represented by

```
selectedProbes = c( Fgf4 = "1420085_at", Gata4 = "1418863_at",
                    Gata6 = "1425463_at",  Sox2 = "1416967_at")
```

To extract data from this representation and convert them into a dataframe, we use the function `melt` from the *reshape2* package.[7]

```
library("reshape2")
genes = melt(exprs(x)[selectedProbes, ],
             varnames = c("probe", "sample"))
head(genes)

##         probe  sample      value
## 1 1420085_at 1 E3.25 3.027715
## 2 1418863_at 1 E3.25 4.843137
## 3 1425463_at 1 E3.25 5.500618
## 4 1416967_at 1 E3.25 1.731217
## 5 1420085_at 2 E3.25 9.293016
## 6 1418863_at 2 E3.25 5.530016
```

For good measure, we also add a column that provides the gene symbol along with the probe identifiers.

```
genes$gene =
    names(selectedProbes)[match(genes$probe, selectedProbes)]
```

3.6.1   Barplots

A popular way to display data such as in our dataframe `genes` is through barplots (Figure 3.15).

```
ggplot(genes, aes( x = gene, y = value)) +
    stat_summary(fun.y = mean, geom = "bar")
```

In Figure 3.15, each bar represents the mean of the values for that gene. Such plots are commonly used in the biological sciences, as well as in the popular media. However, summarizing the data into only a single number, the mean, loses much of the information, and given the amount of space it takes, a barplot tends to be a poor way to visualize data.[8]

Sometimes we want to add error bars, and one way to achieve this in *ggplot2* is as follows.

```
library("Hmisc")
ggplot(genes, aes( x = gene, y = value, fill = gene)) +
  stat_summary(fun.y = mean, geom = "bar") +
  stat_summary(fun.data = mean_cl_normal, geom = "errorbar",
               width = 0.25)
```

Here we see again the principle of layered graphics: we use two summary functions, `mean` and `mean_cl_normal`, and two associated geometric objects, `bar` and `errorbar`. The function `mean_cl_normal` is from the *Hmisc* package and computes the standard error (or confidence limits) of the mean; it's a simple function, and we could also compute it ourselves using base R expressions if we wished to do so. We have also colored the bars to make the plot more visually pleasing.

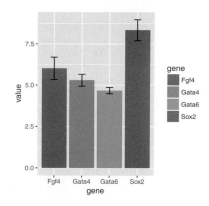

Figure 3.16: Barplots with error bars indicating standard error of the mean.

3.6.2   Boxplots

Boxplots take up a similar amount of space as barplots, but are much more informative.

```
p = ggplot(genes, aes( x = gene, y = value, fill = gene))
p + geom_boxplot()
```

In Figure 3.17 we see that two of the genes (Gata4, Gata6) have relatively concentrated distributions, with only a few data points venturing out in the direction of higher values. For Fgf4, we see that the distribution is right-skewed: the median, indicated by the horizontal black bar within the box, is closer to the lower (or left) side of the box. Conversely, for Sox2 the distribution is left-skewed.

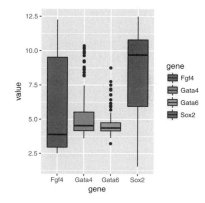

Figure 3.17: Boxplots.

3.6.3   Violin plots

A variation on the boxplot idea, but with an even more direct representation of the shape of the data distribution, is the violin plot (Figure 3.18). Here the shape of the violin gives a rough impression of the distribution density.

```
p + geom_violin()
```

3.6.4   Dot plots and beeswarm plots

If the number of data points is not too large, it is possible to show the data points directly, and it is good practice to do so, rather than using the summaries we saw above. However, plotting the data directly will often lead to overlapping points, which can be visually unpleasant, or even obscure the data. We can try to lay out the points so that they are as near as possible to their proper locations without overlap (Wilkinson, 1999).

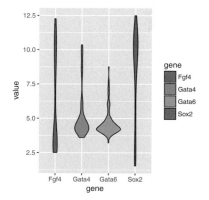

Figure 3.18: Violin plots.

```
p + geom_dotplot(binaxis = "y", binwidth = 1/6,
    stackdir = "center", stackratio = 0.75,
    aes(color = gene))
```

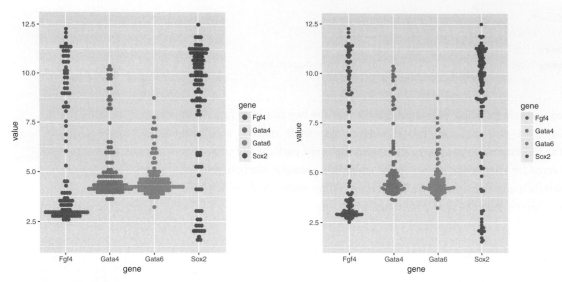

Figure 3.19: Left: Dot plots, made using `geom_dotplot` from *ggplot2*. Right: Beeswarm plots, made using `geom_beeswarm` from *ggbeeswarm*.

The plot is shown in the left-hand panel of Figure 3.19. The *y*-coordinates of the points are discretized into bins (above we chose a bin size of $\frac{1}{6}$), and then they are stacked next to each other.

An alternative is provided by the package *ggbeeswarm*, which provides the function `geom_beeswarm`.

```
library("ggbeeswarm")
p + geom_beeswarm(aes(color = gene))
```

The plot is shown in the right-hand panel of Figure 3.19. The layout algorithm aims to avoid overlaps between the points. If a point were to overlap an existing point, it is shifted along the *x*-axis by a small amount sufficient to avoid overlap. Some tweaking of the layout parameters is usually needed for each new dataset to make a dot plot or a beeswarm plot look good.

3.6.5   Density plots

Yet another way of representing the same data is by density plots. Here we try to estimate the underlying data-generating density by smoothing out the data points (Figure 3.20).

```
ggplot(genes, aes( x = value, color = gene)) + geom_density()
```

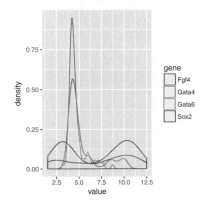

Figure 3.20: Density plots.

Density estimation has, however, a number of complications, in particular, the need to choose a smoothing window. A window size that is small enough to capture peaks in the dense regions of the data may lead to instable ("wiggly") estimates elsewhere. On the other hand, if the window is made bigger, pronounced features of the density, such as sharp peaks, may be smoothed out. Moreover, the density lines do not convey the information on how much data was used to estimate them, and plots like Figure 3.20 can be especially problematic if the sample sizes for the curves differ.

3.6.6   ECDF plots

The mathematically most convenient way to describe the distribution of a one-dimensional random variable X is its **cumulative distribution function (CDF)**, i.e., the function defined by

$$F(x) = P(X \leqslant x), \tag{3.1}$$

where x takes all values along the real axis. The density of X is then the derivative of F, if it exists.[9] The finite sample version of the probability (3.1) is called the **empirical cumulative distribution function (ECDF)**,

$$\widehat{F}_n(x) = \frac{\text{number of } i \text{ for which } x_i \leqslant x}{n} = \frac{1}{n} \sum_{i=1}^{n} \mathbb{1}(x \leqslant x_i), \tag{3.2}$$

where $x_1, \ldots, x_n$ denote a sample of n draws from X and $\mathbb{1}$ is the indicator function, i.e., the function that takes the value 1 if the expression in its argument is true and 0 otherwise. If this sounds abstract, we can get a perhaps more intuitive understanding from the following example (Figure 3.21).

```
simdata = rnorm(70)
tibble(index = seq(along = simdata),
       sx = sort(simdata)) %>%
ggplot(aes(x = sx, y = index)) + geom_step()
```

Plotting the sorted values against their ranks gives the essential features of the ECDF (Figure 3.21). In practice, we do not need to do the sorting and the other steps in the above code manually and will instead use the `stat_ecdf()` geometric object. The ECDFs of our data are shown in Figure 3.22.

```
ggplot(genes, aes( x = value, color = gene)) + stat_ecdf()
```

The ECDF has several nice properties:

- It is lossless: the ECDF $\widehat{F}_n(x)$ contains all the information contained in the original sample $x_1, \ldots, x_n$, except for the order of the values, which is assumed to be unimportant.
- As n grows, the ECDF $\widehat{F}_n(x)$ converges to the true CDF $F(x)$. Even for limited sample sizes n, the difference between the two functions tends to be small. Note that this is not the case for the empirical density! Without smoothing, the empirical density of a finite sample would be a sum of Dirac delta functions (probability distributions that have all their mass at 0), which is difficult to visualize and quite different from any underlying smooth, true density. With smoothing, the difference can be less pronounced, but is difficult to control, as we discussed above.

▶ Task **Tibbles.** In the above code we saw the `tibble` for the first time. Have a look at the vignette of the *tibble* package to see what it does.   ◀

3.6.7   The effect of transformations on densities

It is tempting to look at histograms or density plots and inspect them for evidence of **bimodality** (or multimodality) as an indication of some underlying biological

[9] By its definition, F tends to 0 for small x ($x \to -\infty$) and to 1 for large x ($x \to +\infty$).

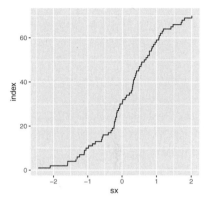

Figure 3.21: Sorted values of `simdata` versus their index. This is the empirical cumulative distribution function of `simdata`.

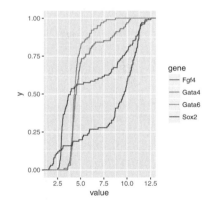

Figure 3.22: Empirical cumulative distribution functions (ECDFs).

Figure 3.23: Part of Figure 1 from Lawrence et al. (2013). Each dot corresponds to a tumor-normal pair, with vertical position indicating the total frequency of somatic mutations in the exome. The resulting curves are, in essence, ECDF plots, and conceptually this plot is similar to Figure 3.22, except that the graphs are rotated by 90 degrees (i.e., the roles of the x- and y-axis are exchanged) and the curves for the individual tumor types are horizontally displaced to keep them better separated.

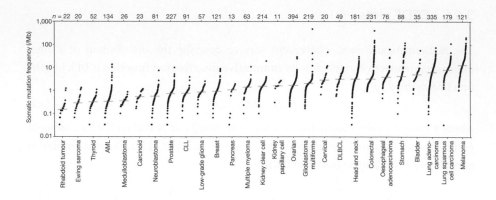

phenomenon. Before doing so, it is important to remember that the number of modes of a density depends on scale transformations of the data, via the **chain rule**. For instance, let's look at the data from one of the arrays in the Hiiragi dataset (Figure 3.24).

```
ggplot(dfx, aes(x = `64 E4.5 (EPI)`)) + geom_histogram(bins = 100)
ggplot(dfx, aes(x = 2 ^ `64 E4.5 (EPI)`)) +
  geom_histogram(binwidth = 20) + xlim(0, 1500)
```

▶ Question **3.5** (Advanced) Consider a random variable X and a nonlinear 1:1 transformation $f : x \mapsto y$ that defines the transformed random variable $Y = f(X)$. Suppose the density function of Y is $p(y)$. What is the density of X? How is the mode (or modes) of X related to the mode(s) of Y?

Hint: note that a mode of a function p is a root of its derivative $p' = dp/dx$. Is it generally true that if x_0 is a mode of X, then $y_0 = f(x_0)$ is a mode of Y?   ◀

▶ Solution **3.5**   By the chain rule, $p(y) \, dy = p(f(x)) \, f'(x) \, dx$, so the density of X is $\tilde{p}(x) = p(f(x)) \, f'(x)$. The modes of $\tilde{p}$ are roots of its derivative $d\tilde{p}/dx$, i.e., they obey $p'(f(x)) \, f'^2(x) + p(f(x))f''(x) = 0$. The second term in the sum vanishes if f is affine linear ($f'' \equiv 0$), but in general there is no simple relationship between the roots of the two densities, and therefore between the modes of X and Y.   □

Figure 3.24: Histograms of the same data, with and without logarithm transform. On the left, the data are shown on the scale on which they are stored in the data object x, which resulted from logarithm (base 2) transformation of the microarray fluorescence intensities (Irizarry et al., 2003); on the right, after re-exponentiating them back to the fluorescence scale. For better use of space, we capped the x-axis range at 1500.

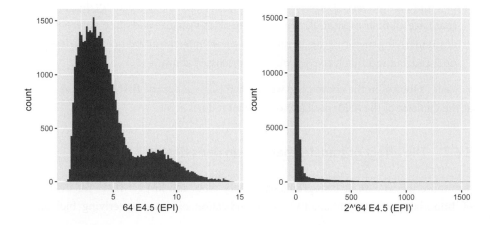

3.7 Visualizing data in 2D: scatterplots

Scatterplots are useful for visualizing treatment–response comparisons (as in Figure 3.3), associations between variables (as in Figure 3.10), or paired data (e.g., a disease biomarker in several patients before and after treatment). We use the two dimensions of our plotting paper, or screen, to represent the two variables. Let's take a look at differential expression between a wild-type and an FGF4-KO sample.

```
scp = ggplot(dfx, aes(x = `59 E4.5 (PE)` ,
                      y = `92 E4.5 (FGF4-KO)`))
scp + geom_point()
```

The labels 59 E4.5 (PE) and 92 E4.5 (FGF4-KO) refer to column names (sample names) in the dataframe dfx, which we created above. Since they contain special characters (spaces, parentheses, hyphen) and start with numerals, we need to enclose them with the downward-sloping quotes to make them syntactically digestible for R. The plot is shown in Figure 3.25. We get a dense point cloud that we can try to interpret on the outskirts of the cloud, but we really have no idea visually how the data are distributed within the denser regions of the plot.

One easy way to ameliorate the overplotting is to adjust the transparency (alpha value) of the points by modifying the alpha parameter of geom_point (Figure 3.26).

```
scp  + geom_point(alpha = 0.1)
```

This is already better than Figure 3.25, but in the more dense regions even the semi-transparent points quickly overplot to a featureless black mass, while the more isolated outlying points are getting faint. An alternative is a contour plot of the 2D density, which has the added benefit of not rendering all of the points on the plot, as in Figure 3.27.

```
scp + geom_density2d()
```

However, we see in Figure 3.27 that the point cloud at the bottom right (which contains a relatively small number of points) is no longer represented. We can somewhat overcome this by tweaking the bandwidth and binning parameters of geom_density2d (Figure 3.28, *left*).

```
scp + geom_density2d(h = 0.5, bins = 60)
```

We can fill in each space between the contour lines with the relative density of points by explicitly calling the function stat_density2d (for which geom_density2d is a wrapper) and using the geometric object *polygon*, as in the right-hand panel of Figure 3.28.

```
library("RColorBrewer")
colorscale = scale_fill_gradientn(
    colors = rev(brewer.pal(9, "YlGnBu")),
    values = c(0, exp(seq(-5, 0, length.out = 100))))

scp + stat_density2d(h = 0.5, bins = 60,
        aes( fill = ..level..), geom = "polygon") +
    colorscale + coord_fixed()
```

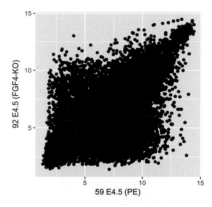

Figure 3.25: Scatterplot of 45,101 expression measurements for two of the samples.

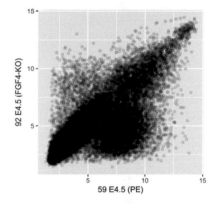

Figure 3.26: As Figure 3.25, but with semi-transparent points to resolve some of the overplotting.

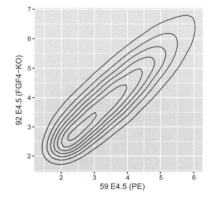

Figure 3.27: As Figure 3.25, but rendered as a contour plot of the 2D density estimate.

Figure 3.28: Left: As Figure 3.27, but with smaller smoothing bandwidth and tighter binning for the contour lines. Right: With color filling.

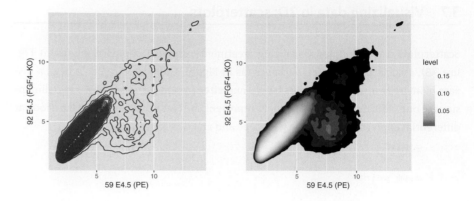

We used the function `brewer.pal` from the package *RColorBrewer* to define the color scale, and we added a call to `coord_fixed` to fix the aspect ratio of the plot, to make sure that the mapping of data range to *x*- and *y*-coordinates is the same for the two variables. Both of these issues merit a deeper look, and we'll talk more about plot shapes in Section 3.7.1 and colors in Section 3.9.

The density-based plotting methods in Figure 3.28 are more visually appealing and interpretable than the overplotted point clouds of Figures 3.25 and 3.26, though we have to be careful in using them, as we lose much of the information on the outlier points in the sparser regions of the plot. One possible remedy is to use `geom_point` to add such points back in.

But arguably the best alternative, which avoids the limitations of smoothing, is hexagonal binning (Carr et al., 1987); see Figure 3.29.

```
scp + geom_hex() + coord_fixed()
scp + geom_hex(binwidth = c(0.2, 0.2)) + colorscale +
  coord_fixed()
```

3.7.1   Plot shapes

Choosing the proper shape for your plot is important in ensuring that the information is conveyed well. By default, the shape parameter – that is, the ratio between the height of the graph and its width – is chosen by *ggplot2* based on the available space in the current plotting device. The width and height of the device are specified when it is opened in R, either explicitly by you or through default parameters.[10] Moreover, the graph dimensions also depend on the presence or absence of additional decorations, like the color scale bars in Figure 3.29.

There are two simple rules that you can apply to scatterplots:

- If the variables on the two axes are measured in the **same units**, then make sure that the same mapping of data space to physical space is used – i.e., use `coord_fixed`. In the scatterplots above, both axes are the logarithm to base 2 of expression-level measurements; that is, a change by one unit has the same meaning on both axes

[10] See, for example, the manual pages of the `pdf` and `png` functions.

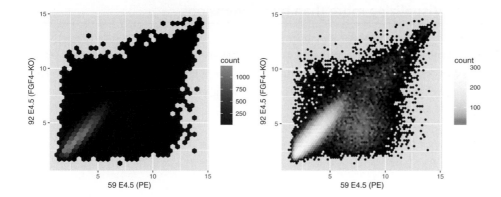

Figure 3.29: Hexagonal binning. Left: Default parameters. Right: Finer bin sizes and customized color scale.

(a doubling of the expression level). Another case is principal component analysis (PCA), where the x-axis typically represents component 1 and the y-axis component 2. Since the axes arise from an orthonormal rotation of input data space, we want to make sure their scales match. Since the variance of the data is (by definition) smaller along the second component than along the first component (or, at most, equal), well-made PCA plots are usually wider than they are tall.

- If the variables on the two axes are measured in **different units**, then we can still relate them to each other by comparing their dimensions. The default in many plotting routines in R, including *ggplot2*, is to look at the range of the data and map it to the available plotting region. However, particularly when the data more or less follow a line, looking at the typical slope of the line can be useful. This technique is called **banking** (Cleveland et al., 1988).

To illustrate banking, let's use the classic sunspot data from Cleveland's paper.

```
library("ggthemes")
sunsp = tibble(year   = time(sunspot.year),
               number = as.numeric(sunspot.year))
sp = ggplot(sunsp, aes(x = year, y = number)) + geom_line()
sp
```

The resulting plot is shown in the upper panel of Figure 3.30. We can clearly see long-term fluctuations in the amplitude of sunspot activity cycles, with particularly low maximum activities in the early 1700s, early 1800s, and around the turn of the 20th century. But now let's try banking.

```
ratio = with(sunsp, bank_slopes(year, number))
sp + coord_fixed(ratio = ratio)
```

How does the algorithm work? It aims to make the slopes in the curve be around 1. In particular, `bank_slopes` computes the median absolute slope, and then, with the call to `coord_fixed`, we set the aspect ratio of the plot such that this quantity becomes 1. The result is shown in the lower panel of Figure 3.30. Quite counterintuitively, even though the plot takes much less space, we see more on it! In particular, we can see the sawtooth shape of the sunspot cycles, with sharp rises and more gradual declines.

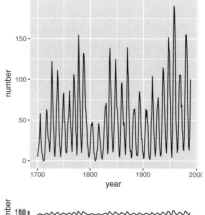

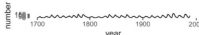

Figure 3.30: Sunspot data. In the upper panel, the plot shape is roughly quadratic, a frequent default choice. In the lower panel, a technique called *banking* is used to choose the plot shape. Here the default placement of the tick labels is not great and would benefit from customization.

3.8   Visualizing more than two dimensions

Sometimes we want to show the relationships between more than two variables. Obvious choices for including additional dimensions are plot symbol shapes and colors. The `geom_point` geometric object offers the following aesthetics (beyond `x` and `y`):

- `fill`
- `color`
- `shape`
- `size`
- `alpha`

They are explored on the manual page of the `geom_point` function; `fill` and `color` refer to the fill and outline color of an object, and `alpha` to its transparency level. In Figures 3.26–3.29, we used color or transparency to reflect point density and avoid the obscuring effects of overplotting. We can also use these properties to show other dimensions of the data. In principle, we could use all five aesthetics listed above simultaneously to show up to seven-dimensional data; however, such a plot would be hard to decipher. Usually we are better off limiting ourselves to only one or two of these aesthetics and varying them to show one or two additional dimensions in the data.

3.8.1   Faceting

This slicing is also called *trellis* or *lattice* graphics, in an allusion to how these arrays of plots look. The first major R package to implement faceting was *lattice*. In this book, we'll use the faceting functionalities provided through *ggplot2*.

Another way to show additional dimensions of the data is to show multiple plots that result from repeatedly subsetting (or "slicing") the data based on one (or more) of the variables, so that we can visualize each part separately. This is called **faceting** and it enables us to visualize data in up to four or five dimensions. So we can, for instance, investigate whether the observed patterns among the other variables are the same or different across the range of the faceting variable. Let's look at an example:

```
library("magrittr")
dftx$lineage %<>% sub("^$", "no", .)
dftx$lineage %<>% factor(levels = c("no", "EPI", "PE", "FGF4-KO"))

ggplot(dftx, aes( x = X1426642_at, y = X1418765_at)) +
  geom_point() + facet_grid( . ~ lineage )
```

The first three lines of this code chunk are not necessary – they're just reformatting the `lineage` column of the `dftx` dataframe to make it more concise.

The result is shown in Figure 3.31. We used R's formula language to specify the variable by which we want to split the data, and that the separate panels should be in

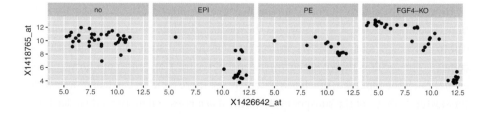

Figure 3.31: *Faceting*: the same data as in Figure 3.9, but now split by the categorical variable `lineage`.

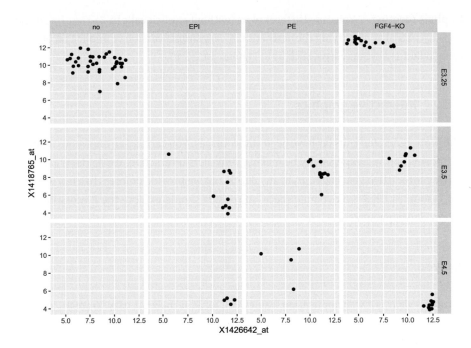

Figure 3.32: *Faceting*: the same data as in Figure 3.9, split by the categorical variables `Embryonic.day` (rows) and `lineage` (columns).

different columns: `facet_grid( . ~ lineage )`. In fact, we can specify two faceting variables, as follows (the result is shown in Figure 3.32).

```
ggplot( dftx,
  aes( x = X1426642_at, y = X1418765_at)) + geom_point() +
  facet_grid( Embryonic.day ~ lineage )
```

Another useful function is `facet_wrap`: if the faceting variable has too many levels for all the plots to fit in one row or one column, then this function can be used to wrap them into a specified number of columns or rows. So far we have seen faceting by categorical variables, but we can also use it with continuous variables by discretizing them into levels. The function `cut` is useful for this purpose.

```
ggplot(mutate(dftx, Tdgf1 = cut(X1450989_at, breaks = 4)),
  aes( x = X1426642_at, y = X1418765_at)) + geom_point() +
  facet_wrap( ~ Tdgf1, ncol = 2 )
```

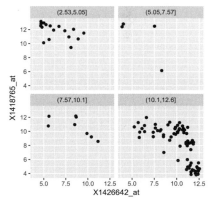

We see in Figure 3.33 that the numbers of points in the four panels are different. This is because `cut` splits into bins of equal length, not equal number of points. If we want the latter, then we can use `quantile` in conjunction with `cut`, or cut on the ranks of the variable's values.

Figure 3.33: *Faceting*: the same data as in Figure 3.9, split by the continuous variable `X1450989_at` and arranged by `facet_wrap`.

Axis scales.   In Figures 3.31–3.33, the axis scales are the same for all panels. Alternatively, we could let them vary by setting the `scales` argument of the `facet_grid` and `facet_wrap` functions. This argument lets you control whether the *x*-axis and *y*-axis in each panel have the same scale or whether either or both adapt to each panel's data range. There is a trade-off: adaptive axis scales might let us see more detail; on the other hand, the panels are then less comparable across the groupings.

Implicit faceting. You can also facet plots (without explicit calls to `facet_grid` and `facet_wrap`) by specifying the aesthetics. A very simple version of implicit faceting is using a factor as your *x*-axis, such as in Figures 3.15–3.19.

3.8.2   Interactive graphics

The plots generated thus far have been static images. You can add an enormous amount of information and expressivity by making your plots interactive. We do not try here to convey interactive visualizations in any depth, but we provide pointers to a few important resources. This is a dynamic space, so readers should explore the R ecosystem for recent developments.

shiny

Rstudio's *shiny* is a web application framework for R. It makes it easy to create interactive displays with sliders, selectors and other control elements that allow changes to all aspects of the plot(s) shown – since the interactive elements call back directly into the R code that produces the plot(s). See `http://shiny.rstudio.com/gallery/` for some great examples.

As a graphics engine for *shiny*-based interactive visualizations, you can use *ggplot2* and, indeed, base R graphics or any other graphics package. What may be a little awkward here is that the language used for describing the interactive options is separated from the production of the graphics via *ggplot2* and the grammar of graphics. The *ggvis* package aims to overcome this limitation.

ggvis

[11] At the time of writing (summer 2017), it is not clear whether the initial momentum of *ggvis* development will be maintained, and its current functionality and maturity do not yet match *ggplot2*.

The package *ggvis*[11] is an attempt to extend the good features of *ggplot2* into the realm of interactive graphics. In contrast to *ggplot2*, which produces graphics into R's traditional graphics devices (PDF, PNG, etc.), *ggvis* builds upon a JavaScript infrastructure called *Vega*, and its plots are intended to be viewed in an HTML browser. Like *ggplot2*, the *ggvis* package is inspired by grammar of graphics concepts, but uses distinct syntax. It leverages *shiny*'s infrastructure to connect to R to perform the computations needed for the interactivity. As its author put it, "The goal is to combine the best of R (e.g., every modeling function you can imagine) and the best of the web (everyone has a web browser). Data manipulation and transformation are done in R, and the graphics are rendered in a web browser, using Vega."[12]

[12] `http://ggvis.rstudio.com.`

As a consequence of the interactivity in *shiny* and *ggvis*, there needs to be an R interpreter running with the underlying data and code to respond to the user's actions while she views the graphic. This R interpreter can be on the user's local machine or on a server; in both cases, the viewing application is a web browser and the interaction with R goes through web protocols (http or https). That is, of course, different from a graphic stored in a self-contained file, which is produced once by R and can then be viewed in a PDF or HTML viewer without any connection to a running instance of R.

plotly

A great web-based tool for interactive graphic generation is **plotly**. You can view some examples of interactive graphics online at `https://plot.ly/r`. To create your own interactive plots in R, you can use code such as

```
library("plotly")
plot_ly(economics, x = ~ date, y = ~ unemploy / pop)
```

As with *shiny* and *ggvis*, the graphics are viewed in an HTML browser; however, no running R session is required. The graphics are self-contained HTML documents whose "logic" is coded in JavaScript, or more precisely, in the D3.js system.

rgl, webgl

For visualizing 3D objects (say, a geometric structure), there is the package *rgl*. It produces interactive viewer windows (either in a specialized graphics device on your screen or through a web browser) in which you can rotate the scene, zoom and in out, etc. A screenshot of the scene produced by the code below is shown in Figure 3.34.

```
data("volcano")
volcanoData = list(
  x = 10 * seq_len(nrow(volcano)),
  y = 10 * seq_len(ncol(volcano)),
  z = volcano,
  col = terrain.colors(500)[cut(volcano, breaks = 500)]
)
library("rgl")
with(volcanoData, persp3d(x, y, z, color = col))
```

In the code above, the base R function `cut` computes a mapping from the value range of the `volcano` data to the integers between 1 and 500,[13] which we use to index the color scale, `terrain.colors(500)`. For more information, consult the package's excellent vignette.

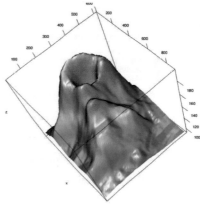

Figure 3.34: *rgl* rendering of the `volcano` data, the topographic information for Maunga Whau (Mt. Eden), one of about 50 volcanoes in the Auckland volcanic field.

[13] More precisely, it returns a factor with as many levels, which we let R autoconvert to integers.

3.9 Color

An important consideration when making plots is the coloring that we use in them. Most R users are likely familiar with the built-in R color scheme, used by base R graphics, as shown in Figure 3.35.

```
pie(rep(1, 8), col=1:8)
```

These color choices date back to 1980s hardware, where graphics cards handled colors by letting each pixel either use or not use each of the three basic color channels of

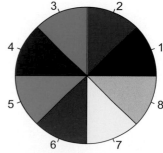

Figure 3.35: Basic R colors. The appearance of colors tends to differ between print and screen.

the display: red, green and blue (RGB). This led to $2^3 = 8$ combinations, which lie at the eight extreme corners of the RGB color cube.[14]

The basic R colors are harsh to the eyes, and there is no longer a good excuse for creating graphics that are based on this palette. Fortunately, the default color palettes used by the more modern visualization-oriented packages (including *ggplot2*) are more appealing. However, often the default is not good enough, and we need to make our own choices.

In Section 3.7 we saw the function `scale_fill_gradientn`, which allowed us to create the color gradient used in Figures 3.28 and 3.29 by interpolating the basic color palette defined by the function `brewer.pal` in the *RColorBrewer* package. This package defines a set of well-designed color palettes. We can see all of them at a glance with the function `display.brewer.all` (Figure 3.36).

```
display.brewer.all()
```

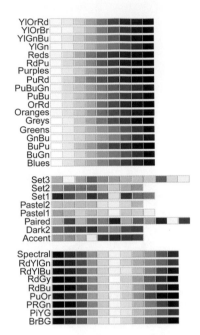

Figure 3.36: RColorBrewer palettes.

We can get information about available color palettes from `brewer.pal.info`.

```
head(brewer.pal.info)
```

```
##       maxcolors category colorblind
## BrBG         11      div       TRUE
## PiYG         11      div       TRUE
## PRGn         11      div       TRUE
## PuOr         11      div       TRUE
## RdBu         11      div       TRUE
## RdGy         11      div      FALSE
```

```
table(brewer.pal.info$category)
```

```
##
## div qual  seq
##   9    8   18
```

The palettes are divided into three categories:

- qualitative: for categorical properties that have no intrinsic ordering; the `Paired` palette supports up to six categories that each divide into two subcategories – such as *before* and *after*, *with* and *without* treatment, etc.;
- sequential: for quantitative properties that go from *low* to *high*; and
- diverging: for quantitative properties for which there is a natural midpoint or neutral value, and whose value can deviate both up and down; we'll see an example in Figure 3.38.

Figure 3.37: A quasi-continuous color palette derived by interpolating between the colors `darkorange3`, `white` and `darkblue`.

To obtain the colors from a particular palette, we use the function `brewer.pal`. Its first argument is the number of colors we want (which can be less than the available maximum number in `brewer.pal.info`).

```
brewer.pal(4, "RdYlGn")
## [1] "#D7191C" "#FDAE61" "#A6D96A" "#1A9641"
```

If we want more than the available number of preset colors (e.g., so we can plot a heatmap with continuous colors) we can interpolate using the `colorRampPalette` function.[15]

```
mypalette  = colorRampPalette(
    c("darkorange3", "white","darkblue")
  )(100)
head(mypalette)
## [1] "#CD6600" "#CE6905" "#CF6C0A" "#D06F0F" "#D17214" "#D27519"
par(mai = rep(0.1, 4))
image(matrix(1:100, nrow = 100, ncol = 10), col = mypalette,
        xaxt = "n", yaxt = "n", useRaster = TRUE)
```

3.10 Heatmaps

Heatmaps are a powerful way of visualizing large, matrix-like datasets and providing a quick overview of the patterns that might be in the data. There are a number of heatmap drawing functions in R; one that is convenient and produces good-looking output is the function `pheatmap` from the eponymous package.[16] In the code below, we first select the top 500 most variable genes in the dataset x and define a function `rowCenter` that centers each gene (row) by subtracting the mean across columns. By default, `pheatmap` uses the *RdYlBu* color palette from *RcolorBrewer* in conjuction with the `colorRampPalette` function to interpolate the 11 colors into a smooth-looking palette (Figure 3.38).

[16] A very versatile and modular alternative is the *ComplexHeatmap* package.

```
library("pheatmap")
topGenes = order(rowVars(exprs(x)), decreasing = TRUE)[1:500]
rowCenter = function(x) { x - rowMeans(x) }
pheatmap( rowCenter(exprs(x)[ topGenes, ] ),
  show_rownames = FALSE, show_colnames = FALSE,
  breaks = seq(-5, +5, length = 101),
  annotation_col =
    pData(x)[, c("sampleGroup", "Embryonic.day", "ScanDate") ],
  annotation_colors = list(
    sampleGroup = groupColor,
    genotype = c(`FGF4-KO` = "chocolate1", `WT` = "azure2"),
    Embryonic.day = setNames(brewer.pal(9, "Blues")[c(3, 6, 9)],
                        c("E3.25", "E3.5", "E4.5")),
    ScanDate = setNames(brewer.pal(nlevels(x$ScanDate), "YlGn"),
                        levels(x$ScanDate))
  ),
  cutree_rows = 4
)
```

Let's take a minute to deconstruct this rather massive-looking call to `pheatmap`. The options `show_rownames` and `show_colnames` control whether the row and column names are printed at the sides of the matrix. Because our matrix is large in relation to the available plotting space, the labels would not be readable, and we suppress them. The `annotation_col` argument takes a dataframe that carries additional information about the samples. The information is shown in the colored bars at the top of the heatmap. There is also a similar `annotation_row` argument, which we haven't used here, for colored bars at the side. The argument `annotation_colors` is a list of

Figure 3.38: A heatmap of relative expression values, i.e., logarithmic fold change compared to the average expression of that gene (row) across all samples (columns). The color scale uses a diverging palette whose midpoint is at 0.

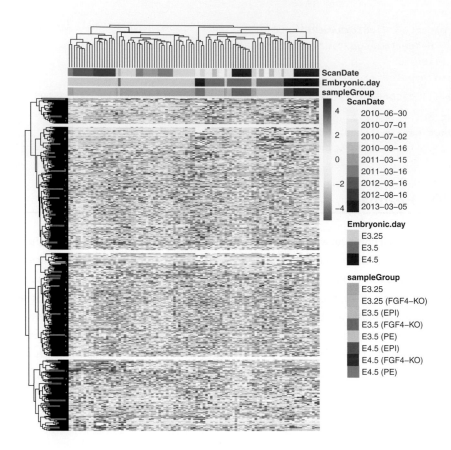

named vectors by which we can override the default choice of colors for the annotation bars. Finally, with the `cutree_rows` argument we cut the row dendrogram into four (an arbitrarily chosen number) clusters, and the heatmap shows them by leaving a bit of white space in between. The `pheatmap` function has many further options, and if you want to use it for your own data visualizations, it's worth studying them.

3.10.1   Dendrogram ordering

In Figure 3.38, the trees at the left and the top represent the result of a hierarchical clustering algorithm and are also called **dendrograms**. The ordering of the rows and columns is based on the dendrograms and has an enormous effect on the visual impact of the heatmap. However, it can be difficult to decide which of the apparent patterns are real and which are consequences of arbitrary tree layout decisions.[17] Let's keep in mind that:

[17] We will learn about clustering and methods for evaluating cluster significance in Chapter 5.

- Ordering the rows and columns by cluster dendrogram (as in Figure 3.38) is an arbitrary choice, and you could just as well make others.
- Even if you settle on dendrogram ordering, there is an essentially arbitrary choice at each internal branch, as each branch could be flipped without changing the topology of the tree (see Figure 5.17, for example).

▶ **Question 3.6** How does the `pheatmap` function deal with the decision about which branches of the subtree go left and right? ◀

▶ **Solution 3.6** This is described in the manual page of the `hclust` function in the *stats* package, which, by default, is used by `pheatmap`. □

▶ **Question 3.7** What other ordering methods can you think of? ◀

▶ **Solution 3.7** Among the methods proposed is the travelling salesman problem (McCormick Jr et al., 1972) or projection on the first principal component (for instance, see the examples on the manual page of `pheatmap`). □

▶ **Question 3.8** Check the argument `clustering_callback` of the `pheatmap` function. ◀

3.10.2 Color spaces

Color perception in humans (von Helmholtz, 1867) is three dimensional.[18] There are different ways of parameterizing this space. We've already encountered the RGB color model, which uses three values in $[0, 1]$, for instance at the beginning of Section 3.4, where we printed out the contents of `groupColor`.

```
groupColor[1]
##      E3.25
## "#CAB2D6"
```

Here, CA is the hexadecimal representation for the strength of the red color channel, B2 of the green and D6 of the blue. In decimal, these numbers are 202, 178 and 214, respectively. The range of these values goes from to 0 to 255, so by dividing by this maximum value, an RGB triplet can also be thought of as a point in the three-dimensional unit cube.

The function `hcl` uses a different coordinate system. Again this consists of three coordinates: hue H, an angle in the range $[0, 360]$, chroma C, a positive number, and luminance L, a value in $[0, 100]$. The upper bound for C depends on on hue and luminance.

The `hcl` function corresponds to polar coordinates in the CIE–LUV[19] and is designed for area fills. By keeping chroma and luminance coordinates constant and only varying hue, it is easy to produce color palettes that are harmonious and avoid irradiation illusions that make light-colored areas look bigger than dark ones. Our attention also tends to get drawn to loud colors, and fixing the value of chroma makes the colors equally attractive to our eyes.

There are many ways of choosing colors from a color wheel. *Triads* are three colors chosen equally spaced around the color wheel; for example, $H = 0$, 120, 240 gives red, green, blue. *Tetrads* are four equally spaced colors around the color wheel, and some graphic artists describe the effect as "dynamic". *Warm colors* are a set of equally spaced colors close to yellow, *cool colors* a set of equally spaced colors close to blue. *Analogous color* sets contain colors from a small segment of the color wheel, for example, yellow,

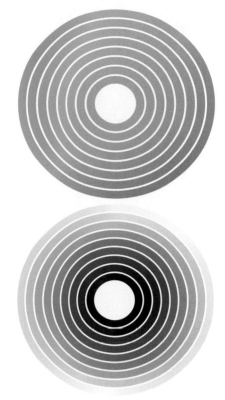

Figure 3.39: Circles in HCL colorspace. Upper panel: The luminance L is fixed at 75, while the angular coordinate H (hue) varies from 0 to 360 and the radial coordinate $C = 0, 10, \ldots, 60$. Lower panel: Constant chroma $C = 50$, H as above, and varying luminance $L = 10, 20, \ldots, 90$.

[18] Physically, there is an infinite number of wavelengths of light and an infinite number of ways of mixing them, so other species, or robots, can perceive fewer, or more, than three colors.

[19] CIE: Commission Internationale de l'Éclairage – see, e.g., Wikipedia for more information.

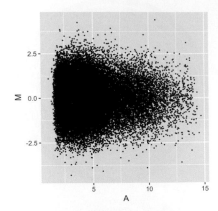

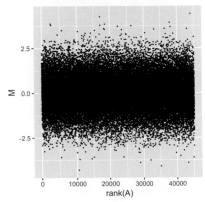

Figure 3.40: The effect of rank transformation on the visual perception of dependency.

[20] We used it implicitly, since the data in the *ExpressionSet* object x already come log-transformed.

orange and red, or green, cyan and blue. *Complementary colors* are colors diametrically opposite each other on the color wheel. A tetrad is two pairs of complementaries. *Split complementaries* are three colors consisting of a pair of complementaries, with the partners split equally to each side, for example, $H = 60, 240-30, 240+30$. This is useful to emphasize the difference between a pair of similar categories and a third different one. More thorough discussions are provided in Mollon (1995) and Ihaka (2003).

Lines versus areas

For lines and points, we want a strong contrast to the background, so on a white background, we want them to be relatively dark (low luminance L). For area fills, lighter, more pastel-type colors with low to moderate chromatic content are usually more pleasant.

3.11   Data transformations

Plots in which most points are huddled in one area, with much of the available space sparsely populated, are difficult to read. If the histogram of the marginal distribution of a variable has a sharp peak and then long tails to one or both sides, transforming the data can be helpful. These considerations apply both to x and y aesthetics and to color scales. The plots in this chapter that involve microarray data use the logarithmic transformation[20] – not only in scatterplots like Figure 3.25 for the x- and y-coordinates, but also in Figure 3.38 for the color scale that represents the expression fold changes. The logarithm transformation is attractive because it has a definitive meaning – a move up or down by the same amount on a log-transformed scale corresponds to the same multiplicative change on the original scale: $\log(ax) = \log a + \log x$.

Sometimes, however, the logarithm is not good enough, for instance when the data include zero or negative values, or when even on the logarithmic scale the data distribution is highly uneven. From the upper panel of Figure 3.40, it is easy to take away the impression that the distribution of M depends on A, with higher variances for lower A. However, this is entirely a visual artifact, as the lower panel confirms: the distribution of M is independent of A, and the apparent trend we saw in the upper panel was caused by the higher point density at smaller A.

```
gg = ggplot(tibble(A = exprs(x)[, 1], M = rnorm(length(A))),
       aes(y = M))
gg + geom_point(aes(x = A), size = 0.2)
gg + geom_point(aes(x = rank(A)), size = 0.2)
```

▶ Question **3.9** Can the visual artifact be avoided by using a density- or binning-based plotting method, as in Figure 3.29?   ◀

▶ Question **3.10** Can the rank transformation also be applied when choosing color scales, for example for heatmaps? What does *histogram equalization* in image processing do?   ◀

3.12 Mathematical symbols and other fonts

We can use mathematical notation in plot labels, using a notation that is a mix of R syntax and LaTeX-like notation (see `help("plotmath")` for details).

```
volume = function(rho, nu)
            pi^(nu/2) * rho^nu / gamma(nu/2+1)

ggplot(tibble(nu    = 1:15,
  Omega = volume(1, nu)), aes(x = nu, y = Omega)) +
geom_line() +
xlab(expression(nu)) + ylab(expression(Omega)) +
geom_text(label =
"Omega(rho,nu)==frac(pi^frac(nu,2)~rho^nu, Gamma(frac(nu,2)+1))",
  parse = TRUE, x = 6, y = 1.5)
```

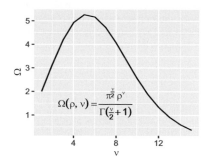

Figure 3.41: Volume Ω of the ν-dimensional sphere with radius $\rho = 1$, for $\nu = 1, \ldots, 15$.

The result is shown in Figure 3.41. It's also easy to switch to other fonts, for instance the serif font Times (Figure 3.42).

```
ggplot(genes, aes( x = value, color = gene)) + stat_ecdf() +
  theme(text = element_text(family = "Times"))
```

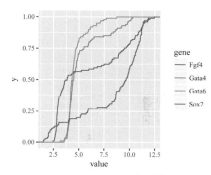

Figure 3.42: As Figure 3.22, with a different font.

In fact, the set of fonts that can be used with a standard R installation is limited, but luckily there is the package *extrafont*, which facilitates using fonts other than R's standard set of PostScript fonts. There's some extra work needed before we can use it, since fonts external to R first need to be made known to it. Fonts could come shipped with your operating system, with a word processor or with another graphics application. The fonts available and their physical location are therefore not standardized, but will depend on your operating system and further configurations. In the first session after attaching the *extrafont* package, you will need to run the function `font_import` to import fonts and make them known to the package. Then, in each session in which you want to use them, you need to call the `loadfonts` function to register the fonts with one or more of R's graphics devices. Finally, you can use the `fonttable` function to list the available fonts. You will need to refer to the documentation of the *extrafonts* package to see how to make this work on your machine.

▶ Task   Use the package *extrafont* to produce a version of Figure 3.42 with the font Bauhaus 93 (or another one available on your system).   ◀

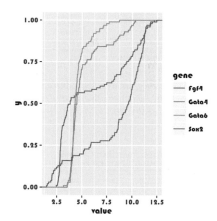

Figure 3.43: As Figure 3.22, with font Bauhaus 93.

3.13 Genomic data

To visualize genomic data, in addition to the general principles we have discussed in this chapter, there are some specific considerations. The data are usually associated with genomic coordinates. In fact, genomic coordinates offer a great organizing principle for the integration of genomic data. You probably have seen genome browser displays such as in Figure 3.44. Here we will briefly show how to produce such plots programmatically,

Figure 3.44: Screenshot from Ensembl genome browser, showing gene annotation of a genomic region as well as a read pile-up visualization of an RNA-Seq experiment.

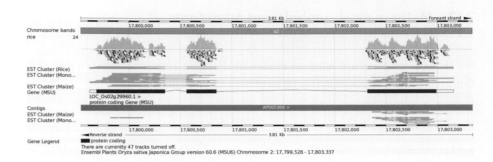

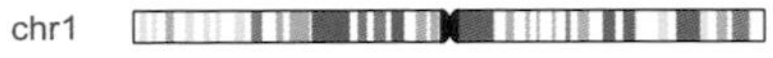

Figure 3.45: Chromosome 1 of the human genome: ideogram plot.

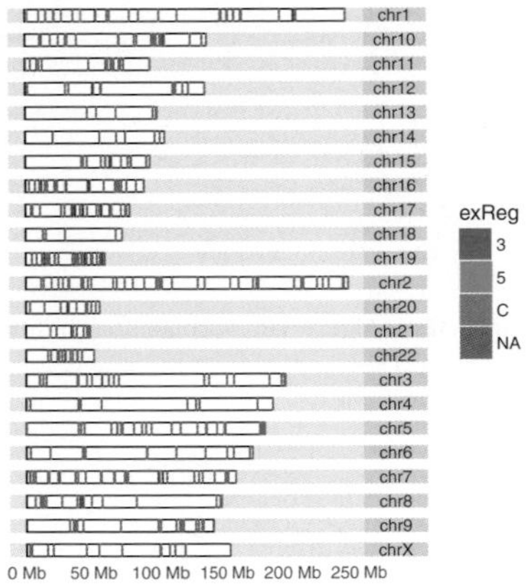

Figure 3.46: Karyogram with RNA editing sites. `exReg` indicates whether a site is in the coding region (C), 3'- or 5'-UTR.

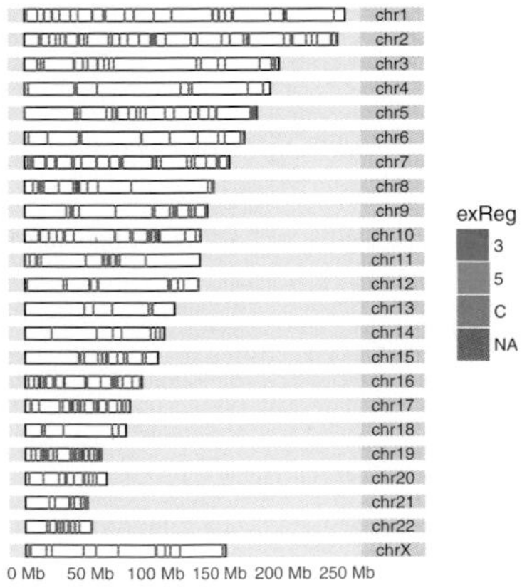

Figure 3.47: Improved version of Figure 3.46.

using your data as well as public annotation. It will be a short glimpse, and we refer to resources such as *Bioconductor* for a fuller picture.

The main challenge of genomic data visualization is the size of genomes. We need visualizations at multiple scales, from whole genome down to the nucleotide level. It should be easy to zoom in and out, and we may need different visualization strategies for the different size scales. It can be convenient to visualize biological molecules (genomes, genes, transcripts, proteins) in a linear manner, although their embedding in the 3D physical world can matter (a great deal).

Let's start with some fun examples, an ideogram plot of human chromosome 1 (Figure 3.45) and a plot of the genome-wide distribution of RNA editing sites (Figure 3.46).

```
library("ggbio")
data("hg19IdeogramCyto", package = "biovizBase")
plotIdeogram(hg19IdeogramCyto, subchr = "chr1")
```

The `darned_hg19_subset500` lists a selection of 500 RNA editing sites in the human genome. It was obtained from the *Database of RNA Editing in Flies, Mice and Humans* (DARNED, `http://darned.ucc.ie`). The result is shown in Figure 3.46.

```
library("GenomicRanges")
data("darned_hg19_subset500", package = "biovizBase")
autoplot(darned_hg19_subset500, layout = "karyogram",
        aes(color = exReg, fill = exReg))
```

▶ Question **3.11** How do you fix the ordering of the chromosomes in Figure 3.46 and get rid of the warning about chromosome lengths? ◀

▶ Solution **3.11** The information on chromosome lengths in the hg19 assembly of the human genome is (for instance) stored in the `ideoCyto` dataset. We use the function `keepSeqlevels` to reorder the chromosomes. See Figure 3.47.

```
data("ideoCyto", package = "biovizBase")
dn = darned_hg19_subset500
seqlengths(dn) = seqlengths(ideoCyto$hg19)[names(seqlengths(dn))]
dn = keepSeqlevels(dn, paste0("chr", c(1:22, "X")))
autoplot(dn, layout = "karyogram", aes(color = exReg, fill = exReg))□
```

▶ Question **3.12** What type of object is `darned_hg19_subset500`? ◀

▶ **Solution 3.12**

```
darned_hg19_subset500[1:2,]
## GRanges object with 2 ranges and 10 metadata columns:
##       seqnames               ranges strand |      inchr
##          <Rle>            <IRanges>  <Rle> | <character>
##   [1]     chr5 [86618225, 86618225]      - |           A
##   [2]     chr7 [99792382, 99792382]      - |           A
##            inrna         snp        gene       seqReg
##        <character> <character> <character> <character>
##   [1]            I        <NA>        <NA>           O
##   [2]            I        <NA>        <NA>           O
##            exReg      source        ests        esta      author
##        <character> <character>   <integer>   <integer> <character>
##   [1]         <NA>    amygdala           0           0    15342557
##   [2]         <NA>        <NA>           0           0    15342557
##   -------
##   seqinfo: 23 sequences from an unspecified genome; no seqlengths
```

It is a *GRanges* object, that is, a specialized class from the Bioconductor project for storing data that are associated with genomic coordinates. The first three columns are obligatory: `seqnames`, the name of the containing biopolymer (in our case, these are names of human chromosomes); `ranges`, the genomic coordinates of the intervals (in this case, the intervals all have length 1, as they each refer to a single nucleotide); and the DNA `strand` from which the RNA is transcribed. You can find out more on how to use this class and its associated infrastructure in the documentation, e.g., the vignette of the *GenomicRanges* package. Learning it is worth the effort if you want to work with genome-associated datasets, as it enables convenient, efficient and safe manipulation of these data and provides many powerful utilities.   □

3.14   Summary of this chapter

Visualizing data, either "raw" or along the various steps of processing, summarization and inference, is one of the most important activities in applied statistics and, indeed, in science. It sometimes gets short shrift in textbooks since there is not much deductive theory. However, there are many good (and bad) practices, and once you pay attention to it, you will quickly see whether a certain graphic is effective in conveying its message, or what choices you could make to create powerful and aesthetically attractive data visualizations. Among the important options are the plot type (what is called a `geom` in *ggplot2*), proportions (including aspect ratios) and colors. The *grammar of graphics* is a powerful set of concepts for reasoning about graphics and communicating to a computer our intentions for a data visualization.

Avoid *laziness* – just using the software's defaults without thinking about the options – and avoid *getting carried away* – adding lots of visual candy that just clutters up the plot but has no real message. Creating your own visualizations is in many ways like good writing. It is extremely important to get your message across (in talks, in papers), but there is no simple recipe for it. Look carefully at lots of visualizations made by others;

experiment with making your own visualizations to learn the ropes, and then decide what is your style.

3.15   Further reading

The most useful resources about *ggplot2* are the second edition of Wickham (2016) and the *ggplot2* website. There are many *ggplot2* code snippets online, which you will find through search engines after some practice. But be critical and check your sources: sometimes code examples that you find online refer to outdated versions of the package, and sometimes they are of poor quality.

The foundation of the system lies in the work of Wilkinson (2005) and the ideas of Tukey (1977) and Cleveland (1988).

3.16   Exercises

▶ **Exercise 3.1** Use *themes* to change the visual appearance of your plots. Start by running the following example.

```
ggcars = ggplot(mtcars, aes(x = hp, y = mpg)) + geom_point()
ggcars
ggcars + theme_bw()
ggcars + theme_minimal()
```

What other themes are there? (Hint: have a look at the section on themes in the online documentation of *ggplot2*.[21]) Are these all the themes? (Hint: have a look at the *ggthemes* package.) Make a version of the example plot in the style of *The Economist* magazine. Add a smoothing line. ◀

[21] http://ggplot2.tidyverse.org/reference.

▶ **Exercise 3.2** What are admissible *color names* in R? Have a look at the manual page of the `colors` function in the *grDevices* package, and run the examples and the demo.

Use an internet search engine to search for "R color names" and explore some of the resources that come up, e.g., cheat sheets with all the colors displayed.

Produce a version of the heatmap in Figure 3.38 that uses a color palette from the R package *beyonce*.[22] ◀

[22] https://github.com/dill/beyonce.

▶ **Exercise 3.3** Create plots in the style of the xkcd webcomic. Look at

- a thread on Stackoverflow titled *How can we make xkcd style graphs?*
- the R source code of this book for the code that produces the chapter's opening figure, and
- the vignette of the *xkcd* package. ◀

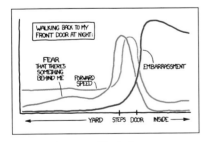

Image credit: xkcd.com.

▶ **Exercise 3.4** Check out the *shiny* tutorials on the RStudio website. Write a *shiny app* that displays one of the plots from this chapter, but with interactive elements to control, e.g., which genes are displayed (Figures 3.31–3.33). ◀

▶ **Exercise 3.5** What options are there for *serializing* a graphic, i.e., for storing a graphic in a file that you can save for later use or load in another software? How can you serialize interactive graphics? ◀

CHAPTER 4

Mixture Models

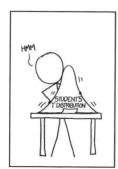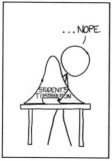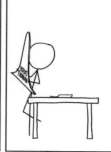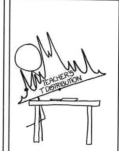

One of the main challenges of biological data analysis is dealing with heterogeneity. The quantities we are interested in often do not show a simple, unimodal "textbook" distribution. For example, in Chapter 2 we saw how the histogram of sequence scores in Figure 2.25 had two separate modes, one for CpG islands and one for non-islands. We can see the data as a simple mixture of a few (in this case, two) components. We call these *finite mixtures*. Other mixtures can involve almost as many components as we have observations. These we call *infinite mixtures*.[1]

In Chapter 1 we saw how a simple generative model with a Poisson distribution led us to make useful inference in the detection of an epitope. Unfortunately, a satisfactory fit to real data with such a simple model is often out of reach. However, simple models such as the normal or Poisson distribution can serve as building blocks for more realistic models using the mixing framework that we cover in this chapter. Mixtures occur naturally for flow cytometry data, biometric measurements, RNA-Seq, ChIP-Seq, microbiome and many other types of data collected using modern biotechnologies. In this chapter we will learn from simple examples how to build more realistic models of distributions using mixtures.

[1] We will see that, as for so many modeling choices, the correct complexity of the mixture is in the eye of the beholder and often depends on the amount of data and the resolution and smoothness we want to attain.

4.1 Goals for this chapter

In this chapter we will:

- Generate our own mixture model data from distributions composed of two normal populations.
- See how the expectation–maximization (EM) algorithm allows us to "reverse engineer" the underlying mixtures in a dataset.
- Use a special type of mixture called zero-inflation on ChIP-Seq data that has many extra zeros in it.
- Explore the empirical cumulative distribution, a special mixture that we can build from observed data. This will enable us to see how we can simulate the variability of our estimates using the bootstrap.

- Build the Laplace distribution as an instance of an infinite mixture model. We will use it to model promoter lengths and microarray intensities.
- Have our first encounter with the gamma–Poisson distribution, a hierarchical model useful for RNA-Seq data. We will see that it arises naturally from mixing different Poisson-distributed sources.
- See how mixture models enable us to choose data transformations.

4.2 Finite mixtures

4.2.1 Simple examples and computer experiments

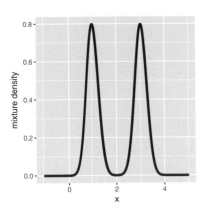

Figure 4.1: Histogram of 10,000 random draws from a fair mixture of two normals. The left-hand part of the histogram is dominated by numbers generated from (A), that on the right from (B).

To start, we'll make an example of a **mixture model** with two equal-sized components. The generating process consists of two steps:

Flip a fair coin.

A. If it comes up heads Generate a random number from a normal distribution with mean 1 and variance 0.25.

B. If it comes up tails Generate a random number from a normal distribution with mean 3 and variance 0.25.

The histogram shown in Figure 4.1 was produced by repeating these two steps 10,000 times using the following code.

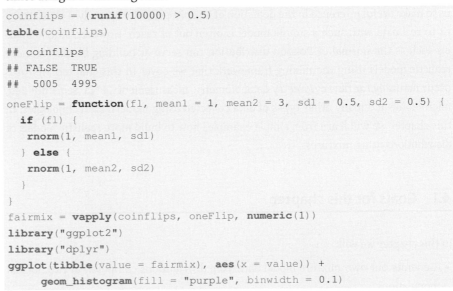

```
coinflips = (runif(10000) > 0.5)
table(coinflips)

## coinflips
## FALSE   TRUE
##  5005   4995

oneFlip = function(fl, mean1 = 1, mean2 = 3, sd1 = 0.5, sd2 = 0.5) {
  if (fl) {
    rnorm(1, mean1, sd1)
  } else {
    rnorm(1, mean2, sd2)
  }
}
fairmix = vapply(coinflips, oneFlip, numeric(1))
library("ggplot2")
library("dplyr")
ggplot(tibble(value = fairmix), aes(x = value)) +
    geom_histogram(fill = "purple", binwidth = 0.1)
```

Figure 4.2: The theoretical density of the mixture.

▶ Question **4.1** How can you use R's vectorized syntax to remove the `vapply` loop and generate the `fairmix` vector more efficiently?   ◀

▶ **Solution 4.1**

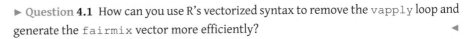

```
means = c(1, 3)
sds   = c(0.25, 0.25)
values = rnorm(length(coinflips),
```

```
        mean = ifelse(coinflips, means[1], means[2]),
        sd   = ifelse(coinflips, sds[1],   sds[2]))
```

▶ Question **4.2** Using your improved code, perform one million coin flips and make a histogram with 500 bins. What do you notice? ◀

▶ **Solution 4.2**

```
fair = tibble(
  coinflips = (runif(1e6) > 0.5),
  values = rnorm(length(coinflips),
            mean = ifelse(coinflips, means[1], means[2]),
            sd   = ifelse(coinflips, sds[1],   sds[2])))
ggplot(fair, aes(x = values)) +
    geom_histogram(fill = "purple", bins = 500)
```

As we increase the number of observations and bins, the histogram gets nearer to a smooth curve. This smooth limiting curve is called the **density function** of the random variable `fair$values`.

The density function for a normal $N(\mu, \sigma)$ random variable can be written explicitly; we usually call it $\phi(x)$ and it is given by $\phi(x) = \frac{1}{\sigma\sqrt{2\pi}} e^{-\frac{1}{2}(\frac{x-\mu}{\sigma})^2}$.

▶ Question **4.3** (a) Plot a histogram only of those values of `fair$values` for which `coinflips` is `TRUE`. Hint: use `y = ..density..` in the call to `aes` (to specify that the vertical axis shows the proportion of counts) and set the binwidth to 0.01. (b) Overlay the line corresponding to $\phi(z)$. ◀

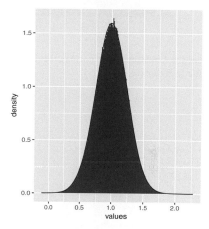

Figure 4.3: In purple: histogram of half a million draws from the normal distribution $N(\mu = 1, \sigma^2 = 0.25)$. The curve is the theoretical density $\phi(x)$ calculated using the function `dnorm`.

▶ **Solution 4.3**

```
ggplot(filter(fair, coinflips), aes(x = values)) +
    geom_histogram(aes(y = ..density..), fill = "purple",
                binwidth = 0.01) +
    stat_function(fun = dnorm,
            args = list(mean = means[1], sd = sds[1]), color = "red")
```

We can write the formula for the density of all of `fair$values` (the limiting curve that the histogram approaches) as a sum of the two densities:

$$f(x) = \frac{1}{2}\phi_1(x) + \frac{1}{2}\phi_2(x), \qquad (4.1)$$

where ϕ_1 is the density of the normal $N(\mu_1 = 1, \sigma^2 = 0.25)$ and ϕ_2 is the density of the normal $N(\mu_2 = 3, \sigma^2 = 0.25)$. Figure 4.2 was generated by the following code.

```
fairtheory = tibble(
  x = seq(-1, 5, length.out = 1000),
  f = 0.5 * dnorm(x, mean = means[1], sd = sds[1]) +
      0.5 * dnorm(x, mean = means[2], sd = sds[2]))
ggplot(fairtheory, aes(x = x, y = f)) +
  geom_line(color = "red", size = 1.5) + ylab("mixture density")
```

In this case the mixture model is extremely visible, as the two component distributions have little overlap. Figure 4.2 shows two distinct peaks: we call this a **bimodal** distribution. In many cases, however, the separation is not so clear.

▶ **Question 4.4** Figure 4.4 is a histogram of a fair mixture of two normals with the same variances. Can you guess the two *mean* parameters of the component distributions? Hint: you can use trial and error, and simulate various mixtures to see if you can make a matching histogram. Looking at the R code for the chapter will show you exactly how the data were generated – in this case, you can look inside the black box.   ◀

▶ **Solution 4.4** The following code colors in red those points generated from *heads* coin flips and in blue those from *tails*. Its output, in Figure 4.5, shows the two underlying distributions.

```
head(mystery, 3)

## # A tibble: 3 x 2
##   coinflips values
##   <lgl>     <dbl>
## 1 F         2.09
## 2 T         0.518
## 3 F         0.992
br = with(mystery, seq(min(values), max(values), length.out = 30))
ggplot(mystery, aes(x = values)) +
  geom_histogram(data = dplyr::filter(mystery, coinflips),
    fill = "red", alpha = 0.2, breaks = br) +
  geom_histogram(data = dplyr::filter(mystery, !coinflips),
    fill = "darkblue", alpha = 0.2, breaks = br)
```

In Figure 4.5, the bars from the two component distributions are plotted on top of each other. A different way of showing the components is Figure 4.6, produced by the code below.

```
ggplot(mystery, aes(x = values, fill = coinflips)) +
  geom_histogram(breaks = br, alpha = 0.2) +
  scale_fill_manual(values = c(`TRUE` = "red", `FALSE` = "darkblue"),
                    guide = FALSE)
```

In Figures 4.5 and 4.6, we are able to use the `coinflips` column in the data to disentangle the components, or groups, by looking at the colors. In real data, this information is missing.

4.2.2 Discovering the hidden group labels

We use a method called the **expectation–maximization (EM) algorithm** to infer the hidden groups that are mixed together in the data.[2] The expectation–maximization algorithm is a popular iterative procedure that alternates between

- pretending we know the probability with which each observation belongs to a group or component and estimating the distribution parameters of the components, and
- pretending we know the parameters of the component distributions and estimating the probability with which each observation belongs to the components.

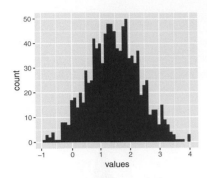

Figure 4.4: A mixture of two normals that is harder to recognize.

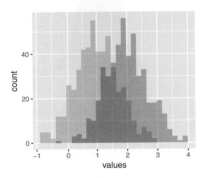

Figure 4.5: The mixture from Figure 4.4, but with the two components colored in red and blue.

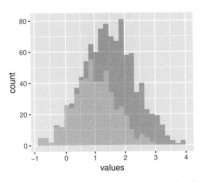

Figure 4.6: As Figure 4.5, with stacked bars for the two mixture components.

[2] Such groups in the data are often called *classes*.

Let's start with a simple example. We measure a variable Y on a series of objects that we think come from two groups, although we do not know the group labels. We start by *augmenting*[3] the data with a variable for the unobserved (latent) group label, which we'll call U.

[3] Adding another variable that was not measured, called a hidden or **latent variable**.

We are interested in finding the values of U and the unknown parameters of the underlying densities. We will use the maximum likelihood approach introduced in Chapter 2 to estimate the parameters that make the data Y the most likely. We will use the notion of **bivariate distribution** here because we are going to look at the distribution of "couples" (Y, U). We can write the probability densities under the parametric model:

$$f_\theta(y, u) = f_\theta(y \mid u) f_\theta(u), \qquad (4.2)$$

where θ stands for the tuple of parameters of the underlying density. In the example in Section 4.2.1, θ would be the two means, the two standard deviations and the **mixture fraction** $\lambda = 0.5$; thus $\theta = (\mu_1, \mu_2, \sigma_1, \sigma_2, \lambda)$.

▶ Question **4.5** Suppose we have two unfair coins, whose probabilities of heads are $p_1 = 0.125$ and $p_2 = 0.25$. With probability π we pick coin 1, and with probability $1 - \pi$, coin 2. We then toss that coin twice and record the number of heads K.
(a) Simulate 100 instances of this procedure with $\pi = \frac{1}{8}$, and compute the contingency table of K.
(b) Do the same with $\pi = \frac{1}{4}$.
(c) If you were not told p_1, p_2 and π, could you infer them from the contingency table?

◀

▶ **Solution 4.5**

```
probHead = c(0.125, 0.25)
for (pi in c(1/8, 1/4)) {
  whCoin = sample(2, 100, replace = TRUE, prob = c(pi, 1-pi))
  K = rbinom(length(whCoin), size = 2, prob = probHead[whCoin])
  print(table(K))
}

## K
##  0  1  2
## 60 34  6
## K
##  0  1  2
## 65 31  4
```

This question alerts you to the issue of **identifiability**: the same observed values could have several explanations in terms of values of p_1, p_2 and π. This occurs when there are too many degrees of freedom in the parameters.[4]   □

[4] We see this issue again in Section 10.4.1.

Mixture of normals.   Suppose we have a mixture of two normals with mean parameters unknown and standard deviation 1; thus, our tuple is $(\mu_1 = ?, \mu_2 = ?, \sigma_1 = \sigma_2 = 1)$. Here is an example of data generated according to such a model. The labels are u.

The situation is similar to the "black box" we tackled visually in Section 4.2.1. There the label was `coinflips`.

```
mus = c(-0.5, 1.5)
u = sample(2, 100, replace = TRUE)
y = rnorm(length(u), mean = mus[u])
duy = tibble(u, y)
head(duy)

## # A tibble: 6 x 2
##       u        y
##   <int>    <dbl>
## 1     1   -0.257
## 2     2    1.74
## 3     2   -0.835
## 4     1   -1.47
## 5     2    2.05
## 6     1   -2.37
```

In Section 4.2.1 we knew the labels: TRUE and
FALSE.

If we know the labels u, we can estimate the means using separate MLEs for each group. The overall MLE is obtained by maximizing

$$f(y, u \mid \theta) = \prod_{\{i:\, u_i = 1\}} \phi_1(y_i) \prod_{\{i:\, u_i = 2\}} \phi_2(y_i), \tag{4.3}$$

or its logarithm. The maximization can be split into two independent pieces and solved as if we had two different MLEs to find.

```
group_by(duy, u) %>% summarize(mean(y))

## # A tibble: 2 x 2
##       u  `mean(y)`
##   <int>      <dbl>
## 1     1     -0.537
## 2     2      1.54
```

▶ Question **4.6** Suppose we know the mixing fraction is $\lambda = \frac{1}{2}$, so that the density is as in Equation (4.1), namely $\frac{1}{2}\phi_1 + \frac{1}{2}\phi_2$. Try writing out the (log-)likelihood. What prevents us from solving for the MLE explicitly here?   ◀

▶ Solution **4.6** See Chapter 19 (Equations 19.8–19.12) in Shalizi (2017) for the computation of the likelihood of a finite mixture of normals: "If we try to estimate the mixture model, then we're doing weighted maximum likelihood, with weights given by the posterior label probabilities. These, to repeat, depend on the parameters we are trying to estimate, so there seems to be a vicious circle."   □

In reality, we do not know the labels u, nor do we know the mixture proportion λ. We have to start with an initial guess for the labels, estimate the parameters and go through several iterations of the algorithm, updating at each step our current best guess of the group labels and the parameters until we see no substantial improvement in our optimizations.

In fact, we can do something more elaborate and replace the "hard" labels u for each observation (it is in either group 1 or 2) by membership probabilities that sum up to 1. The probability $p(u, x \mid \theta)$ serves as a weight or "participation" of observation x in the likelihood function.[5] The **marginal likelihood** for the observed y is the sum over all

[5] This is sometimes called "soft" averaging (Slonim et al., 2005). We create weighted averages where each point's probability serves as the weight, so we don't have to make a hard decision that a point belongs to this or that group.

possible values of u of the densities at (y, u):

$$\text{marglike}(\theta; y) = f(y \mid \theta) = \sum_u f(y, u \mid \theta) \, du.$$

At each iteration (we mark the present values with an asterisk, $*$), the current best guesses for the unknown parameters (for instance μ_1^* and μ_2^*) are combined into $\theta^* = (\mu_1^*, \mu_2^*, \lambda^*)$. We use these to compute the so-called **e**xpectation[6] function $E^*(\theta)$:

$$E^*(\theta) = E_{\theta^*, Y}[\log p(u, y \mid \theta^*)] = \sum_u p(u \mid y, \theta^*) \log p(u, y \mid \theta^*).$$

[6] The term *expectation* here means that we average, or integrate, over all possible values of u.

The value of θ that maximizes E^* is found in what is known as the **m**aximization step. These two iterations (**E** and **M**) are repeated until increases in E^* are small; this is a numerical indication that we are close to a flattening of the likelihood and so have reached a local maximum.[7] It's good practice to repeat the procedure several times from different starting points and check that we always get the same answer.

[7] The path that the iteration follows will depend on the starting point, but, as in an uphill hike, while the intermediate points may be different, we always end up on top of the same hill – as long as there is only one hilltop and not several.

▶ **Question 4.7** Several R packages implement the EM algorithm, including *mclust*, *EMcluster* and *EMMIXskew*. Choose one and run the EM function several times with different starting values. Then use the function `normalmixEM` from the *mixtools* package to compare the outputs.   ◀

▶ **Solution 4.7** Here we show the output from *mixtools*.

```
library("mixtools")
y = c(rnorm(100, mean = -0.2, sd = 0.5),
      rnorm( 50, mean =  0.5, sd =   1))
gm = normalmixEM(y, k = 2, lambda = c(0.5, 0.5),
     mu = c(-0.01, 0.01), sigma = c(1, 1))
## number of iterations= 159
gm$lambda
## [1] 0.4077652 0.5922348
gm$mu
## [1] -0.5031351  0.3508157
gm$sigma
## [1] 0.3748884 0.8297709
gm$loglik
## [1] -171.4799
```

The EM algorithm is very instructive:

1. It shows us how we can tackle a difficult problem with too many unknowns by alternating between solving simpler problems. In this way, we eventually find estimates of **hidden variables**.

2. It provides a first example of **soft** averaging, i.e., where we don't decide whether an observation belongs to one group or another, but allow it to participate in several groups by using probabilities of membership as weights, and thus obtain more nuanced estimates.

3. The method used here can be extended to the more general case of **model averaging** (Hoeting et al., 1999). It can sometimes be beneficial to consider several models simultaneously if we are unsure which one is relevant for our data. We can combine them together into a weighted model. The weights are provided by the likelihoods of the models.

4.2.3   Models for zero-inflated data

Ecological and molecular data often come in the form of counts. For instance, this may be the number of individuals from each of several species at each of several locations. Such data can often be seen as a mixture of two scenarios. If the species is not present, the count is necessarily zero. If the species is present, the number of individuals we observe varies, with a random sampling distribution, and this distribution may also include zeros. We model this as a mixture:

$$f_{zi}(y) = \lambda\,\delta(y) + (1 - \lambda)\,f_{count}(y),$$

where δ is the Dirac delta function, which represents a probability distribution that has all its mass at 0. The zeros from the first mixture component, δ, are called "structural"; in our example, they occur because certain species do not live in certain habitats. The second component, f_{count}, may also include zeros and other small numbers; in our example, a random sample happened not to find members of a species in some locations. The R packages *pscl* (Zeileis et al., 2008) and *zicounts* provide many examples and functions for working with such **zero-inflated** counts.

Example: ChIP-Seq data

Let's consider the example of ChIP-Seq data. These data are sequences of pieces of DNA that are obtained from chromatin immunoprecipitation (ChIP). This technology enables the mapping of the locations along genomic DNA of transcription factors, nucleosomes, histone modifications, chromatin remodeling enzymes, chaperones, polymerases and other proteins. It was the main technology used by the Encyclopedia of DNA Elements (ENCODE) Project. Here we use an example (Kuan et al., 2011) from the *mosaicsExample* package, which shows data measured on chromosome 22 from a ChIP-Seq of antibodies for the STAT1 protein and the H3K4me3 histone modification applied to the GM12878 cell line.

Here we do not show the code used to construct the `binTFBS` object that contains the binding sites for one chromosome (22); it is shown in the source code file for this chapter and follows the vignette of the *mosaics* package.

```
binTFBS

## Summary: bin-level data (class: BinData)
## ----------------------------------------
## - # of chromosomes in the data: 1
## - total effective tag counts: 462479
```

```
##   (sum of ChIP tag counts of all bins)
## - control sample is incorporated
## - mappability score is NOT incorporated
## - GC content score is NOT incorporated
## - uni-reads are assumed
## ----------------------------------------
```

From this object, we can create the histogram of per-bin counts.

```
bincts = print(binTFBS)
ggplot(bincts, aes(x = tagCount)) +
  geom_histogram(binwidth = 1, fill = "forestgreen")
```

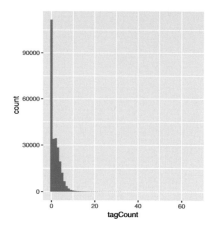

Figure 4.7: The number of binding sites found in 200nt windows along chromosome 22 in a ChIP-Seq dataset.

Figure 4.7 shows many zeros, although from this plot it is not immediately obvious whether the number of zeros is really extraordinary, given the frequencies of the other small numbers $(1, 2, \ldots)$.

▶ **Question 4.8** (a) Redo the histogram of counts using a logarithm base 10 scale on the y-axis.

(b) Estimate π_0, the proportion of bins with zero counts. ◀

▶ **Solution 4.8**

```
ggplot(bincts, aes(x = tagCount)) + scale_y_log10() +
  geom_histogram(binwidth = 1, fill = "forestgreen")
```
□

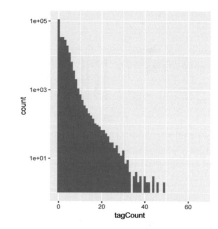

Figure 4.8: As Figure 4.7, but using a logarithm base 10 scale on the y-axis. The fraction of zeros seems elevated compared to that of ones, twos, ...

4.2.4 More than two components

So far we have looked at mixtures of two components. We can extend our description to cases where there may be more. For instance, when weighing N=7000 nucleotides obtained from mixtures of deoxyribonucleotide monophosphates (each type has a different weight, measured with the same standard deviation sd=3), we might observe the histogram, shown in Figure 4.9, generated by the following code.

```
masses = c(A =   331, C =   307, G =   347, T =   322)
probs  = c(A = 0.12, C = 0.38, G = 0.36, T = 0.14)
N  = 7000
sd = 3
nuclt   = sample(length(probs), N, replace = TRUE, prob = probs)
quadwts = rnorm(length(nuclt),
                mean = masses[nuclt],
                sd   = sd)
ggplot(tibble(quadwts = quadwts), aes(x = quadwts)) +
  geom_histogram(bins = 100, fill = "purple")
```

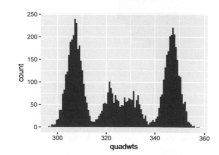

Figure 4.9: Simulation of 7000 nucleotide mass measurements.

▶ **Question 4.9** Repeat this simulation experiment with N=1000 nucleotide measurements. What do you notice in the histogram? ◀

▶ **Question 4.10** What happens when N=7000 but the standard deviation is 10? ◀

▶ **Question 4.11** Plot the theoretical density curve for the distribution simulated in Figure 4.9. ◀

In this case, as we have enough measurements with good enough precision, we are able to distinguish the four nucleotides and decompose the distribution shown in Figure 4.9. With fewer data points and/or more noisy measurements, the four modes and the distribution components might be less clear.

4.3   Empirical distributions and the nonparametric bootstrap

In this section, we consider an extreme case of mixture model, where we model our sample of n data points as a mixture of n point masses. We could use almost any set of data here; to be concrete, we use Darwin's *Zea mays* data[8] in which he compared the heights of 15 pairs of *Zea mays* plants (15 self-hybridized versus 15 crossed). The data are available in the *HistData* package, and we plot the distribution of the 15 differences in height, shown in Figure 4.10.

[8] Darwin collected the data and asked his cousin Francis Galton to analyze them. R.A. Fisher reanalyzed the same data using a paired *t*-test (Bulmer, 2003). We will come back to this example in Chapter 13.

```
library("HistData")
ZeaMays$diff
```
```
##  [1]  6.125 -8.375  1.000  2.000  0.750  2.875  3.500  5.125
##  [9]  1.750  3.625  7.000  3.000  9.375  7.500 -6.000
```
```
ggplot(ZeaMays, aes(x = diff, ymax = 1/15, ymin = 0)) +
  geom_linerange(size = 1, col = "forestgreen") + ylim(0, 0.1)
```

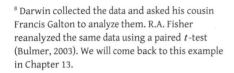

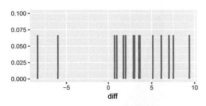

Figure 4.10: The observed sample can be seen as a mixture of point masses at each of the values (real point masses would be bars without any width whatsoever).

In Section 3.6.6 we saw that the **empirical cumulative distribution function (ECDF)** for a sample of size n is

$$\widehat{F}_n(x) = \frac{1}{n}\sum_{i=1}^{n} \mathbb{1}(x \leqslant x_i), \tag{4.4}$$

and we saw ECDF plots in Figure 3.22. We can also write the **density** of our sample as

$$\hat{f}_n(x) = \frac{1}{n}\sum_{i=1}^{n} \delta_{x_i}(x). \tag{4.5}$$

In general, the density of a probability distribution is the derivative (if it exists) of the distribution function. We have applied this principle here: the density of the distribution defined by Equation (4.4) is Equation (4.5). We can do this because one can consider the function δ_a the "derivative" of the step function $\mathbb{1}(x \leqslant a)$: it is completely flat almost everywhere, except at the one point a where there is the step, where its value is "infinite".[9] Equation (4.5) highlights that our data sample can be considered a mixture of n **point masses**, one at each of the observed values $x_1, x_2, \ldots, x_n$, as in Figure 4.10.

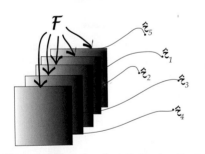

Figure 4.11: The value of a statistic τ is estimated from data (the gray matrices) generated from an underlying distribution F. Different samples from F lead to different data, and so to different values of the estimate $\hat{\tau}$; this is called *sampling variability*. The distribution of all the $\hat{\tau}$s is the *sampling distribution*.

[9] Some advanced mathematics (beyond standard calculus) that is outside the scope of our treatment is required for this to make sense.

Statistics of our sample, such as the mean, minimum or median, can now be written as a function of the ECDF; for instance, $\bar{x} = \int \delta_{x_i}(x)\, dx$. As another instance, if n is an odd number, the median is $x_{(\frac{n+1}{2})}$ or $\widehat{F}_n^{-1}(0.5)$, the value right in the middle of the ordered list.

The true **sampling distribution** of a statistic $\hat{\tau}$ is often hard to know as it requires many different data samples from which to compute the statistic; the situation is illustrated in Figure 4.11.

The **bootstrap** principle approximates the true sampling distribution of $\hat{\tau}$ by creating new samples drawn from the empirical distribution built from the original sample (Figure 4.12). We *reuse* the data (by considering it a mixture distribution of δs) to create new "datasets" by taking samples and looking at the sampling distribution of the statistics $\hat{\tau}^*$ computed on them. This is called the **nonparametric bootstrap** resampling approach; see Efron and Tibshirani (1994) for a complete treatment. It is a versatile and powerful method that can be applied to almost any statistic, no matter how complicated it is. We will see example applications of this method, in particular to clustering, in Chapter 5.

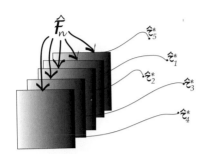

Figure 4.12: The bootstrap simulates the sampling variability by drawing samples not from the underlying true distribution F (as in Figure 4.11), but from the empirical distribution function $\hat{F}_n$.

Using these ideas, let's try to estimate the sampling distribution of the median of the *Zea mays* differences in Figure 4.10. We use simulation. Draw $B = 1000$ samples of size 15 from the 15 values (each being a component in the 15-component mixture). Compute the median of each of these samples of 15 values, then look at the distribution of the 1000 medians: this is the bootstrap sampling distribution of the median, shown in Figure 4.13.

```
B = 1000
meds = replicate(B, {
  i = sample(15, 15, replace = TRUE)
  median(ZeaMays$diff[i])
})
ggplot(tibble(medians = meds), aes(x = medians)) +
  geom_histogram(bins = 30, fill = "purple")
```

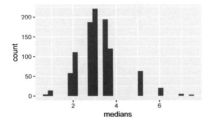

Figure 4.13: The bootstrap sampling distribution of the median of the *Zea mays* differences.

▶ Question **4.12** Estimate a 99% confidence interval for the median based on these simulations. What can you conclude from looking at the overlap between this interval and 0?   ◀

▶ Question **4.13** Use the *bootstrap* package to redo the analysis using the function `bootstrap` for both `median` and `mean`. What differences do you notice between the sampling distributions of the mean and the median?   ◀

▶ Solution **4.13**

```
library("bootstrap")
bootstrap(ZeaMays$diff, B, mean)
bootstrap(ZeaMays$diff, B, median)
```
□

Despite their name, nonparametric methods do use parameters; all statistical methods estimate unknown quantities.

Why nonparametric?   In theoretical statistics, **nonparametric methods** are those that allow *infinitely many* degrees of freedom or numbers of unknown parameters.

In practice, we do not wait for infinity; when the number of parameters becomes as large as or larger than the amount of data available, we say the method is nonparametric. The bootstrap uses a mixture with n components, so with a sample of size n, it qualifies as a nonparametric method.

When using nonparametric methods, we often replace analytical calculations by simulations. The bootstrap is no exception: instead of generating all possible samples from the empirical distribution (in theory this is possible, since there is a finite number of them), we use Monte Carlo simulations to make bootstrap resamples of the data.

▶ Question **4.14** If a sample is composed of $n = 3$ different values, how many different bootstrap resamples are possible? Answer the same question with $n = 15$.   ◀

▶ Solution **4.14**   The set of all bootstrap resamples is equivalent to the set of all vectors of n integers whose sum is n. Denote by $\boldsymbol{k} = (k_1, k_2, \ldots, k_n)$ the number of times the observations $x_1, x_2, \ldots, x_n$ occur in a bootstrap sample. We can think of each k_i as a box (as in the multinomial distribution), and there are n boxes in which to drop n balls. We can count the number of configurations by counting the number of ways of separating n balls into the boxes, i.e., by writing down n times a ∘ (for the balls) and $n - 1$ times a separator | between them. So we have $2n - 1$ positions to fill, for which we must choose either ∘ (a ball) or | (a separator). For $n = 3$, a possible placement would be ∘∘||∘, which corresponds to $\boldsymbol{k} = (2, 0, 1)$. In general, this number is $\binom{2n-1}{n-1}$, and thus the answers for $n = 3$ and 15 are

```
c(N3 = choose(5, 3), N15 = choose(29, 15))

##       N3         N15
##       10  77558760
```

▶ **Question 4.15** What are the two types of error that can occur when using the bootstrap as it is implemented in the *bootstrap* package? Which parameter can you modify to improve one of them? ◀

▶ **Solution 4.15** Monte Carlo simulations of subsets of data by random resampling approximate the exhaustive bootstrap (Diaconis and Holmes, 1994). Increasing the size of the `nboot` argument in the `bootstrap` function reduces the Monte Carlo error; however, the exhaustive bootstrap is still not exact: we are still using an approximate distribution function, that of the data instead of the true distribution. If the sample size is small or the original sample biased, the approximation can still be quite poor, no matter how large we choose `nboot`. □

4.4 Infinite mixtures

Mixtures can be useful even if we don't aim to assign a label to each observation or, to put it differently, if we allow as many "labels" as there are observations. If the number of mixture components is as big as (or bigger than) the number of observations, we say we have an **infinite mixture**. Let's look at some examples.

4.4.1 Infinite mixture of normals

Consider the following two-level data-generating scheme:

Level 1 Create a sample of ws from an exponential distribution.

```
w = rexp(10000, rate = 1)
```

Level 2 The ws serve as the variances of normal variables with mean μ generated using `rnorm`.

```
mu   = 0.3
lps = rnorm(length(w), mean = mu, sd = sqrt(w))
ggplot(data.frame(lps), aes(x = lps)) +
  geom_histogram(fill = "purple", binwidth = 0.1)
```

A book-long treatment on the subject of finite mixtures is McLachlan and Peel (2004).

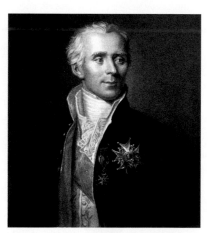

Figure 4.14: Laplace knew already that the probability density

$$f_Y(y) = \frac{1}{2\phi} \exp\left(-\frac{|y - \theta|}{\phi}\right), \qquad \phi > 0$$

has the median as its location parameter θ and the median absolute deviation (MAD) as its scale parameter ϕ. Image credit: traveler1116/E+/Getty Images.

This turns out to be a rather useful distribution. It has well-understood properties and is named after **Laplace**, who proved that the median is a good estimator of its location parameter θ and that the median absolute deviation can be used to estimate its scale parameter ϕ. From the formula in the Figure 4.14 caption, we see that the L_1 distance (absolute value of the difference) holds a similar position in the Laplace density as the L_2 (square of the difference) does in the normal density.

Conversely, in Bayesian regression, having a Laplace distribution as a prior on the coefficients amounts to an L_1 penalty, called the *lasso* (Tibshirani, 1996), while a normal distribution as a prior leads to an L_2 penalty, called *ridge regression*.[10]

[10] Don't worry if you are not familiar with the lasso or ridge regression; just skip this sentence.

▶ **Question 4.16** Write a random variable whose distribution is the symmetric Laplace as a function of normal and exponential random variables. ◀

▶ **Solution 4.16** We can write the hierarchical model with variances generated as exponential variables, W, as

$$Y = \sqrt{W} \cdot Z, \qquad W \sim \text{Exp}(1), \qquad Z \sim N(0,1). \qquad \square$$

Asymmetric Laplace

In the Laplace distribution, the variances of the normal components depend on W, while the means are unaffected. A useful extension adds another parameter θ that controls the locations or centers of the components. We generate data `alps` from a hierarchical model with W an exponential variable; the output shown in Figure 4.16 is a histogram of normal $N(\theta + w\mu, \sigma w)$ random numbers, where the ws themselves were randomly generated from an exponential distribution with mean 1, as shown in the following code.

```
mu = 0.3; sigma = 0.4; theta = -1
w   = rexp(10000, 1)
alps = rnorm(length(w), theta + mu * w, sigma * sqrt(w))
ggplot(tibble(alps), aes(x = alps)) +
  geom_histogram(fill = "purple", binwidth = 0.1)
```

Such hierarchical mixture distributions, where every instance of the data has its own mean and variance, are useful models in many biological settings. Examples are shown in Figure 4.17.

▶ **Question 4.17** Looking at the log-ratio of gene expression values from a microarray, one gets a distribution as shown on the right of Figure 4.17. How would one explain that the data have a histogram of this form? ◀

Studying the Laplace distribution shows us that considering the generative process can indicate how the variance and mean are linked. The expectation and variance of an asymmetric Laplace distribution $AL(\theta, \mu, \sigma)$ are

$$E(Y) = \theta + \mu \qquad \text{and} \qquad \text{var}(Y) = \sigma^2 + \mu^2. \tag{4.6}$$

The variance depends on the mean μ, unless $\mu = 0$ (the case of the symmetric Laplace

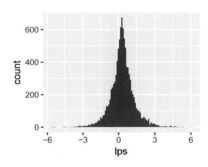

Figure 4.15: Data sampled from a Laplace distribution.

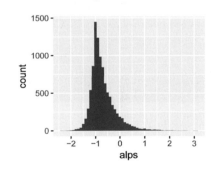

Figure 4.16: Histogram of data generated from an asymmetric Laplace distribution – a scale mixture of many normals whose means and variances are dependent. We write $X \sim AL(\theta, \mu, \sigma)$.

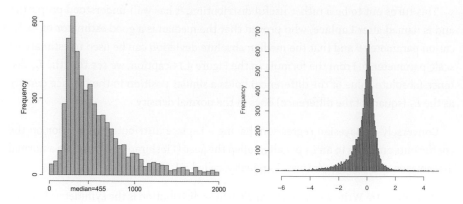

Figure 4.17: Histogram of real data. On the left, the lengths of the promoters shorter than 2000bp from Saccharomyces cerevisiae as studied by Kristiansson et al. (2009). On the right, the log-ratios of microarray gene expression measurements for 20,000 genes (Purdom and Holmes, 2005). Both distributions can be modeled by asymmetric Laplace distributions.

distribution). This feature of the distribution makes it useful. Mean–variance dependence is very common in physical measurements, be they microarray fluorescence intensities, peak heights from a mass spectrometer or read counts from high-throughput sequencing, as we'll see in the next section.

4.4.2 Infinite mixtures of Poisson variables

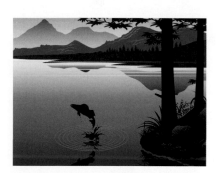

Figure 4.18: How to count the fish in a lake? Image credit: johnwoodcock/Vetta/Getty Images.

A similar two-level hierarchical model is often also needed to model real-world count data. At the lower level, simple Poisson and binomial distributions serve as the building blocks, but their parameters may depend on some underlying (latent) process. In ecology, for instance, we might be interested in variations of fish species in all the lakes in a region. We sample the fish species in each lake to estimate their true abundances, and that could be modeled by a Poisson. But the true abundances will vary from lake to lake. And if we want to see whether, for example, changes in climate or altitude play a role, we need to disentangle such systematic effects from random lake-to-lake variation. The different Poisson rate parameters λ can be modeled as coming from a distribution of rates. Such a hierarchical model also enables us to add supplementary steps in the hierarchy; for instance, we could be interested in many different types of fish, or in modeling the effects of altitude and other environmental factors separately.

Further examples of sampling schemes that are well modeled by mixtures of Poisson variables include applications of high-throughput sequencing, such as RNA-Seq, which we will cover in detail in Chapter 8, and 16S rRNA-Seq data used in microbial ecology.

4.4.3 Gamma distribution: two parameters (shape and scale)

Now we'll explore a distribution that we haven't seen before. The **gamma distribution** is an extension of the (one-parameter) exponential distribution; it has two parameters, which makes it more flexible. It is often useful as a building block for the upper level of a hierarchical model. The gamma distribution is positive valued and continuous. While the density of the exponential has its maximum at zero and then simply decreases toward 0 as the value goes to infinity, the density of the gamma distribution has its maximum at some finite value. Let's explore it by simulation examples. The histograms in Figure 4.19 were generated by the following lines of code.

```
ggplot(tibble(x = rgamma(10000, shape = 2, rate = 1/3)),
   aes(x = x)) + geom_histogram(bins = 100, fill= "purple")
ggplot(tibble(x = rgamma(10000, shape = 10, rate = 3/2)),
   aes(x = x)) + geom_histogram(bins = 100, fill= "purple")
```

Gamma–Poisson mixture: a hierarchical model

We again use a two-level scheme:

Level 1 Generate a set of parameters, $\lambda_1, \lambda_2, \ldots$, from a gamma distribution.
Level 2 Use these to generate a set of Poisson(λ_i) random variables, one for each λ_i.

```
lambda = rgamma(10000, shape = 10, rate = 3/2)
gp = rpois(length(lambda), lambda = lambda)
ggplot(tibble(x = gp), aes(x = x)) +
  geom_histogram(bins = 100, fill= "purple")
```

The resulting values are said to come from a **gamma–Poisson mixture**. Figure 4.20 shows the histogram of gp.

▶ Question **4.18** (a) Are the values generated from a gamma–Poisson mixture continuous or discrete?
(b) What is another name for this distribution? Hint: try the different distributions provided by the goodfit function from the *vcd* package.   ◀

▶ Solution **4.18**

```
library("vcd")
ofit = goodfit(gp, "nbinomial")
plot(ofit, xlab = "")
ofit$par

## $size
## [1] 10.10145
##
## $prob
## [1] 0.6052424
```

In R, and in some other places, the gamma–Poisson distribution travels under the alias **negative binomial distribution**. The two names are synonyms: "negative binomial" alludes to the fact that the formula for its distribution – in Equation (4.7) – bears some formal similarities to that for a binomial distribution; "gamma–Poisson" is more indicative of the distribution's generating mechanism, and that's the term we will use in the rest of the book. It is a discrete distribution, which means that it takes values only on the natural numbers (in contrast to the gamma distribution, which covers the whole positive real axis). Its probability distribution is

$$P(K = k) = \binom{k + a - 1}{k} p^a (1 - p)^k, \qquad (4.7)$$

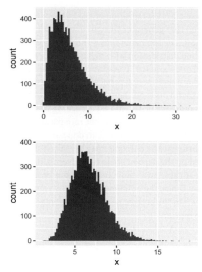

Figure 4.19: Histograms of random samples from gamma distributions. The upper histogram shows a Gamma($2, \frac{1}{3}$), the lower a Gamma($10, \frac{3}{2}$) distribution. The gamma is a flexible two-parameter distribution; the second parameter can be chosen to be the *shape* or its inverse, called the *rate*. See *gamma distribution* on Wikipedia.

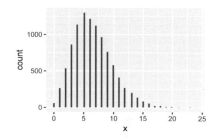

Figure 4.20: Histogram of gp, generated via a gamma–Poisson hierarchical model.

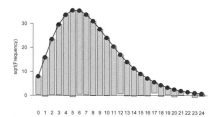

Figure 4.21: Goodness-of-fit plot. The *rootogram* shows the theoretical probabilities of the gamma–Poisson distribution (aka negative binomial) as red dots and the square roots of the observed frequencies as the height of the rectangular bars. The bars all end close to the horizontal axis, which indicates a good fit to the negative binomial distribution.

Figure 4.22: Visualization of the hierarchical model that generates the gamma–Poisson distribution. The top panel shows the density of a gamma distribution with mean 50 (vertical black line) and variance 30. Assume that in one particular experimental replicate, the value 60 is realized. This is our latent variable. The observable outcome is distributed according to the Poisson distribution with that rate parameter, shown in the middle panel. In one particular experiment the outcome may be, say, 55, indicated by the dashed green line. Overall, if we repeat these two subsequent random processes many times, the outcomes will be distributed as shown in the bottom panel – the gamma–Poisson distribution.

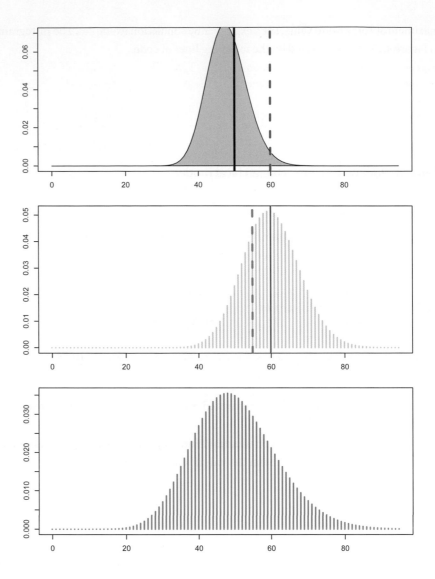

which depends on the two parameters $a \in \mathbb{R}^+$ and $p \in [0, 1]$. Equivalently, the two parameters can be expressed by the mean $\mu = pa/(1 - p)$ and a parameter called the **dispersion** $\alpha = 1/a$. The variance of the distribution depends on these parameters, and is $\mu + \alpha\mu^2$.

▶ Question **4.19** If you are more interested in analytical derivations than illustrative simulations, try writing out the mathematical derivation of the gamma–Poisson probability distribution. ◀

▶ Solution **4.19** Recall that the final distribution is the result of a two-step process:

1. Generate a Gamma(a, b)-distributed number, call it x, from the density

$$f_\Gamma(x, a, b) = \frac{b^a}{\Gamma(a)}\, x^{a-1}\, e^{-bx}, \tag{4.8}$$

where Γ is the so-called Γ-function,[11] $\Gamma(a) = \int_0^\infty x^{a-1}\, e^{-x}\, \mathrm{d}x$.

[11] Not to be confused with the gamma distribution, even though there is this incidental relation.

2. Generate a number k from the Poisson distribution with rate x. The probability distribution is

$$f_{\text{Pois}}(k, \lambda = x) = \frac{x^k e^{-x}}{k!}.$$

If x only took on a finite set of values, we could solve the problem simply by summing over all the possible cases, each weighted by its probability according to f_Γ. But x is continuous, so we have to write the sum as an integral instead of a discrete sum. We call the distribution of K the marginal. Its probability mass function is

$$P(K = k) = \int_{x=0}^{\infty} f_{\text{Pois}}(k, \lambda = x)\, f_\Gamma(x, a, b)\, dx$$

$$= \int_{x=0}^{\infty} \frac{x^k e^{-x}}{k!} \frac{b^a}{\Gamma(a)} x^{a-1} e^{-bx}\, dx.$$

Collect terms and move terms independent of x outside the integral:

$$P(K = k) = \frac{b^a}{\Gamma(a)\, k!} \int_{x=0}^{\infty} x^{k+a-1} e^{-(b+1)x} dx.$$

Since the gamma density sums to 1, we get $\int_0^{\infty} x^{k+a-1} e^{-(b+1)x} dx - \frac{\Gamma(k+a)}{(b+1)^{k+a}}$.

$$P(K = k) = \frac{\Gamma(k + a)}{\Gamma(a)\Gamma(k + 1)} \frac{b^a}{(b + 1)^a (b + 1)^k} = \binom{k + a - 1}{k} \left(\frac{b}{b + 1}\right)^a \left(1 - \frac{b}{b + 1}\right)^k,$$

where we used the fact that $\Gamma(v + 1) = v!$. This expression is the same as (4.7) for a gamma–Poisson with size parameter a and probability $p = \frac{b}{b+1}$. □

4.4.4 Variance-stabilizing transformations

A key issue we need to control when we analyze experimental data is how much variability there is between repeated measurements of the same underlying true value, i.e., between replicates. How successful we are will determine whether and how well we can see any true differences, i.e., between different conditions. Data that arise through the type of hierarchical models we have studied in this chapter often turn out to have very heterogeneous variances, and this can be a challenge. We will see how in such cases **variance-stabilizing transformations** can help (Anscombe, 1948). Let's start with a series of Poisson variables with rates `lambdas`.

```
lambdas = seq(100, 900, by = 100)
simdat = lapply(lambdas, function(l)
    tibble(y = rpois(n = 40, lambda=l), lambda = l)
  ) %>% bind_rows
library("ggbeeswarm")
ggplot(simdat, aes(x = lambda, y = y)) +
  geom_beeswarm(alpha = 0.6, color = "purple")
ggplot(simdat, aes(x = lambda, y = sqrt(y))) +
  geom_beeswarm(alpha = 0.6, color = "purple")
```

Note how we construct the dataframe (or, more precisely, the *tibble*) `simdat`: the output of the `lapply` loop is a list of *tibbles*, one for each value of `lambdas`. With the pipe operator % > %, we send it to the function `bind_rows` (from the *dplyr* package). The result is a dataframe of all the list elements neatly stacked on top of each other.

Figure 4.23: Poisson-distributed measurement data, with a range of means from 100 to 900. In the left panel the y-axis is proportional to the data; in the right panel it is on a square-root scale. Note how the shapes of the beeswarm clouds change on the left, but not on the right.

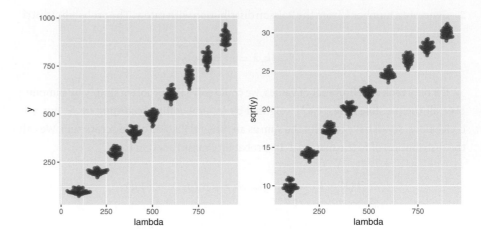

The data that we see in the left-hand panel of Figure 4.23 display what is called **heteroscedasticity**: the standard deviations (or, equivalently, the variance) of our data are different in different regions of our data space. In particular, they increase along the x-axis, with the mean. For the Poisson distribution, we indeed know that the standard deviation is the square root of the mean; for other types of data, there may be other dependencies. The changing variance can be a problem if we want to apply subsequent analysis techniques (for instance, regression or a statistical test) that assume the variances are the same. In Figure 4.23, the number of replicates going into each beeswarm, 40, is quite large. With fewer replicates, heteroscedasticity may be harder to see, even though it is there. However, as we see in the right-hand panel of Figure 4.23, if we apply the square-root transformation to the y-variables, then the transformed variables will have approximately the same variance. In the following code, we use the transformation $y \mapsto 2\sqrt{y}$, which yields variance approximately equal to 1.

```
summarise(group_by(simdat, lambda), sd(y), sd(2*sqrt(y)))
## # A tibble: 9 x 3
##   lambda `sd(y)` `sd(2 * sqrt(y))`
##    <dbl>   <dbl>            <dbl>
## 1    100    11.3             1.13
## 2    200    11.0             0.777
## 3    300    18.3             1.05
## 4    400    19.2             0.957
## 5    500    21.6             0.982
## 6    600    22.7             0.922
## 7    700    30.8             1.17
## 8    800    28.9             1.03
## 9    900    32.2             1.07
```

▶ Question **4.20** Repeat the computation in the code chunk above for a version of `simdat` with a number of replicates larger than 40.   ◀

Another example, now using the gamma–Poisson distribution, is shown in Figure 4.24. We generate gamma–Poisson variables u and plot the 95% confidence intervals around the mean.[12]

[12]To catch a greater range of values for the mean value mu without creating too dense a sequence, we use a geometric series: $\mu_{i+1} = 2\mu_i$.

```
muvalues = 2^seq(0, 10, by = 1)
simgp = lapply(muvalues, function(mu) {
 u = rnbinom(n = 1e4, mu = mu, size = 4)
 tibble(mean = mean(u), sd = sd(u),
        lower = quantile(u, 0.025),
        upper = quantile(u, 0.975),
        mu = mu)
 } ) %>% bind_rows
head(as.data.frame(simgp), 2)
## mean      sd lower upper mu
## 1 0.9995 1.121974    0     4  1
## 2 1.9895 1.725598    0     6  2
ggplot(simgp, aes(x = mu, y = mean, ymin = lower, ymax = upper)) +
 geom_point() + geom_errorbar()
```

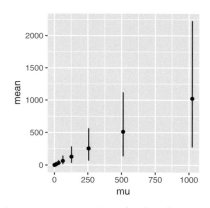

Figure 4.24: Gamma–Poisson-distributed measurement data for a range of μ from 1 to 1024.

▶ Question **4.21** How can we find a transformation for these data that stabilizes the variance, similar to the square-root function for the Poisson-distributed data?   ◀

▶ Solution **4.21** If we divide the values that correspond to `mu[1]` (and are centered around `simgp$mean[1]`) by their standard deviation `simgp$sd[1]`, the values that correspond to `mu[2]` (and are centered around `simgp$mean[2]`) by their standard deviation `simgp$sd[2]`, and so on, then the resulting values will have, by construction, a standard deviation (and thus variance) of 1. And rather than defining 11 separate transformations, we can achieve our goal by defining one single piecewise-linear *and* continuous function that has the appropriate slopes at the appropriate values.   □

```
simgp = mutate(simgp,
  slopes = 1 / sd,
  trsf   = cumsum(slopes * mean))
ggplot(simgp, aes(x = mean, y = trsf)) +
  geom_point() + geom_line() + xlab("")
```

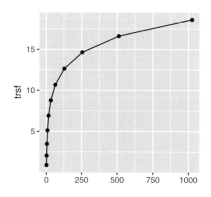

Figure 4.25: Piecewise-linear function that stabilizes the variance of the data in Figure 4.24.

We see in Figure 4.25 that this function has some resemblance to a square-root function, in particular at its lower end. At the upper end, it seems to look more like a logarithm. The more mathematically inclined will see that an elegant extension of these numerical calcuations can be done through a little calculus known as the **delta method**, as follows.

[13] That's not a very strong assumption. Pretty much any function that we might consider reasonable here is differentiable.

Call our transformation function g, and assume it's differentiable.[13] Also call our random variables X_i, with means μ_i and variances v_i, and we assume that v_i and μ_i are related by a functional relationship $v_i = v(\mu_i)$. Then, for values of X_i in the neighborhood of its mean μ_i,

$$g(X_i) = g(\mu_i) + g'(\mu_i)(X_i - \mu_i) + \cdots , \tag{4.9}$$

where the dots stand for higher order terms that we can neglect. The variances of the transformed values are then

$$\text{var}(g(X_i)) \simeq g'(\mu_i)^2 \, \text{var}(X_i) = g'(\mu_i)^2 \, v(\mu_i), \tag{4.10}$$

where we have used the rules $\text{var}(X - c) = \text{var}(X)$ and $\text{var}(cX) = c^2 \, \text{var}(X)$ that hold whenever c is a constant number. Requiring that this be constant leads to the differential equation

$$g'(x) = \frac{1}{\sqrt{v(x)}}. \tag{4.11}$$

For any given mean–variance relationship $v(\mu)$, we can solve (4.11) for the function g. Let's check for some simple cases:

- If $v(\mu) = \mu$ (Poisson), we recover $g(x) = \sqrt{x}$, the square-root transformation.
- If $v(\mu) = c\,\mu^2$, solving the differential equation (4.11) gives $g(x) = \log(x)$. This explains why the logarithm transformation is so popular in data analysis applications: it acts as a variance-stabilizing transformation whenever the data have a constant coefficient of variation, that is, when the standard deviation is proportional to the mean.

▶ Question **4.22** What is the variance-stabilizing transformation associated with $v(\mu) = \mu + c\,\mu^2$? ◀

4.5   Summary of this chapter

We have given motivating examples and ways of using mixtures to model biological data. We have seen how the EM algorithm is an interesting example of solving a difficult optimization problem by iteratively pretending we know one part of the solution to compute the other part, then alternating to pretend the other component is known and computing the first part, and so on, until convergence.

Finite-mixture models We have seen how to model mixtures of two or more normal distributions with different means and variances. We have seen how to decompose a given sample of data from such a mixture, even without knowing the latent variable, using the EM algorithm. The EM approach requires that we know the parametric form of the distributions and the number of components.

Common infinite-mixture models Infinite-mixture models are good for constructing new distributions (such as the gamma–Poisson and the Laplace) out of more basic ones (such as binomial, normal, Poisson). Common examples are:

- mixtures of normals (often with a hierarchical model on the means and the variances);
- **beta–binomial** mixtures – where the probability p in the binomial is generated according to a beta(a, b) distribution;
- **gamma–Poisson** for read counts; and
- **gamma–exponential** for PCR.

Applications Mixture models are useful whenever there are several layers of experimental **variability**. For instance, at the lowest layer, our measurement precision may be limited by basic physical detection limits, and these may be modeled by a Poisson distribution in the case of a counting-based assay or a normal distribution in the case of the continuous measurement. On top of these may be one or more layers of instrument-to-instrument variation, variation in the reagents, operator variation, etc. Take PCR for instance: the efficiency of a cycle of PCR is not exactly two, but slightly below, but this bias might vary between different sessions or batches of the experiment depending on slight variations in protocols, timings, temperatures, operators.

Mixture models reflect the case that there are often heterogeneous amounts of variability (variances) in the data. In such situations, suitable data transformations, i.e., variance-stabilizing transformations, tend to be useful before subsequent analysis, or before visualization. We'll study in depth an example for RNA-Seq in Chapter 8; this also proves useful in the normalization of next-generation reads in microbial ecology (McMurdie and Holmes, 2014).

Another important application of mixture modeling is the two-component model in multiple testing – we will come back to this in Chapter 6.

The ECDF and bootstrapping   We saw that by using the observed sample as a mixture, we could generate many simulated samples that inform us about the sampling distribution of an estimate. This method is called the bootstrap, and we will return to it several times as it provides a way of evaluating estimates even when an analytic formula is not available (we say it is nonparametric).

Relation between mixture models and clustering   We will see in the next chapter how we can try to tease out mixture components and assign a group membership to each (or most) of the observations even without making explicit assumptions about the distributions: this is called *clustering*.

4.6   Further reading

A useful book-long treatment of finite-mixture models is by McLachlan and Peel (2004); for the EM algorithm, see also the book by McLachlan and Krishnan (2007). A recent book that presents all EM-type algorithms within the Majorize–Minimization (MM) framework is by Lange (2016).

There are, in fact, mathematical reasons why many natural phenomena can be seen as mixtures; this occurs when the observed events are exchangeable (the order in which they occur doesn't matter). The theory underlying this is quite mathematical, and a good way to start is to look at the Wikipedia entry and the paper by Diaconis and Freedman (1980).

We use mixtures for high-throughput data. You will see examples in Chapters 8 and 11.

The bootstrap can be used in many situations and is a very useful tool to know about. A friendly treatment is given in Efron and Tibshirani (1994).

A historically interesting paper is the original article on variance stabilization by Anscombe (1948), who proposed ways of making variance-stabilizing transformations for Poisson and gamma–Poisson random variables. Variance stabilization is explained using the delta method in many standard texts on theoretical statistics, e.g., those by Rice (2006, Chapter 6) and Kéry and Royle (2015, page 35).

Kéry and Royle (2015) provide a nice exploration of using R to build hierarchical models for abundance estimation in niche and spatial ecology.

4.7 Exercises

► **Exercise 4.1 The EM algorithm step by step.** As an example dataset, we use the values in the file `Myst.rds`. As always, it is a good idea to first visualize the data. The histogram is shown in Figure 4.26. We are going to model these data as a mixture of two normal distributions with unknown means and standard deviations. We'll call the two components A and B.

```
yvar = readRDS("../data/Myst.rds")$yvar
ggplot(tibble(yvar), aes(x = yvar)) + geom_histogram(binwidth=0.025)
str(yvar)
## num [1:1800] 0.3038 0.0596 -0.0204 0.1849 0.2842 ...
```

We start by randomly assigning a "probability of membership" to each of the values in `yvar` for each of the groups, A and B. These are numbers between 0 and 1: `pA` represents the probability of coming from mixture component A; the complementary probability is `pB`.

```
pA = runif(length(yvar))
pB = 1 - pA
```

We also need to set up some housekeeping variables: `iter` counts over the iterations of the EM algorithm; `loglik` stores the current log-likelihood; `delta` stores the change in the log-likelihood from the previous iteration to the current one. We also define the parameters `tolerance`, `miniter` and `maxiter` of the algorithm.

```
iter = 0
loglik = -Inf
delta = +Inf
tolerance = 1e-3
miniter = 50; maxiter = 1000
```

Study the code below and answer the following questions:

1. Which lines correspond to the E-step and which to the M-step?
2. What does the M-step do? What does the E-step do?
3. What are the roles of the algorithm arguments `tolerance`, `miniter`, `maxiter`?
4. Why do we need to compute `loglik`?
5. Compare the result of what we are doing here to the output of the `normalmixEM` function from the *mixtools* package.

```
while((delta > tolerance) && (iter <= maxiter) || (iter < miniter)) {
  lambda = mean(pA)
  muA = weighted.mean(yvar, pA)
  muB = weighted.mean(yvar, pB)
  sdA = sqrt(weighted.mean((yvar - muA)^2, pA))
  sdB = sqrt(weighted.mean((yvar - muB)^2, pB))
```

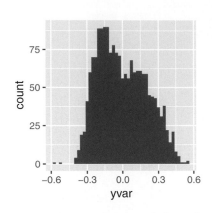

Figure 4.26: Histogram of our example dataset for the EM algorithm.

```
phiA = dnorm(yvar, mean = muA, sd = sdA)
phiB = dnorm(yvar, mean = muB, sd = sdB)
pA   = lambda * phiA
pB   = (1 - lambda) * phiB
ptot = pA + pB
pA   = pA / ptot
pB   = pB / ptot

loglikOld = loglik
loglik = sum(log(pA))
delta = abs(loglikOld - loglik)
iter = iter + 1
}
param = tibble(group = c("A","B"), mean = c(muA,muB), sd = c(sdA,sdB))
param
## # A tibble: 2 x 3
##   group  mean     sd
##   <chr> <dbl>  <dbl>
## 1 A     0.147  0.150
## 2 B    -0.169 0.0983
iter
## [1] 364
```

▶ **Exercise 4.2** Use a QQ-plot to compare the theoretical values of the gamma–Poisson distribution whose parameters are given by the estimates in `ofit$par` in Section 4.4.3 to the data used for the estimation.   ◀

▶ **Exercise 4.3 Mixture modeling examples for regression.** The *FlexMix* package (Grün et al., 2012) enables us to simultaneously cluster and fit regressions to data. The standard M-step `FLXMRglm` of *FlexMix* is an interface to R's generalized linear modeling facilities (the `glm` function). Load the package and an example dataset.

```
library("flexmix")
data("NPreg")
```

a. First, plot the data and try to guess how the points were generated.
b. Fit a two-component mixture model using the commands

```
m1 = flexmix(yn ~ x + I(x^2), data = NPreg, k = 2)
```

c. Look at the estimated parameters of the mixture components and make a truth table that cross-classifies true classes versus cluster memberships. What does the summary of the object `m1` show us?
d. Plot the data again, this time coloring each point according to its estimated class.   ◀

▶ **Exercise 4.4 Other hierarchical noise models.** Find two papers that show the use of other infinite mixtures for modeling molecular biology technological variation.   ◀

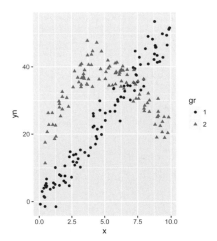

Figure 4.27: Regression example using `flexmix` with the points colored according to their estimated class. You can see that, at the intersection, we have an "identifiability" problem: we cannot distinguish points that belong to the straight line from ones that belong to the parabola.

CHAPTER 5

Clustering

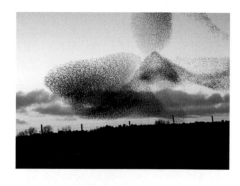

Finding categories of cells, illnesses and organisms and then naming them is a core activity in the natural sciences. In Chapter 4 we saw that some data can be modeled as mixtures from different groups or populations with a clear parametric generative model. We saw how in those examples we could use the EM algorithm to disentangle the components. We are going to extend the idea of unraveling different groups to cases where the clusters do not necessarily have nice elliptical shapes.[1]

[1] Mixture modeling with multivariate normal distributions implies elliptical cluster boundaries.

Clustering takes data (continuous or quasi-continuous) and adds to them a new categorical *group* variable that can often simplify decision making, even if this sometimes comes at the cost of ignoring *intermediate* states. For instance, medical decisions are simplified by replacing possibly complex, high-dimensional diagnostic measurements by simple groupings: a full report of numbers associated with fasting glucose, glycated hemoglobin and plasma glucose two hours after intake is replaced by assigning the patient to a diabetes mellitus "group".

In this chapter we will study how to find meaningful clusters or groups in both low-dimensional and high-dimensional *nonparametric* settings. However, there is a caveat: clustering algorithms are designed to find clusters, so they *will find* clusters even where there are none.[2] Cluster *validation* is therefore an essential component of our process, especially if there is no prior domain knowledge that supports the existence of clusters.

[2] This is reminiscent of humans: we like to see patterns – even in randomness.

5.1 Goals for this chapter

In this chapter we will:

- Study the different types of data that can be beneficially clustered.
- See measures of (dis)similarity and distances that help us define clusters.
- Uncover hidden or latent clustering by partitioning the data into *tight* sets.
- Use clustering when given biomarkers on each of hundreds of thousands cells. We'll see that, for instance, immune cells can be naturally grouped into tight subpopulations.

- Run nonparametric algorithms such as k-means and k-medoids on real single-cell data.
- Experiment with recursive approaches to clustering that combine observations and groups into a hierarchy of sets; these methods are known as hierarchical clustering.
- Study how to validate clusters by using resampling-based bootstrap approaches that we will demonstrate on some single-cell data.

5.2   What are the data and why do we cluster them?

5.2.1   Clustering can sometimes lead to discoveries

John Snow made a map of cholera cases and identified *clusters* of cases. He then collected additional information about the situation of the water pumps. The proximity of dense clusters of cases to the Broadstreet pump pointed to the water as a possible culprit. He collected separate sources of information that enabled him to infer the source of the cholera outbreak.

Now let's look at another map of London, shown in Figure 5.2. The red dots mark locations that were bombed during World War II. Many theories were put forward during the war by analytical teams. They attempted to find a rational explanation for the bombing patterns (proximity to utility plants, arsenals, . . .). In fact, after the war it was revealed that the bombings were randomly distributed without any attempt to hit particular targets.

Clustering is a useful technique for understanding complex multivariate data; it is an **unsupervised** method.[3] Exploratory techniques show groupings that can be important in interpreting the data.

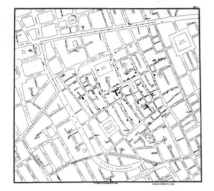

Figure 5.1: John Snow's map of cholera cases: a small barchart at each house indicates a clustering of diagnosed cases. Image credit: Wikicommons.

David Freedman has a wonderful detailed account of all the steps that led to Snow's discovery (Freedman, 1991).

[3] Thus named because all variables have the same **status**; we are not trying to predict or learn the value of one variable (the supervisory response) based on information from explanatory variables.

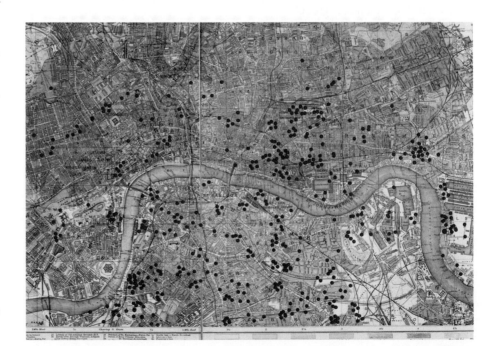

Figure 5.2: Here is a map of the locations of the bombs that were dropped on London on September 7th, 1940, as depicted by the website of the British National Archives. Background map is from nicoolay/E+/Getty Images, reproduced with permission.

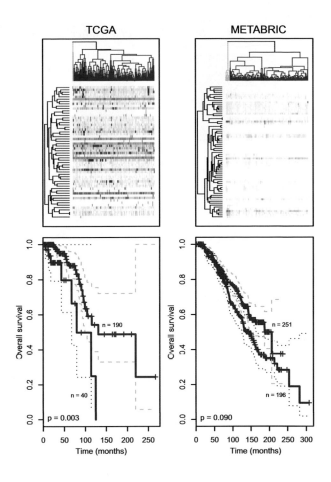

Figure 5.3: The breast cancer samples (shown from The Cancer Genome Atlas (TCGA) and the Molecular Taxonomy of Breast Cancer International Consortium (METABRIC)) can be split into groups using their miRNA expression (Aure et al., 2017). The authors show in the lower plots that the survival times in different groups were different. Thus these clusters were biologically and clinically relevant. The promise of such analyses is that the groups can be used to provide more specific, optimized treatments.

For instance, clustering has enabled researchers to enhance their understanding of cancer biology. Tumors that appeared to be the same, based on their anatomical location and histopathology, fell into multiple clusters based on their molecular signatures, such as gene expression data (Hallett et al., 2012). Eventually, such clusterings might lead to the definition of new, more relevant disease types. Relevance is evidenced, e.g., by the fact that they are associated with different patient outcomes. What we aim to do in this chapter is understand how pictures like Figure 5.3 are constructed and how to interpret them.

In Chapter 4, we studied one technique for uncovering groups, the EM algorithm. The techniques we explore in this chapter are more general and can be applied to more complex data. Many of them are based on distances between pairs of observations (this can be all versus all, or sometimes all versus some), and they make no explicit assumptions that the generative mechanism of the data involves particular families of distributions, such as the normal, gamma–Poisson, etc. There is a proliferation of clustering algorithms in the literature and in the scientific software landscape; this can be intimidating. In fact, it is linked to the diversity of the types of data and the objectives pursued in different domains.

▶ **Task** Look up the *BiocViews Clustering* or the *Cluster view on CRAN* and count the number of packages providing clustering tools. ◀

Figure 5.4: We decompose the choices made in a clustering algorithm according to the steps taken: starting from an observations-by-features rectangular table X, we choose an observations-to-observations distance measure and compute the distance matrix, here schematized by the triangle. The distances are used to construct the clusters. On the left, we schematize agglomerative methods that build a *hierarchical clustering* tree, and on the right, *partitioning methods* that separate the data into subsets. Both types of methods require a choice to be made: the number k of clusters. For partitioning approaches such as k-means, this choice has to be made at the outset; for hierarchical clustering, this can be deferred to the end of the analysis.

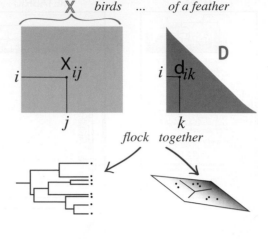

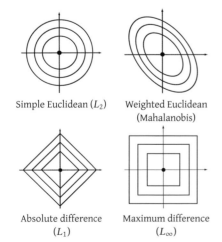

Of a feather. How the distances are measured and similarities between observations defined has a strong impact on the clustering result.

Simple Euclidean (L_2)

Weighted Euclidean (Mahalanobis)

Absolute difference (L_1)

Maximum difference (L_∞)

Figure 5.5: Equal-distance contour plots according to four distances: points on any one curve are all the same distance from the center point.

5.3 How do we measure similarity?

Our first step is to decide what we mean by *similar*. There are multiple ways of comparing birds to define a **distance** between them: for instance, a distance using size and weight will give a different clustering than one using diet or habitat. Once we have chosen the relevant features, we have to decide how we combine differences between the multiple features into a single number. Here is a selection of choices; some of them are illustrated in Figure 5.5.

Euclidean The simple Euclidean (L_2) distance between two points $A = (a_1, \ldots, a_p)$ and $B = (b_1, \ldots, b_p)$ in a p-dimensional space (for the p features) is the square root of the sum of squares of the differences in all p coordinate directions:

$$d(A, B) = \sqrt{(a_1 - b_1)^2 + (a_2 - b_2)^2 + \ldots + (a_p - b_p)^2}.$$

Manhattan The Manhattan, City Block, Taxicab or L_1 distance takes the sum of the *absolute* differences in all coordinates:

$$d(A, B) = |a_1 - b_1| + |a_2 - b_2| + \ldots + |a_p - b_p|.$$

Maximum The maximum of the absolute differences between coordinates is also called the L_∞ distance:

$$d_\infty(A, B) = \max_i |a_i - b_i|.$$

Weighted Euclidean distance This generalization of the ordinary Euclidean distance gives different directions in feature space different weights. We have already encountered one example of a weighted Euclidean distance in Chapter 2, the χ^2 distance. It is used to compare rows in contingency tables, and the weight of each feature is the inverse of the expected value. The *Mahalanobis* distance is another weighted Euclidean distance that takes into account the fact that different features may have different dynamic ranges, and that some features may be positively or negatively correlated with each other. The weights in this case are derived from the covariance matrix of the features. See also Question 5.1.

Minkowski Allowing the exponent to be m instead of 2, as in the Euclidean distance, gives the Minkowski distance:

$$d(A, B) = \left((a_1 - b_1)^m + (a_2 - b_2)^m + \cdots + (a_p - b_p)^m\right)^{1/m}.$$

Edit, Hamming This distance is the simplest way to compare character sequences. It simply counts the number of differences between two character strings. This could be applied to nucleotide or amino acid sequences – although in that case, the different character substitutions are usually associated with different contributions to the distance (to account for physical or evolutionary similarity), and deletions and insertions may also be allowed.

Binary When the two vectors have binary bits as coordinates, we can think of the non-zero elements as "on" and the zero elements as "off". The binary distance is the proportion of features having only one bit on among those features that have at least one bit on.

Jaccard distance Occurrence of traits or features in ecological or mutation data can be translated into presence and absence and encoded as 1s and 0s. In such situations, **co-occurrence** is often more informative than co-absence. For instance, when comparing mutation patterns in HIV, the co-existence of a mutation in two different strains tends to be a more important observation than its co-absence. For this reason, biologists use the **Jaccard index**. Let's call our two observation vectors S and T, f_{11} the number of times a feature co-occurs in S and T, f_{10} (and f_{01}) the number of times a feature occurs in S but not in T (and vice versa), and f_{00} the number of times a feature is co-absent. The Jaccard index is

$$J(S, T) = \frac{f_{11}}{f_{01} + f_{10} + f_{11}} \tag{5.1}$$

(i.e., it ignores f_{00}), and the **Jaccard dissimilarity** is

$$d_J(S, T) = 1 - J(S, T) = \frac{f_{01} + f_{10}}{f_{01} + f_{10} + f_{11}}. \tag{5.2}$$

Correlation-based distance

$$d(A, B) = \sqrt{2(1 - \text{cor}(A, B))}.$$

▶ Question **5.1** Which of the two cluster centers in Figure 5.6 is the red point closest to? ◀

▶ Solution **5.1** A naive answer would use the Euclidean metric and decide that the point is closer to the left cluster. However, as we see that the features have different ranges and correlations, and that these even differ between the two clusters, it makes sense to use cluster-specific Mahalanobis distances. The figure shows contour lines for both clusters. These were obtained from a density estimate; the Mahalanobis distance approximates these contours with ellipses. The distance between the red point and each of the cluster centers corresponds to the number of contour lines crossed. We see that, as the group on the right is more spread out, the red point is in fact closer to it. □

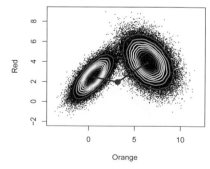

Figure 5.6: An example of the use of Mahalanobis distances to measure the distance of a new data point (red) from two cluster centers.

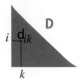

Figure 5.7: The lower triangle of distances can be computed by any of a hundred different functions in various R packages (vegdist in *vegan*, daisy in *cluster*, genetic_distance in *gstudio*, dist.dna in *ape*, Dist in *amap*, distance in *ecodist*, dist.multiPhylo in *distory*, shortestPath in *gdistance*, dudi.dist and dist.genet in *ade4*).

5.3.1   Computations related to distances in R

The dist function in R is designed to use less space than the full n^2 positions a complete $n{\times}n$ distance matrix between n objects would require. The function computes one of six choices of distance (euclidean, maximum, manhattan, canberra, binary, minkowski) and outputs a vector of values sufficient to reconstruct the complete distance matrix. The function returns a special object of class dist that encodes the relevant vector of size $n \times (n-1)/2$. Here is the output for a 3×3 matrix.

```
mx  = c(0, 0, 0, 1, 1, 1)
my  = c(1, 0, 1, 1, 0, 1)
mz  = c(1, 1, 1, 0, 1, 1)
mat = rbind(mx, my, mz)
dist(mat)

##           mx        my
## my 1.732051
## mz 2.000000 1.732051

dist(mat, method = "binary")

##           mx        my
## my 0.6000000
## mz 0.6666667 0.5000000
```

In order to access a particular distance (for example, the distance between observations 1 and 2), one has to turn the dist class object back into a matrix.

```
load("../data/Morder.RData")
sqrt(sum((Morder[1, ] - Morder[2, ])^2))

## [1] 5.593667

as.matrix(dist(Morder))[2, 1]

## [1] 5.593667
```

Let's look at how we would compute the Jaccard distance we defined above between HIV strains.

```
mut = read.csv("../data/HIVmutations.csv")
mut[1:3, 10:16]

##   p32I p33F p34Q p35G p43T p46I p46L
## 1    0    1    0    0    0    0    0
## 2    0    1    0    0    0    1    0
## 3    0    1    0    0    0    0    0
```

▶ Question 5.2 Compare the Jaccard distance (available as the function vegdist in the R package *vegan*) between mutations in the HIV data mut to the correlation-based distance.   ◀

▶ Solution 5.2

```
library("vegan")
mutJ = vegdist(mut, "jaccard")
mutC = sqrt(2 * (1 - cor(t(mut))))
mutJ
```

```
##        1     2     3     4
## 2 0.800
## 3 0.750 0.889
## 4 0.900 0.778 0.846
## 5 1.000 0.800 0.889 0.900
as.dist(mutC)
##        1     2     3     4
## 2 1.19
## 3 1.10 1.30
## 4 1.32 1.13 1.30
## 5 1.45 1.19 1.30 1.32                    □
```

It can also be interesting to compare complex objects that are not traditional vectors or real numbers using dissimilarities or distances. Gower's distance for data of mixed modalities (both categorical factors and continuous variables) can be computed with the `daisy` function. In fact, distances can be defined between any pairs of objects, not just points in $\mathbb{R}^p$ or character sequences. For instance, the `shortest.paths` function from the *igraph* package that we will see in Chapter 10 computes the distance between vertices on a graph, and the function `cophenetic` computes the distance between leaves of a tree, as illustrated in Figure 5.8. We can compute the distance between trees using `dist.multiPhylo` in the *distory* package.

The Jaccard index between graphs can be computed by looking at two graphs built on the same nodes and counting the number of co-occurring edges. This is implemented in the function `similarity` in the *igraph* package. Distances and dissimilarities are also used to compare images, sounds, maps and documents. A distance can usefully encompass domain knowledge and, if carefully chosen, can lead to the solution of many hard problems involving heterogeneous data. Asking yourself what is the *relevant* notion of "closeness" or similarity for your data can provide useful ways of representing them, as we will explore in Chapter 9.

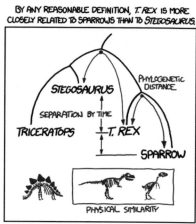

Figure 5.8: An example of computing the cophenetic distance. Image credit: xkcd.com.

5.4 Nonparametric mixture detection

5.4.1 k-methods: k-means, k-medoids and PAM

Partitioning or iterative relocation methods work well in high-dimensional settings, where we cannot[4] easily use probability densities, the EM algorithm and parametric mixture modeling, as we did in Chapter 4. Besides the distance measure, the main choice to be made is the number of clusters k. The PAM (partitioning around medoids; Kaufman and Rousseeuw (2009)) method is as follows:

1. Start from a matrix of p features measured on a set of n observations.
2. Randomly pick k distinct *cluster centers* out of the n observations ("seeds").
3. Assign each of the remaining observations to the group to whose center it is the closest.

[4] This limitation is due to the so-called curse of dimensionality. We will discuss the curse in more detail in Chapter 12.

The centers of the groups are sometimes called medoids, thus the name PAM (partitioning around medoids).

Figure 5.9: An example run of the *k*-means algorithm. The initial randomly chosen centers (black circles) and groups (colors) are shown in the left panel. The group memberships are assigned based on their distance to centers. At each iteration, the group centers are redefined and the points reassigned to the cluster centers.

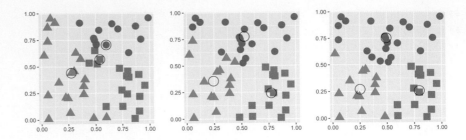

4. For each group, choose a new center from the observations in the group, such that the sum of the distances of group members to the center is minimal; this is called the *medoid*.

5. Repeat Steps 3 and 4 until the groups stabilize.

Each time the algorithm is run, different initial seeds will be picked in Step 2, and in general, this can lead to different final results. A popular implementation is the `pam` function in the package *cluster*.

A slight variation of the method replaces the medoids by the arithmetic means (centers of gravity) of the clusters and is called *k*-means. Whereas in PAM the centers are observations, this is not, in general, the case with *k*-means. The function `kmeans` comes with every installation of R in the *stats* package; an example run is shown in Figure 5.9.

These so-called *k*-methods are the most common off-the-shelf methods for clustering; they work particularly well when the clusters are of comparable size and convex (blob-shaped). On the other hand, if the true clusters are very different in size, the larger ones will tend to be broken up; the same is true for groups that have pronounced non-spherical or non-elliptical shapes.

▶ Question **5.3** The *k*-means algorithm alternates between computing the average point and assigning the points to clusters. How does this alternating, iterative method differ from an EM algorithm?   ◀

▶ Solution **5.3**   In the EM algorithm, each point participates in the computation of the mean of all the groups through a probabilistic weight assigned to it. In the *k*-means method, the points are either attributed to a cluster or not, so each point participates only, and entirely, in the computation of the center of one cluster.   □

5.4.2   Tight clusters with resampling

There are clever schemes that repeat the process many times using different initial centers or resampled datasets. Repeating a clustering procedure multiple times on the same data but with different starting points creates *strong forms*, according to Diday and Brito (1989). Repeatedly subsampling the dataset and applying a clustering method will result in groups of observations that are "almost always" grouped together; these are called *tight clusters* (Tseng and Wong, 2005). The study of strong forms or tight clusters facilitates the choice of the number of clusters. A recent package developed to combine and compare the output from many different clusterings is *clusterExperiment*. Here we give an example from its vignette. Single-cell RNA-Seq experiments provide counts of reads, representing gene transcripts, from individual cells. The single-cell resolution enables scientists to, among other things, follow cell lineage dynamics. Clustering has proved very useful for analyzing such data.

▶ **Question 5.4** Follow the vignette of the package *clusterExperiment*. Call the ensemble clustering function `clusterMany`, using `pam` for the individual clustering efforts. Set the choice of genes to include either the 60, 100 or 150 most variable genes. Plot the clustering results for *k* varying between 4 and 9. What do you notice?   ◀

▶ **Solution 5.4** The output of the following code is shown in Figure 5.10.

```
library("clusterExperiment")
options(getClass.msg = FALSE)
library("scRNAseq")
data("fluidigm")
se = fluidigm[, fluidigm$Coverage_Type == "High"]
normCounts = round(limma::normalizeQuantiles(assay(se)))
assays(se) = list(normalized_counts = normCounts)
ce = clusterMany(se, clusterFunction = "pam", ks = 5:10, run = TRUE,
   isCount = TRUE, dimReduce = c("var"), nVarDims = c(60, 100, 150))
plotClusters(ce, whichClusters = "workflow", axisLine = -1)
```

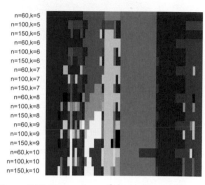

Figure 5.10: Comparison of clustering results (rows) for different numbers of included genes and for varying numbers of clusters, *k*. Each column of the heatmap corresponds to a cell, and the colors represent the cluster assignments.

5.5 Clustering examples: flow cytometry and mass cytometry

Studying measurements on single cells improves both the focus and resolution with which we can analyze cell types and dynamics. Flow cytometry enables the simultaneous measurement of about 10 different cell markers. Mass cytometry expands the collection of measurements to as many as 80 proteins per cell. A particularly promising application of this technology is the study of immune cell dynamics.

You can find reviews of bioinformatics methods for *flow cytometry* in O'Neill et al. (2013) and in the well-kept Wikipedia entry.

5.5.1 Flow cytometry and mass cytometry

At different stages of their development, immune cells express unique combinations of proteins on their surfaces. These protein-markers are called **CDs (clusters of differentiation)** and are collected by flow cytometry (using fluorescence; see Hulett et al., 1969) or mass cytometry (using single-cell atomic mass spectrometry of heavy element reporters; see Bendall et al., 2012). An example of a commonly used CD is CD4; this protein is expressed by helper T cells that are referred to as being "CD4+". Note, however, that some cells express CD4 (thus are CD4+) but are not actually helper T cells. We start by loading some useful Bioconductor packages for cytometry data, *flowCore* and *flowViz*, and read in an exemplary data object `fcsB`.

```
library("flowCore")
library("flowViz")
fcsB = read.FCS("../data/Bendall_2011.fcs")
slotNames(fcsB)

## [1] "exprs"      "parameters"  "description"
```

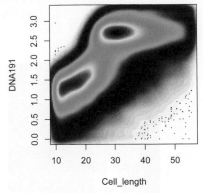

Figure 5.11: Cell measurements that show clear clustering in two dimensions.

Figure 5.11 shows a scatterplot of two of the variables available in the `fcsB` data. (We will see how to make such plots below.) We can see clear bimodality and clustering in these two dimensions.

▶ **Question 5.5** (a) Look at the structure of the `fcsB` object (hint: use the `colnames` function). How many variables were measured?
(b) Subset the data to look at the first few rows (hint: use `exprs(fcsB)`). How many cells were measured?   ◀

5.5.2 Data preprocessing

First we load the table data that reports the mapping between isotopes and markers (antibodies), and then we replace the isotope names in the column names of `fcsB` with the marker names. Changing the column names makes the subsequent analysis and plotting code easier to read.

```
markersB = readr::read_csv("../data/Bendall_2011_markers.csv")
mt = match(markersB$isotope, colnames(fcsB))
stopifnot(!any(is.na(mt)))
colnames(fcsB)[mt] = markersB$marker
```

Now we are ready to generate Figure 5.11.

```
flowPlot(fcsB, plotParameters = colnames(fcsB)[2:3], logy = TRUE)
```

Plotting the data in two dimensions as in Figure 5.11 already shows that the cells can be grouped into subpopulations. Sometimes just one of the markers can be used to define populations on its own; in that case, simple **rectangular gating** is used to separate the populations. For instance, CD4+ cells can be gated by taking the subpopulation with high values for the CD4 marker. Cell clustering can be improved by carefully choosing transformations of the data. The left panel of Figure 5.12 shows a simple one-dimensional histogram before transformation; on the right we see the distribution after transformation. It reveals bimodality and the existence of two cell populations.

Figure 5.12: The left plot shows the histogram of the CD3all variable: the cells are clustered around 0 with a few large values. On the right, we see that after an asinh transformation, the cells cluster and fall into two groups or types.

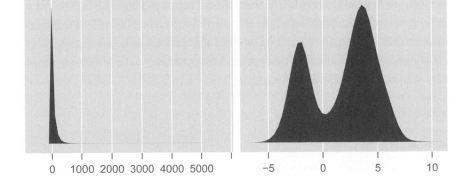

Data transformation: hyperbolic arcsine (asinh).   It is standard to transform both flow and mass cytometry data using one of several special functions. We take the example of the inverse hyperbolic arcsine (asinh):

$$\text{asinh}(x) = \log\left(x + \sqrt{x^2 + 1}\right).$$

From this equation we can see that for large values of x, asinh(x) behaves like the log and is practically equal to $\log(x) + \log(2)$; for small x the function is close to linear in x.

▶ Task   Try running the following code to see the two main regimes of the transformation: small values and large values.

```
v1 = seq(0, 1, length.out = 100)
plot(log(v1), asinh(v1), type = 'l')
plot(v1, asinh(v1), type = 'l')
v3 = seq(30, 3000, length = 100)
plot(log(v3), asinh(v3), type= 'l')                                    ◀
```

This is another example of a variance-stabilizing transformation, also discussed in Chapters 4 and 8. Figure 5.12 is produced by the following code, which uses the *flowCore* package.

```
asinhtrsf = arcsinhTransform(a = 0.1, b = 1)
fcsBT = transform(fcsB,
  transformList(colnames(fcsB)[-c(1, 2, 41)], asinhtrsf))
densityplot( ~'CD3all', fcsB)
densityplot( ~'CD3all', fcsBT)
```

▶ Question 5.6 How many dimensions does the following code use to split the data into two groups using k-means?

```
kf = kmeansFilter("CD3all" = c("Pop1","Pop2"), filterId="myKmFilter")
fres = flowCore::filter(fcsBT, kf)
summary(fres)

## Pop1: 33429 of 91392 events (36.58%)
## Pop2: 57963 of 91392 events (63.42%)

fcsBT1 = flowCore::split(fcsBT, fres, population = "Pop1")
fcsBT2 = flowCore::split(fcsBT, fres, population = "Pop2")       ◀
```

Figure 5.13, generated by the following code, shows a naive projection of the data into the two dimensions spanned by the CD3 and CD56 markers.

```
library("flowPeaks")
fp = flowPeaks(exprs(fcsBT)[, c("CD3all", "CD56")])
plot(fp)
```

When plotting points that densely populate an area, we should try to avoid overplotting. We saw some of the preferred techniques in Chapter 3; here we use contours and shading, produced by the following code.

```
flowPlot(fcsBT, plotParameters = c("CD3all", "CD56"), logy = FALSE)
contour(fcsBT[, c(40, 19)], add = TRUE)
```

The result is Figure 5.14, a more informative version of Figure 5.13.

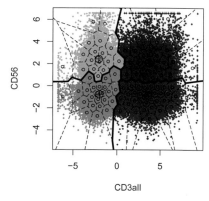

Figure 5.13: After transformation, these cells were clustered using `kmeans`.

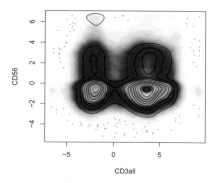

Figure 5.14: Like Figure 5.13, but using contours.

▶ Task Using the more recent Bioconductor package *ggcyto*, plot each patient in a different facet using `ggplot`. Try comparing the output using this approach to what we did above, using the following.

```
library("ggcyto")
library("labeling")
ggcd4cd8=ggcyto(fcsB,aes(x=CD4,y=CD8))
ggcd4=ggcyto(fcsB,aes(x=CD4))
ggcd8=ggcyto(fcsB,aes(x=CD8))
p1=ggcd4+geom_histogram(bins=60)
p1b=ggcd8+geom_histogram(bins=60)
asinhT = arcsinhTransform(a=0,b=1)
transl = transformList(colnames(fcsB)[-c(1,2,41)], asinhT)
fcsBT = transform(fcsB, transl)
p1t=ggcyto(fcsBT,aes(x=CD4))+geom_histogram(bins=90)
p2t=ggcyto(fcsBT,aes(x=CD4,y=CD8))+geom_density2d(colour="black")
p3t=ggcyto(fcsBT,aes(x=CD45RA,y=CD20))+geom_density2d(colour="black")
```
◀

5.5.3 Density-based clustering

Datasets such as flow cytometry, which contain only a few markers and a large number of cells, are amenable to density-based clustering. This method looks for regions of high density separated by sparser regions. It has the advantage of being able to cope with clusters that are not necessarily convex. One implementation of such a method is called **dbscan**. Let's look at an example by running the following code.

```
library("dbscan")
mc5 = exprs(fcsBT)[, c(15,16,19,40,33)]
res5 = dbscan::dbscan(mc5, eps = 0.65, minPts = 30)
mc5df = data.frame(mc5, cluster = as.factor(res5$cluster))
table(mc5df$cluster)

##
##     0     1     2     3     4     5     6     7     8
## 75954  4031  5450  5310   259   257    63    25    43

ggplot(mc5df, aes(x=CD4,    y=CD8,    col=cluster))+geom_density2d()
ggplot(mc5df, aes(x=CD3all, y=CD20, col=cluster))+geom_density2d()
```

The output is shown in Figure 5.15. The overlaps of the clusters in the 2D projections enable us to appreciate the multidimensional nature of the clustering.

▶ Question 5.7 Try increasing the dimension to six by adding one CD marker variable from the input data. Then vary `eps`, and try to find four clusters such that at least two of them have more than 100 points.
Repeat this with seven CD marker variables; what do you notice?   ◀

▶ Solution 5.7 An example with the following six markers:

```
mc6 = exprs(fcsBT)[, c(15, 16, 19, 33, 25, 40)]
res = dbscan::dbscan(mc6, eps = 0.65, minPts = 20)
mc6df = data.frame(mc6, cluster = as.factor(res$cluster))
table(mc6df$cluster)
```

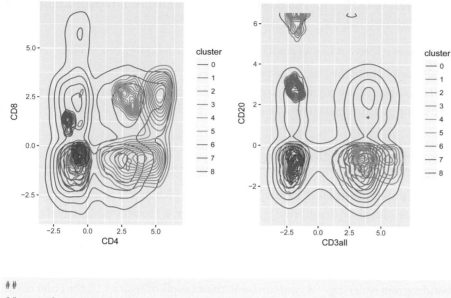

Figure 5.15: These two plots show the results of clustering with dbscan using five markers. Here we show only the projections of the data into the CD4-CD8 and C3all-CD20 planes.

```
##
##      0      1      2      3      4      5      6
## 91068     34     61     20     67    121     21
```

We see that with eps=0.75 it is easier to find large enough clusters than if we take eps=0.65, and with eps=0.55 it is impossible. As we increase the dimensionality to seven, we have to make eps even larger.

```
mc7 = exprs(fcsBT)[, c(11, 15, 16, 19, 25, 33, 40)]
res = dbscan::dbscan(mc7, eps = 0.95, minPts = 20)
mc7df = data.frame(mc7, cluster = as.factor(res$cluster))
table(mc7df$cluster)
```

```
##
##      0      1      2      3      4      5      6      7      8      9
## 90249     21    102    445    158    119     19    224     17     20
##     10
##     18
```

This shows the so-called **curse of dimensionality** in action, of which more in Chapter 12. ☐

How does density-based clustering (dbscan) work?

The dbscan method clusters points in dense regions according to the *density-connectedness* criterion. It looks at small neighborhood spheres of radius ϵ to see if points are connected.

The building block of dbscan is the concept of **density-reachability**: a point q is *directly density-reachable* from a point p if it is not farther away than a given threshold ϵ, and if p is surrounded by sufficiently many points such that one may consider p (and q) to be part of a dense region. We say that q is *density-reachable* from p if there is a sequence of points $p_1, \ldots, p_n$ with $p_1 = p$ and $p_n = q$, so that each p_{i+1} is directly

It is important that the method looks for a high density of points in a neighborhood. Other methods exist that try to define clusters by a void, or "missing points" between clusters. But these are vulnerable to the curse of dimensionality: they can create spurious "voids".

density-reachable from p_i. Two points are density-connected if there is a third point from which each is density-reachable.

A *cluster* is then a subset of points that satisfies the following properties:

1. all points within the cluster are mutually density-connected;
2. if a point is density-connected to any point of the cluster, it is also part of the cluster;
3. a group of points must have at least `MinPts` points for it to be a cluster.

5.6   Hierarchical clustering

Hierarchical clustering is a bottom-up approach, by which similar observations and sub-classes are assembled iteratively. Figure 5.16 shows how Linnæus made nested clusters of organisms according to specific characteristics. Such hierarchical organization has been useful in many fields and goes back to Aristotle, who postulated a *ladder of nature*.

Dendrogram ordering.   As you can see in the example of Figure 5.17, the order of the labels does not matter within sibling pairs. Horizontal distances are usually meaningless, while the vertical distances do encode some information. These properties are important to remember when making interpretations about neighbors that are not monophyletic (i.e., not in the same subtree or clade), but appear as neighbors in the plot (for instance, B and D in the right-hand tree are non-monophyletic neighbors).

Top-down hierarchies.   An alternative, top-down, approach takes all the objects and splits them sequentially according to a chosen criterion. Such so-called **recursive partitioning** methods are often used to make decision trees. They can be useful for prediction (say, survival time, given a medical diagnosis): we are hoping in those instances to split heterogeneous populations into more homogeneous subgroups by partitioning. In this chapter, we concentrate on bottom-up approaches. We will return to partitioning when we talk about supervised learning and classification in Chapter 12.

5.6.1   How to compute (dis)similarities between aggregated clusters?

When creating a hierarchical clustering by aggregation, we will need more than just the distances between all pairs of individual objects; we also need a way to calculate distances between the aggregates. There are different choices of how to define them, based on the object-object distances, and each choice results in a different type of hierarchical clustering.

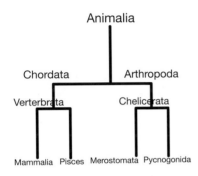

Figure 5.16: A snippet of Linnæus' taxonomy that clusters organisms according to feature similarities.

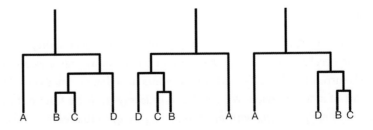

Figure 5.17: Three representations of the *same* hierarchical clustering tree.

Method	Pros	Cons
Single linkage	number of clusters	comblike trees
Complete linkage	compact classes	one obs. can alter groups
Average linkage	similar size and variance	not robust
Centroid	robust to outliers	smaller number of clusters
Ward's	minimizes inertia	classes small if high variability

Table 5.1: Advantages and disadvantages of various distances between aggregates (Chakerian and Holmes, 2012).

A hierarchical clustering algorithm is easy enough to get started, by grouping the most similar observations together. But once an aggregation has occurred, one is required to say what the distance between a newly formed cluster and all other points is computed, or between two clusters.

- The **minimal jump** method, also called the **single linkage** or nearest neighbor method, computes the distance between clusters as the smallest distance between any two points in the two clusters (as shown on the left in Figure 5.18):

$$d_{12} = \min_{i \in C_1, i \in C_2} d_{ij}.$$

This method tends to create clusters that look like contiguous strings of points. The cluster tree often looks like a comb.

- The **maximum jump** (or **complete linkage**) method defines the distance between clusters as the largest distance between any two objects in the two clusters, as represented on the right in Figure 5.18:

$$d_{12} = \max_{i \in C_1, i \in C_2} d_{ij}.$$

- The **average linkage** method is halfway between the two above:

$$d_{12} = \frac{1}{|C_1||C_2|} \sum_{i \in C_1, i \in C_2} d_{ij}.$$

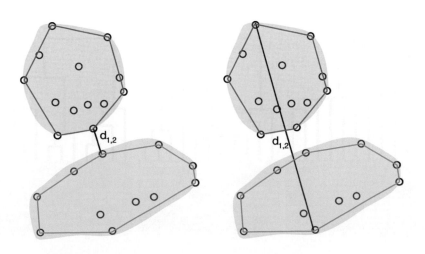

Figure 5.18: Left: In the single linkage method, the distance between groups C_1 and C_2 is defined as the distance between the closest two points from the groups. Right: In the complete linkage method, the distance between groups C_1 and C_2 is defined as the maximum distance between pairs of points from the two groups.

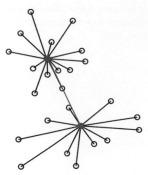

Figure 5.19: Ward's method maximizes the between-groups sum of squares (red edges) while minimizing the sums of squares within groups (black edges).

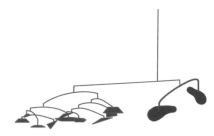

Figure 5.20: Hierarchical clustering output has similar properties to a mobile: the branches can rotate freely from their suspension points.

[5] These will be explained in Chapter 9.

• **Ward's method** takes an analysis of variance approach, where the goal is to minimize the variance within clusters. This method is very efficient; however, it tends to break the clusters up into ones of smaller sizes.

These are the choices we have to make when building hierarchical clustering trees. An advantage of hierarchical clustering compared to the partitioning methods is that it offers a graphical diagnostic of the strength of groupings: the length of the inner edges in the tree.

When we have prior knowledge that the clusters are about the same size, using average linkage or Ward's method of minimizing the within-class variance is the best tactic.

▶ **Question 5.8 Hierarchical clustering for cell populations.** The `Morder` data are gene expression measurements for 156 genes on T cells of three types (naïve, effector, memory) from 10 patients (Holmes et al., 2005). Using the *pheatmap* package, make two simple heatmaps, without dendogram or reordering, for Euclidean and Manhattan distances of these data.   ◀

▶ **Question 5.9** Now look at the differences in orderings in the hierarchical clustering trees with these two distances. What differences are noticeable?   ◀

▶ **Question 5.10** A hierarchical clustering tree is like the Calder mobile in Figure 5.20, which can swing around many internal pivot points, giving many orderings of the tips consistent with a given tree. Look at the tree in Figure 5.22. How many ways are there to order the tip labels and still maintain consistency with that tree?   ◀

It is common to see heatmaps whose rows and/or columns are ordered based on a hierachical clustering tree. Sometimes this makes some clusters look very strong – stronger than what the tree really implies. There are alternative ways of ordering the rows and columns in heatmaps, for instance in the package *NeatMap*, which uses ordination methods[5] to find orderings.

Figure 5.21: Three hierarchical clustering plots made with different agglomeration choices. Note the comb-like structure for single linkage on the left. The average and complete linkage trees only differ by the lengths of their inner branches.

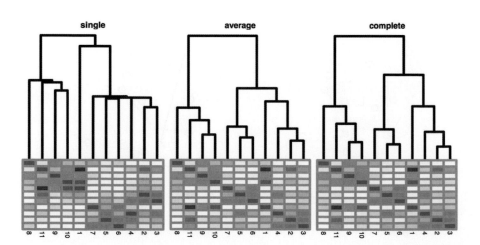

5.7   Validating and choosing the number of clusters

The clustering methods we have described are tailored to deliver good groupings of the data under various constraints. However, keep in mind that clustering methods will always deliver groups, even if there are none. If, in fact, there are no real clusters in the data, a hierarchical clustering tree may show relatively short inner branches, but it is difficult to quantify this. In general, it is important to validate your choice of clusters with more objective criteria.

One criterion to assess the quality of a clustering result is to ask to what extent it maximizes the between-groups differences while keeping the within-groups distances small (maximizing the lengths of red lines and minimizing those of the black lines in Figure 5.19). We formalize this with the within-groups sum of squares (**WSS**) distances:

$$\text{WSS}_k = \sum_{\ell=1}^{k} \sum_{x_i \in C_\ell} d^2(x_i, \bar{x}_\ell). \tag{5.3}$$

Here, k is the number of clusters, C_ℓ is the set of objects in the ℓth cluster and $\bar{x}_\ell$ is the center of mass (the average point) in the ℓth cluster. We state the dependence on k of the WSS in Equation (5.3), as we are interested in comparing this quantity across different values of k for the same cluster algorithm. Stated as it is, however, the WSS is not a sufficient criterion: the smallest value of WSS would simply be obtained by making each point its own cluster. The WSS is a useful building block, but we need more sophisticated ideas than just looking at this number alone.

One idea is to look at WSS_k as a function of k. This will always be a decreasing function, but if there is a pronounced region where it decreases sharply and then flattens out, we call this an *elbow* and might take this as a potential sweet spot for the number of clusters.

▶ Question **5.11 An alternative expression for** WSS_k. Use R to compute the sum of distances between all pairs of points in a cluster and compare it to WSS_k. Can you see how WSS_k can also be written as

$$\text{WSS}_k = \sum_{\ell=1}^{k} \frac{1}{2n_\ell} \sum_{x_i \in C_\ell} \sum_{x_j \in C_\ell} d^2(x_i, x_j), \tag{5.4}$$

where n_ℓ is the size of the ℓth cluster?   ◀

Question 5.11 shows us that the within-clusters sum of squares WSS_k measures both the distances of all points in a cluster to its center, and the average distance between all pairs of points in the cluster.

When looking at the behavior of various indices and statistics that help us decide how many clusters are appropriate for the data, it can be useful to look at cases where we actually know the right answer.

To start, we simulate data coming from four groups. We use the pipe operator (`%>%`) and the `bind_rows` function from *dplyr* to concatenate the four *tibbles* corresponding to each cluster into one big *tibble*.[6]

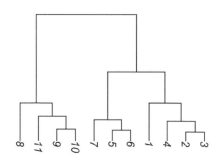

Figure 5.22: This tree can be drawn in many different ways. The ordering of the leaves as it appears here is (8, 11, 9, 10, 7, 5, 6, 1, 4, 2, 3).

[6]The pipe operator passes the value on its left into the function on its right. This can make the flow of data easier to follow in code: `f(x) %>% g(y)` is equivalent to `g(f(x), y)`.

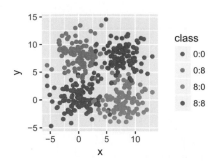

Figure 5.23: The `simdat` data colored by the class labels. Here we know the labels, since we generated the data – usually we do not know them.

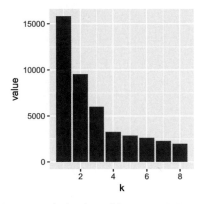

Figure 5.24: The barchart of the WSS statistic as a function of k shows that the last substantial jump is just before $k = 4$. This indicates that the best choice for these data is $k = 4$.

```
library("dplyr")
simdat = lapply(c(0, 8), function(mx) {
  lapply(c(0,8), function(my) {
    tibble(x = rnorm(100, mean = mx, sd = 2),
           y = rnorm(100, mean = my, sd = 2),
           class = paste(mx, my, sep = ":"))
  }) %>% bind_rows
}) %>% bind_rows
simdat
## # A tibble: 400 x 3
##         x       y class
##     <dbl>   <dbl> <chr>
##  1 -2.51    1.96  0:0
##  2  0.802   3.26  0:0
##  3  2.17   -0.562 0:0
##  4  1.76    1.88  0:0
##  5 -0.804  -1.85  0:0
##  6 -0.319  -0.524 0:0
##  7 -1.23   -1.07  0:0
##  8 -2.34    0.286 0:0
##  9  0.709   0.188 0:0
## 10 -1.50   -2.05  0:0
## # ... with 390 more rows
simdatxy = simdat[, c("x", "y")] # without class label
```

```
ggplot(simdat, aes(x = x, y = y, col = class)) + geom_point() +
  coord_fixed()
```

We compute the within-groups sum of squares for the clusters obtained from the k-means method.

```
wss = tibble(k = 1:8, value = NA_real_)
wss$value[1] = sum(scale(simdatxy, scale = FALSE)^2)
for (i in 2:nrow(wss)) {
  km  = kmeans(simdatxy, centers = wss$k[i])
  wss$value[i] = sum(km$withinss)
}
ggplot(wss, aes(x = k, y = value)) + geom_col()
```

▶ Question **5.12** (a) Run the code above several times and compare the `wss` values for different runs. Why are they different?

(b) Create a set of data with uniform instead of normal distributions with the same range and dimensions as `simdat`. Compute the WSS values for for these data. What do you conclude? ◀

▶ Question **5.13** The so-called **Calinski–Harabasz index** uses WSS and **BSS** (between-groups sum of squares). It is inspired by the F-statistic[7] used in analysis of variance:

$$\mathrm{CH}(k) = \frac{\mathrm{BSS}_k}{\mathrm{WSS}_k} \times \frac{N-k}{N-1} \quad \text{where} \quad \mathrm{BSS}_k = \sum_{\ell=1}^{k} n_\ell(\bar{x}_\ell - \bar{x})^2,$$

where $\bar{x}$ is the overall center of mass (average point). Plot the Calinski–Harabasz index for the `simdat` data.   ◄

▶ **Solution 5.13**   Here is the code for generating Figure 5.25.

```
library("fpc")
library("cluster")
CH = tibble(
  k = 2:8,
  value = sapply(k, function(i) {
    p = pam(simdatxy, i)
    calinhara(simdatxy, p$cluster)
  })
)
ggplot(CH, aes(x = k, y = value)) + geom_line() + geom_point() +
  ylab("CH index")
```

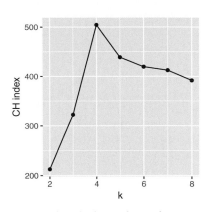

Figure 5.25: The Calinski–Harabasz index, i.e., the ratio of the between- and within-groups variances for different choices of k, computed on the `simdat` data.

5.7.1 Using the gap statistic

Taking the logarithm of the within-groups sum of squares ($\log(\text{WSS}_k)$) and comparing it to averages from simulated data with less structure can be a good way of choosing k. This is the basic idea of the **gap statistic** introduced by Tibshirani et al. (2001). We compute $\log(\text{WSS}_k)$ for a range of values of k, the number of clusters, and compare it to that obtained on reference data of similar dimensions with various possible "non-clustered" distributions. We can use uniformly distributed data as we did above or data simulated with the same covariance structure as our original data.

Algorithm for computing the gap statistic (Tibshirani et al., 2001)

1. Cluster the data with k clusters and compute WSS_k for the various choices of k.
2. Generate B plausible reference datasets using Monte Carlo sampling from a homogeneous distribution, and redo Step 1 above for these new simulated data. This results in B new within-sum-of-squares for simulated data W^*_{kb}, for $b = 1, \ldots, B$.
3. Compute the gap(k) statistic:

$$\text{gap}(k) = \bar{l}_k - \log \text{WSS}_k \quad \text{with} \quad \bar{l}_k = \frac{1}{B}\sum_{b=1}^{B} \log W^*_{kb}.$$

This is a Monte Carlo method that compares the gap statistic $\log(\text{WSS}_k)$ for the observed data to an average over simulations of data with similar structure.

Note that the first term is expected to be bigger than the second one if the clustering is good (i.e., the WSS is smaller); thus the gap statistic will be mostly positive, and we are looking for its highest value.

4. We can use the standard deviation

$$\text{sd}_k^2 = \frac{1}{B-1}\sum_{b=1}^{B}\left(\log(W^*_{kb}) - \bar{l}_k\right)^2$$

to help choose the best k. Several choices are available, for instance choosing the smallest k such that

$$\text{gap}(k) \geqslant \text{gap}(k+1) - s'_{k+1} \quad \text{where } s'_{k+1} = \text{sd}_{k+1}\sqrt{1 + 1/B}.$$

The packages *cluster* and *clusterCrit* provide implementations.

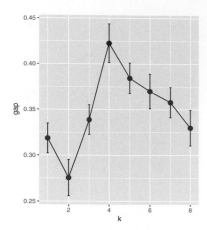

Figure 5.26: The gap statistic; see Question 5.14.

▶ **Question 5.14** Make a function that plots the gap statistic as in Figure 5.26. Show the output for the `simdat` example dataset clustered with the `pam` function. ◀

▶ **Solution 5.14**

```
library("cluster")
library("ggplot2")
pamfun = function(x, k)
  list(cluster = pam(x, k, cluster.only = TRUE))

gss = clusGap(simdatxy, FUN = pamfun, K.max = 8, B = 50,
              verbose = FALSE)
plot_gap = function(x) {
  gstab = data.frame(x$Tab, k = seq_len(nrow(x$Tab)))
  ggplot(gstab, aes(k, gap)) + geom_line() +
    geom_errorbar(aes(ymax = gap + SE.sim,
                      ymin = gap - SE.sim), width=0.1) +
    geom_point(size = 3, col= "red")
}
plot_gap(gss)
```

Let's now use the method on a real example. We load the Hiiragi data that we explored in Chapter 3 (Ohnishi et al., 2014) and see how the cells cluster.

```
library("Hiiragi2013")
data("x")
```

[8] The intention behind this step is to reduce the influence of **technical** (or **batch**) **effects**. Although individually small, when accumulated over all 45,101 features in x, many of which match genes that are weakly or not expressed, without this feature selection step such effects are prone to suppress the biological signal.

We start by choosing the 50 most variable genes (features).[8]

```
selFeats = order(rowVars(exprs(x)), decreasing = TRUE)[1:50]
embmat = t(exprs(x)[selFeats, ])
embgap = clusGap(embmat, FUN = pamfun, K.max = 10, verbose = FALSE)
k1 = maxSE(embgap$Tab[, "gap"], embgap$Tab[, "SE.sim"])
k2 = maxSE(embgap$Tab[, "gap"], embgap$Tab[, "SE.sim"],
        method = "Tibs2001SEmax")
c(k1, k2)

## [1] 9 7
```

The default choice for the number of clusters, `k1`, is the first value of k for which the gap is not larger than the first local maximum minus a standard error s (see the manual page of the `clusGap` function). This gives a number of clusters $k = 9$, whereas the choice recommended by Tibshirani et al. (2001) is the smallest k such that $\text{gap}(k) \geqslant \text{gap}(k+1) - s'_{k+1}$; this gives $k = 7$. Let's plot the gap statistic (Figure 5.27).

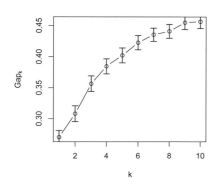

Figure 5.27: The gap statistic for the *Hiiragi2013* data.

```
plot(embgap, main = "")
cl = pamfun(embmat, k = k1)$cluster
table(pData(x)[names(cl), "sampleGroup"], cl)

##                   cl
##                    1  2  3  4  5  6  7  8  9
##   E3.25           23 11  1  1  0  0  0  0  0
##   E3.25 (FGF4-KO)  0  0  1 16  0  0  0  0  0
##   E3.5 (EPI)       2  1  0  0  0  8  0  0  0
##   E3.5 (FGF4-KO)   0  0  8  0  0  0  0  0  0
##   E3.5 (PE)        0  0  0  0  9  2  0  0  0
```

```
##    E4.5 (EPI)           0   0   0   0   0   0   0   4   0
##    E4.5 (FGF4-KO)       0   0   0   0   0   0   0   0   10
##    E4.5 (PE)            0   0   0   0   0   0   4   0   0
```

Above we see the comparison between the clustering that we got from `pamfun` with the sample labels in the annotation of the data.

▶ Question **5.15** How do the results change if you use all the features in `x`, rather than subsetting the top 50 most variable genes?　　　　　　　　　　　　◀

5.7.2   Cluster validation using the bootstrap

We saw the bootstrap principle in Chapter 4: ideally, we would like to use many new samples (sets of data) from the underlying data-generating process, apply our clustering method to each of them, and then see how stable the clusterings are, or how much they change, using an index such as those we used above to compare clusterings. Of course, we don't have these additional samples. So we are, in fact, going to create new datasets simply by taking different random subsamples of the data, looking at the different clusterings we get each time, and comparing them. Tibshirani et al. (2001) recommend using bootstrap resampling to infer the number of clusters using the gap statistic.

We will continue using the *Hiiragi2013* data. Here we follow the investigation of the hypothesis that the inner cell mass (ICM) of the mouse blastocyst on embryonic day 3.5 (E3.5) falls "naturally" into two clusters, corresponding to pluripotent epiblast (EPI) versus primitive endoderm (PE), while the data for embryonic day 3.25 (E3.25) do not yet show this symmetry breaking.

We will not use the true group labels in our clustering and only use them in the final interpretation of the results. We will apply the bootstrap to the two different datasets E3.5 and E3.25 separately. Each step of the bootstrap will generate a clustering of a random subset of the data, and we will need to compare these through a consensus of an ensemble of clusters. There is a useful framework for this in the *clue* package (Hornik, 2005). The function `clusterResampling`, taken from the supplement of

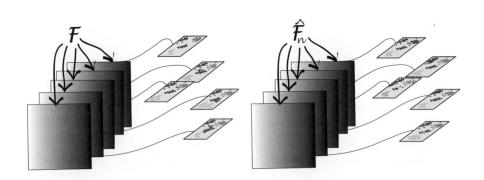

Figure 5.28: Different samples from the same distribution F lead to different clusterings. On the left, we see the true sampling variability. The bootstrap simulates this sampling variability by drawing subsamples using the empirical distribution function $\widehat{F}_n$, as shown on the right.

Ohnishi et al. (2014), implements this approach:

```
clusterResampling = function(x, ngenes = 50, k = 2, B = 250,
                             prob = 0.67) {
  mat = exprs(x)
  ce = cl_ensemble(list = lapply(seq_len(B), function(b) {
    selSamps = sample(ncol(mat), size = round(prob * ncol(mat)),
                      replace = FALSE)
    submat = mat[, selSamps, drop = FALSE]
    sel = order(rowVars(submat), decreasing = TRUE)[seq_len(ngenes)]
    submat = submat[sel,, drop = FALSE]
    pamres = pam(t(submat), k = k)
    pred = cl_predict(pamres, t(mat[sel, ]), "memberships")
    as.cl_partition(pred)
  }))
  cons = cl_consensus(ce)
  ag = sapply(ce, cl_agreement, y = cons)
  list(agreements = ag, consensus = cons)
}
```

The function `clusterResampling` performs the following steps:

1. Draw a random subset of the data (the data are either all E3.25 or all E3.5 samples) by selecting 67% of the samples without replacement.
2. Select the top `ngenes` features by overall variance (in the subset).
3. Apply k-means clustering and predict the cluster memberships of the samples that were not in the subset with the `cl_predict` method from the *clue* package, through their proximity to the cluster centers.
4. Repeat Steps 1–3 B times.
5. Apply consensus clustering (`cl_consensus`).
6. For each of the B clusterings, measure the agreement with the consensus through the function (`cl_agreement`). Here, good agreement is indicated by a value of 1, and less agreement by smaller values. If the agreement is generally high, then the clustering into k classes can be considered stable and reproducible; inversely, if it is low, then no stable partition of the samples into k clusters is evident.

As a measure of between-cluster distance for the consensus clustering, the *Euclidean* dissimilarity of the memberships is used, i.e., the square root of the minimal sum of the squared differences of u and all column permutations of v, where u and v are the cluster membership matrices. As an agreement measure for Step 6, the quantity $1 - d/m$ is used, where d is the Euclidean dissimilarity and m is an upper bound for the maximal Euclidean dissimilarity.

```
iswt = (x$genotype == "WT")
cr1 = clusterResampling(x[, x$Embryonic.day == "E3.25" & iswt])
cr2 = clusterResampling(x[, x$Embryonic.day == "E3.5"  & iswt])
```

The results are shown in Figure 5.29. They confirm the hypothesis that the E3.5 data fall into two clusters, whereas the E3.25 data do not.

```
ag1 = tibble(agreements = cr1$agreements, day = "E3.25")
ag2 = tibble(agreements = cr2$agreements, day = "E3.5")
```

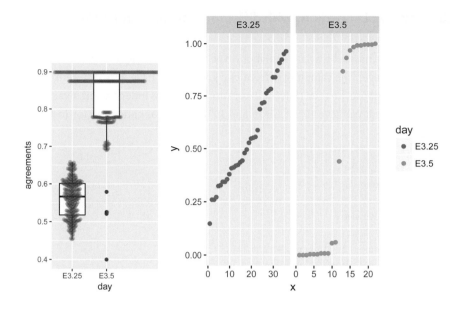

Figure 5.29: Cluster stability analysis with E3.25 and E3.5 samples. Left: Beeswarm plots of the cluster agreements with the consensus, for the B clusterings; 1 indicates perfect agreement, lower values indicate lower degrees of agreement. Right: Membership probabilities of the consensus clustering. For E3.25, the probabilities are diffuse, indicating that the individual clusterings often disagree, whereas for E3.5, the distribution is bimodal, with only one ambiguous sample.

```
ggplot(bind_rows(ag1, ag2), aes(x = day, y = agreements)) +
  geom_boxplot() +
  ggbeeswarm::geom_beeswarm(cex = 1.5, col = "#0000ff40")
```

```
mem1 = tibble(y = sort(cl_membership(cr1$consensus)[, 1]),
              x = seq(along = y), day = "E3.25")
mem2 = tibble(y = sort(cl_membership(cr2$consensus)[, 1]),
              x = seq(along = y), day = "E3.5")
ggplot(bind_rows(mem1, mem2), aes(x = x, y = y, col = day)) +
  geom_point() + facet_grid(~ day, scales = "free_x")
```

Computational and memory issues

It is important to remember that the computation of all-versus-all distances of n objects is an $O(n^2)$ operation (in time and memory). Classic hierarchical clustering approaches (such as `hclust` in the *stats* package) are even $O(n^3)$ in time. For large n, this may become impractical.[9] We can avoid the complete computation of the all-versus-all distance matrix. For instance, k-means has the advantage of only requiring $O(n)$ computations, since it only keeps track of the distances between each object and the cluster centers, whose number remains the same even if n increases.

Fast implementations such as *fastclust* (Müllner, 2013) and *dbscan* have been carefully optimized to deal with large numbers of observations.

5.8   Clustering as a means for denoising

Consider a set of measurements that reflect some underlying true values (say, species represented by DNA sequences from their genomes) but have been degraded by technical **noise**. Clustering can be used to remove such noise.

Computational complexity. An algorithm is said to be $O(n^k)$ if, as n gets larger, the resource consumption (CPU time or memory) grows proportionally to n^k. There may be other (sometimes considerable) baseline costs, or costs that grow proportionally to lower powers of n, but these always become negligible compared to the leading term as $n \to \infty$.

[9] For example, the distance matrix for one million objects, stored as 8-byte floating point numbers, would take up about 4 terabytes, and an `hclust`-like algorithm would run 30 years even under the optimistic assumption that each of the iterations only takes a nanosecond.

5.8.1   Noisy observations with different baseline frequencies

Suppose that we have a bivariate distribution of observations made with the same error variances. However, the sampling is from two groups that have very different baseline frequencies. Suppose, further, that the errors are continuous independent bivariate normally distributed. We have 10^3 of `seq1` and 10^5 of `seq2`, as generated for instance by the code:

```r
library("mixtools")
library("ggplot2")
seq1 = rmvnorm(n = 1e3, mu = -c(1, 1), sigma = 0.5 * diag(c(1, 1)))
seq2 = rmvnorm(n = 1e5, mu =  c(1, 1), sigma = 0.5 * diag(c(1, 1)))
twogr = data.frame(
  rbind(seq1, seq2),
  seq = factor(c(rep(1, nrow(seq1)),
                 rep(2, nrow(seq2))))
)
colnames(twogr)[1:2] = c("x", "y")
ggplot(twogr, aes(x = x, y = y, colour = seq, fill = seq)) +
  geom_hex(alpha = 0.5, bins = 50) + coord_fixed()
```

The observed values would look as in Figure 5.30.

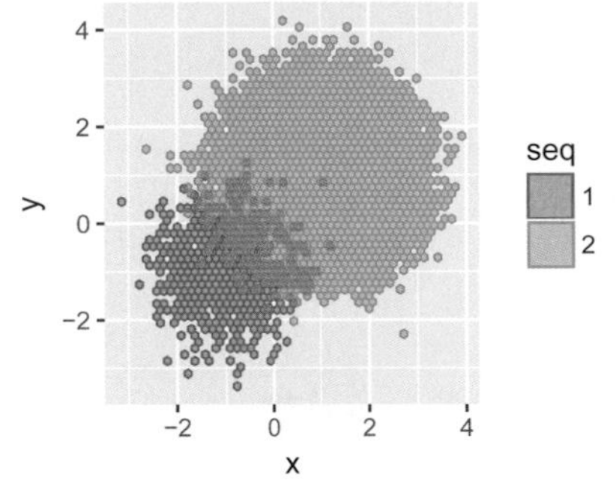

▶ **Question 5.16** Take the data `seq1` and `seq2` and cluster them into two groups according to distance from group center. Do you think the results would depend on the frequencies of each of the two sequence types?   ◀

▶ **Solution 5.16** Such an approach, often used in taxonomic clustering, also called **OTU** (**operational taxonomic unit**) clustering, is suboptimal (Caporaso et al., 2010; Schloss et al., 2009).

The methods based solely on similarities suffer from the **biases** inherent in the **representativeness** heuristic. Let's make a brief digression into the world of cognitive psychology that helps explain how our natural inclination to use only representativeness and a distance-based heuristic in clustering and taxonomic assignment can lead to biased results.

In the 1970s, Tversky and Kahneman (1975) pointed out that we generally assign groups by looking at the most similar *representatives*. In clustering and in group assignments, that would mean assigning a new sequence to the group according to the distance to its center. In fact, this is equivalent to taking balls with the same radius regardless of the differences in prevalence of the different groups. This psychological error was first discussed in an important *Science* paper that covers many different heuristics and biases (Tversky and Kahneman, 1974).   □

▶ **Task** Simulate `n=2000` binary variables of length `len=200` that indicate the quality of n sequencing reads of length `len`. For simplicity, let us assume that sequencing errors occur independently and uniformly with probability `perr=0.001`. That is, we only care whether a base was called correctly (`TRUE`) or not (`FALSE`).

Figure 5.30: Although both groups have noise distributions with the same variances, the apparent radii of the groups are very different. The 10^5 instances in `seq2` have many more opportunities for errors than what we see in `seq1`, of which there are only 10^3. Thus we see that frequencies are important in clustering the data.

See Kahneman (2011) for a book-length treatment of our natural heuristics and the ways in which they can mislead us when we make probability calculations (we recommend especially Chapters 14 and 15).

```
n    = 2000
len  = 200
perr = 0.001
seqs = matrix(runif(n * len) >= perr, nrow = n, ncol = len)
```

Now, compute all pairwise distances between reads.

```
dists = as.matrix(dist(seqs, method = "manhattan"))
```

For various values of number of reads k (from 2 to n), the maximum distance within this set of reads is computed by the code below and shown in Figure 5.31.

```
library("tibble")
dfseqs = tibble(
  k = 10 ^ seq(log10(2), log10(n), length.out = 20),
  diameter = vapply(k, function(i) {
    s = sample(n, i)
    max(dists[s, s])
    }, numeric(1)))
ggplot(dfseqs, aes(x = k, y = diameter)) + geom_point()+geom_smooth()
```

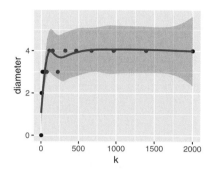

Figure 5.31: The diameter of a set of sequences as a function of the number of sequences.

We will now improve the 16SrRNA-read clustering using a denoising mechanism that incorporates error probabilities.

5.8.2 Denoising 16S rRNA sequences

What are the data?   In the bacterial 16SrRNA gene there are so-called *variable regions* that are taxa-specific. These provide fingerprints that enable *taxon* identification.[10] The raw data are FASTQ-files with quality scored sequences of PCR-amplified DNA regions.[11] We use an iterative alternating approach[12] to build a probabilistic noise model from the data. We call this a *de novo* method, because we use clustering, and we use the cluster centers as our denoised sequence variants (aka amplicon sequence variants, ASVs; see Callahan et al., 2017). After finding all the denoised variants, we create contingency tables of their counts across the different samples. We will show in Chapter 10 how these tables can be used to infer properties of the underlying bacterial communities using networks and graphs.

[10] Calling different groups of bacteria *taxa* rather than *species* highlights the approximate nature of the concept, as the notion of species is more fluid in bacteria than, say, in animals.

[11] See *FASTQ format* on Wikipedia.

[12] Similar to the EM algorithm we saw in Chapter 4.

In order to improve data quality, we often have to start with the raw data and model all the sources of variation carefully. We can think of this as an example of *cooking from scratch* (see the gruesome details in Callahan et al., 2016a, and Exercise 5.5).

▶ **Question 5.17** Suppose that we have two sequences of length 200 (seq1 and seq2) present in our sample at very different abundances. We are told that technological sequencing errors occur as independent Bernoulli(0.0005) random events for each nucleotide.
What is the distribution of the number of errors per sequence?   ◀

▶ **Solution 5.17** Probability theory tells us that the sum of 200 independent Poisson(0.0005) will be Poisson(0.1).

We can also verify this by Monte Carlo simulation.

```
simseq10K = replicate(1e5, sum(rpois(200, 0.0005)))
mean(simseq10K)
## [1] 0.10143
vcd::distplot(simseq10K, "poisson")
```

Figure 5.32 shows us how close the distribution is to being Poisson.

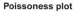

5.8.3   Inferring sequence variants

The DADA method (Divisive Amplicon Denoising Algorithm; Rosen et al., 2012) uses a parameterized model of substitution errors that distinguishes sequencing errors from real biological variation. The model computes the probabilities of base substitutions, such as seeing an A instead of a C. It assumes that these probabilities are independent of the position along the sequence. Because error rates vary substantially between sequencing runs and PCR protocols, the model parameters are estimated from the data themselves using an EM-type approach. A read is classified as noisy or exact given the current parameters, and the noise model parameters are updated accordingly.[13]

The dereplicated sequences are read in, and then divisive denoising and estimation is run with the dada function as in the following code.[14]

```
derepFs = readRDS(file="../data/derepFs.rds")
derepRs = readRDS(file="../data/derepRs.rds")
library("dada2")
ddF = dada(derepFs, err = NULL, selfConsist = TRUE)
ddR = dada(derepRs, err = NULL, selfConsist = TRUE)
```

In order to verify that the error transition rates have been reasonably well estimated, we inspect the fit between the observed error rates (black points) and the fitted error rates (black lines) (Figure 5.33).

```
plotErrors(ddF)
```

Once the errors have been estimated, the algorithm is rerun on the data to find the sequence variants.

```
dadaFs = dada(derepFs, err=ddF[[1]]$err_out, pool = TRUE)
dadaRs = dada(derepRs, err=ddR[[1]]$err_out, pool = TRUE)
```

Note.   The sequence inference function can run in two different modes: independent inference by sample (pool = FALSE), and pooled inference from the sequencing reads combined from all samples. Independent inference has two advantages: as functions of the number of samples, computation time is linear and memory requirements are constant. Pooled inference is more computationally taxing; however, it can improve the detection of **rare variants** that occur just once or twice in an individual sample, but more often across all samples. As this dataset is not particularly large, we performed pooled inference.

Sequence inference removes nearly all substitution and **indel** errors from the data.[15]

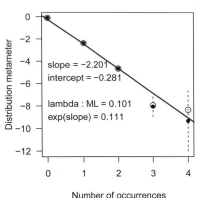

Figure 5.32: `distplot` for the `simseq10K` data.

[13] In the case of a large dataset, the noise model estimation step does not have to be done on the complete set. See `https://benjjneb.github.io/dada2/bigdata.html` for tricks and tools when dealing with large datasets.

[14] F stands for forward strand and R for reverse.

[15] The term *indel* stands for insertion–deletion; when comparing two sequences that differ by a small stretch of characters, it is a matter of viewpoint whether this is an insertion or a deletion, hence the name.

We merge the inferred forward and reverse sequences while removing paired sequences that do not perfectly overlap, as a final control against residual errors.

```
mergers = mergePairs(dadaFs, derepFs, dadaRs, derepRs)
```

We produce a contingency table of counts of ASVs. This is a higher resolution analog of the "OTU table",[16] i.e., a samples-by-features table whose cells contain the number of times each sequence variant was observed in each sample.

[16] Operational taxonomic unit.

```
seqtab.all = makeSequenceTable(mergers[!grepl("Mock",names(mergers))])
```

▶ Question **5.18** Explore the components of the objects `dadaRs` and `mergers`.   ◀

▶ Solution **5.18** `dadaRs` is a list of length 20. Its elements are objects of class *dada* that contain the denoised reads. We will see in Chapter 10 how to align the sequences, assign their taxonomies and combine them with the sample information for downstream analyses.   □

Chimera are sequences that are artificially created during PCR amplification by the melding of two (or, in rare cases, more) of the original sequences. To complete our denoising workflow, we remove them with a call to the function `removeBimeraDenovo`, leaving us with a clean contingency table that we will use later.

```
seqtab = removeBimeraDenovo(seqtab.all)
```

▶ Question **5.19** (a) Why do you think chimera are quite easy to recognize?
(b) What proportion of the reads were chimeric in the `seqtab.all` data?
(c) What proportion of unique sequence variants are chimeric?   ◀

▶ Solution **5.19** Here we observed some sequence variants as chimeric, but these represent only 7% of all reads.   □

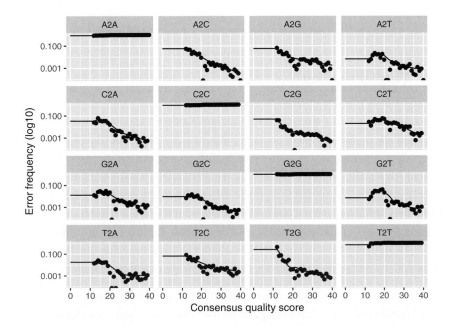

Figure 5.33: Forward transition error rates as provided by `plotErrors(ddF)`. This shows the frequencies of each type of nucleotide transition as a function of quality.

5.9   Summary of this chapter

Of a feather: how to compare observations We saw at the start of the chapter how finding the **right distance** is an essential first step in a clustering analysis; this is a case where the saying *garbage in, garbage out* is in full force. Always choose a distance that is scientifically meaningful and compare output from as many distances as possible; sometimes the same data require different distances when different scientific objectives are pursued.

Two ways of clustering We saw that there are two approaches to clustering:
– iterative partitioning approaches such as k-means and k-medoids (PAM) that alternate between estimating the cluster centers and assigning points to them;
– hierarchical clustering approaches that first agglomerate points, and subsequently the growing clusters, into nested sequences of sets that can be represented by hierarchical clustering *trees*.

Biological examples Clustering is an important tool for finding latent classes in single-cell measurements, especially in immunology and single-cell data analysis. We saw how density-based clustering is useful for lower dimensional data where sparsity is not an issue.

Validating the clusters Clustering algorithms *always* deliver clusters, so we need to be careful when assessing their quality and choosing the number of clusters. These validation steps are performed using visualization tools and repeating the clustering on many resamples of the data. Statistics such as the WSS/BSS or log(WSS) can be calibrated using simulations on data where we understand the group structure. They can provide useful benchmarks for choosing the number of clusters on new data.
Of course, the use of biologically relevant information to inform and confirm the meaning of clusters is always the best validation approach.

Distances and probabilities Finally, distances are not everything. We showed how important it is to take into account baseline frequencies and local densities when clustering. This is essential in cases such as clustering for denoising 16S rRNA sequence reads where the true classes or taxa groups occur at very different frequencies.

5.10   Further reading

For a complete book on *finding groups in data*, see Kaufman and Rousseeuw (2009). The vignette of the *clusterExperiment* package contains a complete workflow for generating clusters using many different techniques, including preliminary dimension reduction (PCA), which we will cover in Chapter 7. There is no consensus on methods for deciding how many clusters are needed to describe data in the absence of contiguous biological information. However, making hierarchical clusters of the *strong forms* is a method that has the advantage of allowing the user to decide how far down to cut the hierarchical tree, being careful not to cut in places where the inner branches are short. See the vignette of *clusterExperiment* for an application to single-cell RNA experimental data.

In analyzing the Hiiragi data, we used cluster probabilities, a concept already mentioned in Chapter 4, where the EM algorithm used them as weights in order to compute expected value statistics. The notion of probabilistic clustering is well developed in the Bayesian nonparametric mixture framework, which enriches the mixture models we covered in Chapter 4 to more general settings. See Dundar et al. (2014) for a real example using this framework for flow cytometry.

Clustering is essential for denoising and assignment of high-throughput sequencing reads to specific strains of bacteria or viruses. In the presence of noise, clustering into groups of *true* strains of very unequal sizes can be challenging. Using the data to create a noise model enables both denoising and cluster assignment concurrently. Denoising algorithms such as those by Rosen et al. (2012) and Callahan et al. (2016b) use an iterative workflow inspired by the EM method (McLachlan and Krishnan, 2007).

5.11 Exercises

▶ Exercise **5.1** We can define the average dissimilarity of a point x_i to a cluster C_k as the average of the distances from x_i to all points in C_k. Let $A(i)$ be the average dissimilarity of all points in the cluster containing x_i. Let $B(i)$ be the lowest average dissimilarity of x_i to any other cluster of which x_i is not a member. The cluster with this lowest average dissimilarity is said to be the **neighboring cluster** of x_i, because it is the next best fit for point x_i. The **silhouette index** is

$$S(i) = \frac{B(i) - A(i)}{\max_i(A(i), B(i))}.$$

a. Compute the silhouette index for the `simdat` data we simulated in Section 5.7.

```
library("cluster")
pam4 = pam(simdatxy, 4)
sil = silhouette(pam4, 4)
plot(sil, col=c("red","green","blue","purple"), main="Silhouette")
```

b. Change the number of clusters k and assess which k gives the best silhouette index.
c. Now repeat this for groups that have uniform (unclustered) data distributions over a whole range of values. ◀

▶ Exercise **5.2**

a. Make a "character" representation of the distance between the 20 locations in the `dune` data from the *vegan* package using the function `symnum`.
b. Make a heatmap plot of these distances. ◀

▶ Exercise **5.3**

a. Load the `spirals` data from the *kernlab* package. Plot the results of using k-means on the data. This should give you something similar to Figure 5.34.
b. You'll notice that the clustering in Figure 5.34 seems unsatisfactory. Show how a different method, such as `specc` or `dbscan`, could cluster `spirals` data more usefully.
c. Repeat the `dbscan` clustering with different parameters. How robust is the number of groups?

Figure 5.34: An example of non-convex clusters. On the left we show the result of k-means clustering with $k = 2$. On the right we have the output from `dbscan`. The colors represent the three clusters found by the algorithm for the settings `eps = 0.16, minPts = 3`.

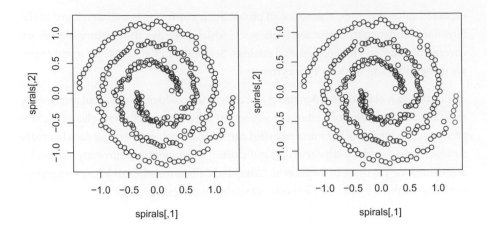

```
data("spirals", package = "kernlab")
res.dbscan = dbscan::dbscan(spirals, eps = 0.16, minPts = 3)
plot(spirals,col=c("blue","red","forestgreen")[res.dbscan$cluster])
```
◄

► **Exercise 5.4** Looking at graphical representations in simple two-dimensional maps can often reveal important clumping patterns. We saw an example of this with the map that enabled Snow to discover the source of the London cholera outbreak. Such clusterings can often indicate important information about hidden variables acting on the observations. Look at a map for breast cancer incidence in the US at: `http://www.huffingtonpost.com/bill-davenhall/post_1663_b_817254.html` (Mandal et al., 2009); the areas of high incidence seem spatially clustered. Can you guess the reason(s) for the clustering and high incidence rates on the West and East coasts and around Chicago?
◄

► **Exercise 5.5 Amplicon bioinformatics: from raw reads to dereplicated sequences.** As a supplementary exercise, we provide the intermediate steps necessary in a full data preprocessing workflow for denoising 16S rRNA sequences. We start by setting the directories and loading the downloaded data.

```
base_dir = "../data"
miseq_path = file.path(base_dir, "MiSeq_SOP")
filt_path = file.path(miseq_path, "filtered")
fnFs = sort(list.files(miseq_path, pattern="_R1_001.fastq"))
fnRs = sort(list.files(miseq_path, pattern="_R2_001.fastq"))
sampleNames = sapply(strsplit(fnFs, "_"), `[`, 1)
if (!file_test("-d", filt_path)) dir.create(filt_path)
filtFs = file.path(filt_path, paste0(sampleNames, "_F_filt.fastq.gz"))
filtRs = file.path(filt_path, paste0(sampleNames, "_R_filt.fastq.gz"))
fnFs = file.path(miseq_path, fnFs)
fnRs = file.path(miseq_path, fnRs)
print(length(fnFs))
## [1] 20
```

The data are highly overlapping Illumina Miseq 2×250 amplicon sequences from the V4 region of the 16S rRNA gene (Kozich et al., 2013). There were originally 360 fecal samples collected longitudinally from 12 mice over their first year of life. These were collected by Schloss et al. (2012) to investigate the development and stabilization of the murine **microbiome**. We selected 20 samples to illustrate how to preprocess the data. We will need to filter out low-quality reads and trim them to a consistent length. While generally recommended **filtering** and trimming parameters serve as a starting point, no two datasets are identical, and therefore it is always worth inspecting the quality of the data before proceeding. We show the sequence quality plots for the two first samples in Figure 5.35. They are generated by

```
plotQualityProfile(fnFs[1:2]) + ggtitle("Forward")
plotQualityProfile(fnRs[1:2]) + ggtitle("Reverse")
```

Note that we also see the background distribution of quality scores at each position in Figure 5.35 as a grayscale heatmap. The dark colors correspond to higher frequencies.

◀

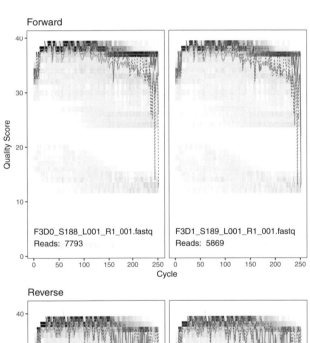
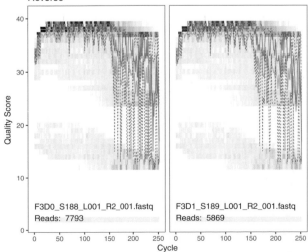

Figure 5.35: Quality scores. The lines show positional summary statistics: green is the mean, orange is the median, and the dashed orange lines are the 25th and 75th quantiles.

▶ Exercise **5.6** Generate similar plots for four randomly selected sets of forward and reverse reads. Compare forward and reverse read qualities; what do you notice?   ◀

▶ Exercise **5.7** Here, the forward reads maintain high quality throughout, while the quality of the reverse reads drops significantly at about position 160. Therefore, we truncate the forward reads at position 240 and trim the first 10 nucleotides, as these positions are of lower quality. The reverse reads are trimmed at position 160. Combine these trimming parameters with standard filtering parameters, and remember to enforce a maximum of two expected errors per read. (Hint: Trim and filter on paired reads jointly; i.e., both reads must pass the filter for the pair to pass. The input arguments should be chosen following the *dada2* vignette carefully. We recommend filtering out any reads with ambiguous nucleotides.)   ◀

CHAPTER 6

Testing

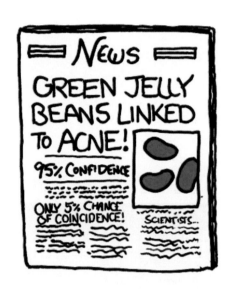

Hypothesis testing is one of the workhorses of science. It is how we can draw conclusions or make decisions based on finite samples of data. For instance, new treatments for a disease are usually approved on the basis of clinical trials that aim to decide whether they have better efficacy compared to the other available options and an acceptable trade-off of side effects. Such trials are expensive and can take a long time. Therefore, the number of patients we can enroll is limited, and we need to base our inference on a limited sample of observed patient responses. The data are noisy, since a patient's response depends not only on the treatment, but on many other factors outside of our control. The sample size needs to be large enough to enable us to make a reliable conclusion. On the other hand, it also must not be too large, so that we do not waste precious resources or time, thereby making drugs more expensive than necessary or denying patients who would benefit from the new drug access to it. The machinery of hypothesis testing was developed largely with such applications in mind, although today it is used much more widely.

In biological data analysis (and in many other fields[1]) we see hypothesis testing applied to screening thousands or millions of possible hypotheses to find the ones that are worth following up. For instance, researchers screen genetic variants for associations with a phenotype, or gene expression levels for associations with disease. Here, "worthwhile" is often interpreted as "statistically significant", although the two concepts are clearly not the same. It is probably fair to say that statistical significance is a necessary condition for making a data-driven decision to find something interesting, but it's clearly not sufficient. In any case, such large-scale association screening is closely related to multiple hypothesis testing.

[1] Detecting credit card fraud, email spam detection,. . .

6.1 Goals for this chapter

In this chapter we will:

- Familiarize ourselves with the statistical machinery of hypothesis testing, its vocabulary, its purpose, and its strengths and limitations.

- Understand what multiple testing means.
- See that multiple testing is not a problem, but rather an opportunity, as it overcomes many of the limitations of single testing.
- Understand the false discovery rate.
- Learn how to make diagnostic plots.
- Use hypothesis weighting to increase the power of our analyses.

6.1.1 Drinking from the firehose

If statistical testing – decision making with uncertainty – seems a hard task when making a single decision, then brace yourself: in genomics, or more generally with "big data", we need to accomplish it not once, but thousands or millions of times. In Chapter 2, we saw the example of epitope detection and the challenges from considering not only one, but several positions. Similarly, in whole genome sequencing, we scan every position in the genome for a difference between the DNA library at hand and a reference (or another library): that's on the order of three billion tests if we are looking at human data! In genetic or chemical compound screening, we test each of the reagents for an effect in the assay compared to a control: that's again tens of thousands, if not millions of tests. In Chapter 8, we will analyze RNA-Seq data for differential expression by applying a hypothesis test to each of the thousands of genes assayed.

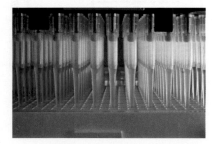

Figure 6.1: High-throughput data in modern biology are being screened for associations with millions of hypothesis tests. Image credit: red_moon_rise/E+/Getty Images.

Yet, in many ways, multiplicity makes the task simpler, not harder. Since we have so much data, and so many tests, we can ask questions like: Are the requirements of the tests actually met by the data? What are the prior probabilities that we should assign to the possible outcomes of the tests? Answers to these questions can be incredibly helpful, and we can address them *because* of the multiplicity. So we should think about it not as a multiple testing "problem", but as an opportunity!

There is a powerful premise in large-scale association screening: we usually expect that most tests will not be rejected. Out of the thousands or millions of tests, we expect that only a small fraction will be interesting. In fact, if that is not the case, if the hits are not rare, then arguably our analysis method – screening each variable separately in turn for association with the outcome – is not suitable for the dataset. We either need better data (a more specific assay) or a different analysis method, e.g., a multivariate model.

So, since we can assume that most of our many null hypotheses are true, we can use the behavior of their test statistics and p-values to empirically understand the null distributions, their correlations, and so on. Rather than having to rely on abstract assumptions, we can check the requirements empirically.

6.1.2 Testing versus classification

Suppose we measured the expression level of a marker gene to decide whether the cells we are studying are from cell type A or B. First, let's consider that we have no prior assumption, and it's equally important to us to get the assignment right no matter whether the true cell type is A or B. This is a *classification* task. We'll cover classification in Chapter 12. In this chapter, we consider the asymmetric case: based on what we already know (we could call this our *prior*), we lean toward calling it an A, and would need strong enough evidence to be convinced otherwise. We can think of this as an application of **Occam's razor**:[2] do not use a complicated explanation if a simpler one does the job. Or maybe the consequences and costs of calling A and B are very different; for instance, A could be healthy and B diseased. In these cases, the machinery of hypothesis testing is right for us.

Formally, there are many similarities between hypothesis testing and classification. In both cases, we aim to use data to choose among several possible decisions. It is even possible to think of hypothesis testing as a special case of classification. However, these two approaches are geared toward different objectives and underlying assumptions, and when you encounter a statistical decision problem, it is good to keep that in mind in your choice of methodology.

6.2   Example: coin tossing

To understand multiple tests, let's first review the mechanics of single **hypothesis testing**. For example, suppose we are flipping a coin to see if it is fair.[3] We flip the coin 100 times and each time record whether it came up heads or tails. So, we have a record that could look something like this:

H H T T H T H T T ...

which we can simulate in R. Let's assume we are flipping a biased coin, so we set `probHead` different from $\frac{1}{2}$.

```
set.seed(0xdada)
numFlips = 100
probHead = 0.6
coinFlips = sample(c("H", "T"), size = numFlips,
  replace = TRUE, prob = c(probHead, 1 - probHead))
head(coinFlips)
## [1] "T" "T" "H" "T" "H" "H"
```

Now, if the coin were fair, we would expect to get heads half the time. Let's see.

```
table(coinFlips)
## coinFlips
##  H  T
## 59 41
```

So that is different from 50/50. Suppose we showed the data to a friend without telling them whether the coin is fair, and their prior assumption, i.e., their null hypothesis, is that coins are, by and large, fair. Would the data be strong enough to make them conclude that this coin isn't fair? They know that random sampling differences are to be expected. To decide, let's look at the *sampling distribution* of our test statistic – the

[2] See also *Occam's razor* on Wikipedia.

[3] We don't look at coin tossing because it's inherently important, but because it is an easy "model system" (just as we use model systems in biology): everything can be calculated easily, and you don't need a lot of domain knowledge to understand what coin tossing is. All the important concepts come up, and we can apply them, only with more additional details, to other applications.

[4] We haven't really defined what we mean be fair – a reasonable definition would be that heads and tails are equally likely, and that the outcome of each coin toss does not depend on the previous ones. For more complex applications, nailing down the most suitable null hypothesis can take some thought.

total number of heads seen in 100 coin tosses – for a fair coin.[4] As we saw in Chapter 1, the number, k, of heads, in n independent tosses of a coin is

$$P(K = k \mid n, p) = \binom{n}{k} p^k (1 - p)^{n-k}, \tag{6.1}$$

where p is the probability of heads (0.5 if we assume a fair coin). We read the left-hand side of the above equation as "the probability that the observed value for K is k, given the values of n and p". Statisticians like to make a difference between all the possible values of a statistic and the one that was observed,[5] and we use the uppercase K for the possible values (so K can be anything between 0 and 100) and the lowercase k for the observed value.

[5] In other words, K is the abstract random variable in our probabilistic model, whereas k is its realization, that is, a specific data point.

We plot Equation (6.1) in Figure 6.2; for good measure, we also mark the observed value `numHeads` with a vertical blue line.

```
library("dplyr")
k = 0:numFlips
numHeads = sum(coinFlips == "H")
binomDensity = tibble(k = k,
    p = dbinom(k, size = numFlips, prob = 0.5))

library("ggplot2")
ggplot(binomDensity) +
  geom_bar(aes(x = k, y = p), stat = "identity") +
  geom_vline(xintercept = numHeads, col = "blue")
```

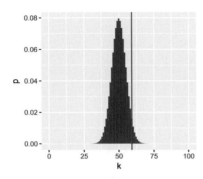

Figure 6.2: The binomial distribution for the parameters $n = 100$ and $p = 0.5$, according to Equation (6.1).

Suppose we didn't know about Equation (6.1). We can still use Monte Carlo simulation to give us something to compare with.

```
numSimulations = 10000
outcome = replicate(numSimulations, {
  coinFlips = sample(c("H", "T"), size = numFlips,
                replace = TRUE, prob = c(0.5, 0.5))
  sum(coinFlips == "H")
})
ggplot(tibble(outcome)) + xlim(0, 100) +
  geom_histogram(aes(x = outcome), binwidth = 1, center = 0) +
  geom_vline(xintercept = numHeads, col = "blue")
```

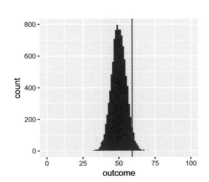

Figure 6.3: An approximation of the binomial distribution from 10^4 simulations (same parameters as Figure 6.2).

[6] More on this in Section 6.3.1.

As expected, the most likely number of heads is 50; that is, half the number of coin flips. But we see that other numbers near 50 are also quite likely. How do we quantify whether the observed value, 59, is among those values that we are likely to see from a fair coin, or whether its deviation from the expected value is already large enough for us to conclude with enough confidence that the coin is biased? We divide the set of all possible k (0 to 100) into two complementary subsets, the **rejection region** and the region of no rejection. Our choice here[6] is to fill up the rejection region with as many k as possible while keeping their total probability, assuming the null hypothesis, below some threshold α (say, 0.05).

```
library("dplyr")
alpha = 0.05
binomDensity = arrange(binomDensity, p) %>%
        mutate(reject = (cumsum(p) <= alpha))

ggplot(binomDensity) +
  geom_bar(aes(x = k, y = p, col = reject), stat = "identity") +
  scale_colour_manual(
    values = c(`TRUE` = "red", `FALSE` = "darkgrey")) +
  geom_vline(xintercept = numHeads, col = "blue") +
  theme(legend.position = "none")
```

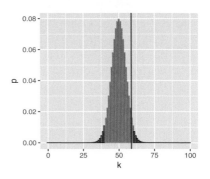

Figure 6.4: As Figure 6.2, with rejection region (red) that has been chosen so that it contains the maximum number of bins whose total area is at most $\alpha = 0.05$.

In the code above, we use the function `arrange` from the *dplyr* package to sort the p-values from lowest to highest, then pass the result to `mutate`, which adds another dataframe column `reject` that is defined by computing the cumulative sum (`cumsum`) of the p-values and thresholding it against `alpha`. The logical vector `reject` therefore marks with `TRUE` a set of `k`s whose total probability is less than `alpha`. These are marked in Figure 6.4, and we can see that our rejection region is not contiguous – it comprises both the very large and the very small values of `k`.

The explicit summation over the probabilities is clumsy: we did it here for pedagogic value. For one-dimensional distributions, R provides functions not only for the densities (e.g., `dbinom`) but also for the cumulative distribution functions (`pbinom`), which are more precise and faster than `cumsum` over the probabilities. These should be used in practice.

▶ Task Do the computations for the rejection region and produce a plot like Figure 6.4 without using `dbinom` and `cumsum`, but using `pbinom` instead.　◀

We see in Figure 6.4 that the observed value, 59, lies in the gray shaded area, so we would *not* reject the null hypothesis of a fair coin from these data at a significance level of $\alpha = 0.05$.

▶ Question **6.1** Does the fact that we don't reject the null hypothesis mean that the coin is fair?　◀

▶ Question **6.2** Would we have a better chance of detecting that the coin is not fair if we did more coin tosses? How many?　◀

▶ Question **6.3** If we repeat the whole procedure and again toss the coin 100 times, might we *then* reject the null hypothesis?　◀

▶ Question **6.4** The rejection region in Figure 6.4 is asymmetric – its left part ends with $k = 40$, while its right part starts with $k = 61$. Why is that? Which other ways of defining the rejection region might be useful?　◀

We have just gone through the steps of a binomial test. In fact, this is such a frequent activity in R that it has been wrapped into a single function, and we can compare its output to our results.

```
binom.test(x = numHeads, n = numFlips, p = 0.5)
##
##   Exact binomial test
##
## data:  numHeads and numFlips
## number of successes = 59, number of trials = 100,
## p-value = 0.08863
## alternative hypothesis: true probability of success
##                         is not equal to 0.5
## 95 percent confidence interval:
##   0.4871442 0.6873800
## sample estimates:
## probability of success
##                   0.59
```

6.3   The five steps of hypothesis testing

Let's summarize the general principles of hypothesis testing:

Null hypothesis: often denoted by H_0.

1. Decide on the effect that you are interested in, design a suitable experiment or study, pick a data summary function and **test statistic**.
2. Set up a **null hypothesis**, which is a simple, computationally tractable model of reality that lets you compute the **null distribution**, i.e., the possible outcomes of the test statistic and their probabilities under the assumption that the null hypothesis is true.
3. Decide on the **rejection region**, i.e., a subset of possible outcomes whose total probability is small.[7]
4. Do the experiment and collect the data;[8] compute the test statistic.
5. Make a decision: reject the null hypothesis[9] if the test statistic is in the rejection region.

[7] More on this in Section 6.3.1.

[8] Or if someone else has already done it, download their data.

[9] That is, conclude that it is unlikely to be true.

Note how, in this idealized **workflow**, we make all the important decisions in Steps 1–3 before we have even seen the data. As we already alluded to in the Introduction (Figures 1 and 2), this is often not realistic. We will also come back to this question in Section 6.6.

There was also some idealization in the null hypothesis that we used in the example above: we postulated that a fair coin should have a probability of exactly 0.5 (not, say, 0.500001) and that there should be absolutely no dependence between tosses. We did not worry about any possible effects of air drag, elasticity of the material on which the coin falls, and so on. This gave us the advantage that the null hypothesis was computationally tractable, namely, with the binomial distribution. Here, these idealizations may not seem very controversial, but in other situations the trade-off between how tractable and how realistic a null hypothesis is can be more substantial. The problem is that if a null hypothesis is too idealized to start with, rejecting it is not all that interesting. The result may be misleading, and certainly we are wasting our time.

The test statistic in our example was the total number of heads. Suppose we observed

50 tails in a row, and then 50 heads in a row. Our test statistic ignores the order of the outcomes, and we would conclude that this is a perfectly fair coin. However, if we used a different test statistic, say, the number of times we see two tails in a row, we might notice that there is something funny about this coin.

▶ Question **6.5** What is the null distribution of this different test statistic?   ◀

▶ Question **6.6** Would a test based on that statistic be generally preferable?   ◀

▶ **Solution 6.6** No, while it has more power to detect such correlations between coin tosses, it has *less* power to detect bias in the outcome.   □

What we have just done is look at two different classes of **alternative hypotheses**. The first class of alternatives was that subsequent coin tosses are still independent of each other, but that the probability of heads differed from 0.5. The second one was that the overall probability of heads may still be 0.5, but that subsequent coin tosses were correlated.

▶ Question **6.7** Recall the concept of *sufficient* statistics from Chapter 1. Is the total number of heads a sufficient statistic for the binomial distribution? Why might it be a good test statistic for our first class of alternatives, but not for the second?   ◀

So let's remember that we typically have multiple possible choices of test statistic (in principle it could be any numerical summary of the data). Making the correct choice is important in getting a test with good power.[10] What the right choice is will depend on what kind of alternatives we expect. This is not always easy to know in advance.

[10] See Sections 1.4.1 and 6.4.

Once we have chosen the test statistic, we need to compute its null distribution. You can do this either with pencil and paper or by computer simulations. The former is parametric and leads to a closed form mathematical expression (like Equation (6.1)), which has the advantage that it holds for a range of model parameters of the null hypothesis (such as n, p). It can also be quickly computed for any specific set of parameters. But it is not always as easy as in the coin tossing example. Sometimes a pencil and paper solution is impossibly difficult to compute. At other times, it may require simplifying assumptions. An example is a null distribution for the t-statistic (which we will see later in this chapter). We can compute this if we assume that the data are independent and normally distributed: the result is called the t-distribution. Such modeling assumptions may be more or less realistic. Simulating the null distribution offers a potentially more accurate, more realistic and perhaps even more intuitive approach. The drawback of simulating is that it can take a rather long time, and we need to do extra work to get a systematic understanding of how varying parameters influence the result. Generally, it is more elegant to use the parametric theory when it applies.[11] When you are in doubt, simulate – or do both.

We can derive null distributions by paper and pencil or by Monte Carlo simulations.

[11] The assumptions don't need to be *exactly* true – it is sufficient that the theory's predictions are an acceptable approximation of the truth.

6.3.1   The rejection region

How do you choose the correct rejection region for your test? First, what should its size be? That is your choice of the **significance level** or false positive rate α, which is the

Some people at some point in time for a particular set of questions colluded on a significance level of $\alpha = 0.05$ as being "small". But there is nothing special about this number, and in any particular case the best choice for a decision threshold may very much depend on context (Wasserstein and Lazar, 2016; Altman and Krzywinski, 2017).

total probability of the test statistic falling into this region even if the null hypothesis is true.

Given the size, the next question is about its shape. For any given size, there are usually multiple possible shapes. It makes sense to require that the probability of the test statistic falling into the rejection region is as large possible if the alternative hypothesis is true. In other words, we want our test to have high **power**, or true positive rate.

The criterion that we used in the code for computing the rejection region for Figure 6.4 was to make the region contain as many k as possible. That is because in the absence of any information about the alternative distribution, one k is as good as any other, and we maximize their total number.

A consequence of this is that in Figure 6.4 the rejection region is split between the two tails of the distribution. This is because we anticipate that unfair coins could have a bias either toward heads or toward tails: we don't know. But if we did, we would instead concentrate our rejection region entirely on the appropriate side, e.g., the right tail if we think the bias would be toward heads. Such choices are also referred to as *two-sided* and *one-sided* tests. More generally, if we have assumptions about the alternative distribution, this can influence our choice of the shape of the rejection region.

6.4   Types of error

Having set out the mechanics of testing, we can assess how well we are doing. Table 6.1 compares reality (whether or not the null hypothesis is in fact true) with our decision whether or not to reject the null hypothesis after we have seen the data.

It's always possible to reduce one of the two error types at the cost of increasing the other one. The real challenge is to find an acceptable trade-off between them. This is exemplified in Figure 6.5. We can always decrease the **false positive rate** (FPR) by shifting the threshold to the right. We can become more *conservative*. But this happens at the price of a higher **false negative rate** (FNR). Analogously, we can decrease the FNR by shifting the threshold to the left. But then this happens at the price of a higher FPR. A bit on terminology: the FPR is the same as the probability α that we mentioned above. $1 - \alpha$ is also called the **specificity** of a test. The FNR is sometimes also called β, and $1 - \beta$ the **power**, **sensitivity** or **true positive rate** of a test.

▶ Question **6.8** At the end of Section 6.3 we learned about one- and two-sided tests. Why does this distinction exist? Why don't we always just use the two-sided test, which is sensitive to a larger class of alternatives?   ◀

Table 6.1: Types of error in a statistical test.

Test vs. reality	Null hypothesis is true	...is false
Reject null hypothesis	Type I error (false positive)	True positive
Do not reject	True negative	Type II error (false negative)

6.5   The *t*-test

Many experimental measurements are reported as rational numbers, and the simplest comparison we can make is between two groups, say, cells treated with a substance compared to cells that are not. The basic test for such situations is the *t*-test. The test statistic is defined as

$$t = c \, \frac{m_1 - m_2}{s},$$ (6.2)

where m_1 and m_2 are the means of the values in the two groups, s is the pooled standard deviation and c is a constant that depends on the sample sizes, i.e., the numbers of observations n_1 and n_2 in the two groups. In formulas,

$$m_g = \frac{1}{n_g} \sum_{i=1}^{n_g} x_{g,i}, \qquad g = 1, 2,$$

$$s^2 = \frac{1}{n_1 + n_2 - 2} \left(\sum_{i=1}^{n_1} \left(x_{1,i} - m_1 \right)^2 + \sum_{j=1}^{n_2} \left(x_{2,j} - m_2 \right)^2 \right),$$

$$c = \sqrt{\frac{n_1 n_2}{n_1 + n_2}},$$ (6.3)

where $x_{g,i}$ is the ith data point in the gth group. Let's try it with the `PlantGrowth` data from R's *datasets* package.

```
library("ggbeeswarm")
data("PlantGrowth")
ggplot(PlantGrowth, aes(y = weight, x = group, col = group)) +
  geom_beeswarm() + theme(legend.position = "none")
tt = with(PlantGrowth,
          t.test(weight[group =="ctrl"],
                 weight[group =="trt2"],
                 var.equal = TRUE))
tt

##
##   Two Sample t-test
##
## data:  weight[group == "ctrl"] and weight[group == "trt2"]
## t = -2.134, df = 18, p-value = 0.04685
## alternative hypothesis: true difference in means is not equal to 0
## 95 percent confidence interval:
##   -0.980338117 -0.007661883
## sample estimates:
## mean of x mean of y
##     5.032     5.526
```

▶ **Question 6.9** What do you get from the comparison with `trt1`? What about for `trt1` versus `trt2`?   ◀

▶ **Question 6.10** What is the significance of the `var.equal = TRUE` in the above call to `t.test`?   ◀

▶ **Solution 6.10** We'll get back to this on page 148.   □

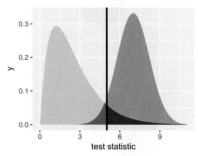

Figure 6.5: The trade-off between type I and II errors. The densities represent the distributions of a hypothetical test statistic under either the null or the alternative hypothesis. The peak on the left (light and dark blue plus dark red) represents the test statistic's distribution under the null. It integrates to 1. Suppose the decision boundary is the black line and the hypothesis is rejected if the statistic falls to the right. The probability of a false positive (the FPR) is then simply the dark red area. Similarly, if the peak on the right (light and dark red plus dark blue area) is the test statistic's distribution under the alternative, the probability of a false negative (the FNR) is the dark blue area.

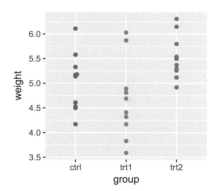

Figure 6.6: The `PlantGrowth` data.

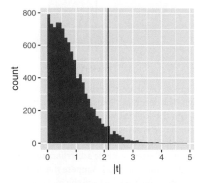

Figure 6.7: The null distribution of the (absolute) *t*-statistic determined by simulations – namely, random permutations of the group labels.

▶ Question **6.11** Rewrite the above call to `t.test` using the formula interface, i.e., using the notation `weight ~ group`.   ◀

To compute the p-value, the `t.test` function uses the asymptotic theory for the *t*-statistic (6.2); this theory states that under the null hypothesis of equal means in both groups, the statistic follows a known mathematical distribution, the so-called *t*-distribution with $n_1 + n_2$ degrees of freedom. The theory uses additional technical assumptions, namely that the data are independent and come from a normal distribution with the same standard deviation. We could be worried about these assumptions. Clearly they do not hold: weights are always positive, while the normal distribution extends over the whole real axis. The question is whether this deviation from the theoretical assumption makes a real difference. We can use a permutation test to figure this out (we will discuss the idea behind permutation tests in a bit more detail in Section 6.5.1).

```
abs_t_null = with(
  filter(PlantGrowth, group %in% c("ctrl", "trt2")),
    replicate(10000,
      abs(t.test(weight ~ sample(group))$statistic)))

ggplot(tibble(`|t|` = abs_t_null), aes(x = `|t|`)) +
  geom_histogram(binwidth = 0.1, boundary = 0) +
  geom_vline(xintercept = abs(tt$statistic), col = "red")
mean(abs(tt$statistic) <= abs_t_null)
## [1] 0.0484
```

▶ Question **6.12** Why did we use the absolute value function (`abs`) in the above code?

◀

▶ Task Plot the (parametric) *t*-distribution with appropriate degrees of freedom.   ◀

The *t*-test comes in multiple flavors, all of which can be chosen through parameters of the `t.test` function. What we did above was to call a two-sided two-sample unpaired test with equal variance. **Two-sided** expresses the fact that we were open to rejecting the null hypothesis if the weight of the treated plants was *either larger or smaller* than that of the untreated ones.

Two-sample[12] indicates that we compared the means of two groups to each other; another option is to compare the mean of one group against a given fixed number.

Unpaired means that there was no direct 1:1 mapping between the measurements in the two groups. If, on the other hand, the data were measured on the same plants before and after treatment, then a paired test would be more appropriate, as it looks at the change of weight within each plant rather than their absolute weights.

Equal variance refers to the way the statistic (6.2) is calculated. That expression is most appropriate if the variances within each group are about the same. If they are very different, an alternative form[13] and an associated asymptotic theory exist.

To explore the **independence assumption**, let's try something peculiar: duplicate the data.

[12] It can be confusing that the term *sample* has a different meaning in statistics than in biology. In biology, a sample is a single specimen on which an assay is performed; in statistics, it is a set of measurements, e.g., the n_1-tuple $(x_{1,1}, \ldots, x_{1,n_1})$ in Equation (6.3), which can comprise several biological samples. In contexts where this double meaning might create confusion, we refer to the data from a single biological sample as an *observation*.

[13] Welch's *t*-test.

```
with(rbind(PlantGrowth, PlantGrowth),
        t.test(weight[group == "ctrl"],
                weight[group == "trt2"],
                var.equal = TRUE))
##
##  Two Sample t-test
##
## data:  weight[group == "ctrl"] and weight[group == "trt2"]
## t = -3.1007, df = 38, p-value = 0.003629
## alternative hypothesis: true difference in means is not equal to 0
## 95 percent confidence interval:
##  -0.8165284 -0.1714716
## sample estimates:
## mean of x mean of y
##     5.032     5.526
```

Note how the estimates of the group means (and thus of the difference) are un-changed, but the p-value is now much smaller! We can conclude two things from this:

- The power of the *t*-test depends on the sample size. Even if the underlying biological differences are the same, a dataset with more observations tends to give more significant results.[14]
- The assumption of independence between the measurements is really important. Blatant duplication of the same data is an extreme form of **dependence**, but to some extent the same thing happens if you mix up different levels of replication. For instance, suppose you had data from eight plants but measured the same thing twice on each one (*technical replicates*), then pretending that these are now 16 independent measurements is wrong.

[14] You can also see this from the way the numbers n_1 and n_2 appear in Equation (6.3).

6.5.1 Permutation tests

What happened above when we contrasted the outcome of the parametric *t*-test with that of the permutation test applied to the *t*-statistic? It's important to realize that these are two different tests, and the similarity of their outcomes is desirable, but coincidental. In the parametric test, the null distribution of the *t*-statistic follows from the assumed null distribution of the data, a multivariate normal distribution with unit covariance in the $(n_1 + n_2)$-dimensional space $\mathbb{R}^{n_1+n_2}$, and is continuous: the *t*-distribution. In contrast, the permutation distribution of our test statistic is discrete, as it is obtained from the finite set of $(n_1 + n_2)!$ permutations[15] of the observation labels, from a single instance of the data (the $n_1 + n_2$ observations). All we assume here is that under the null hypothesis, the variables $X_{1,1}, \ldots, X_{1,n_1}, X_{2,1}, \ldots, X_{2,n_2}$ are exchangeable. Logically, this assumption is implied by that of the parametric test, but is weaker. The permutation test employs the *t*-statistic, but not the *t*-distribution (nor the normal distribution). The fact that the two tests gave us very similar results is a consequence of the Central Limit Theorem.

[15] Or a random subset, in case we want to save computation time.

6.6   P-value hacking

Let's go back to the coin tossing example. We did not reject the null hypothesis (that the coin is fair) at a level of 5% – even though we "knew" that it is unfair. After all, `probHead` was chosen as 0.6 on page 141. Let's suppose we now start looking at different test statistics. Perhaps the number of consecutive series of three or more heads, or the number of heads in the first 50 coin flips, and so on. At some point we will find a test that happens to result in a small p-value, even if just by chance (after all, the probability that the p-value is less than 5% under the null is 0.05, not an infinitesimally small number). We just did what is called **p-value hacking**[16] (Head et al., 2015). You see what the problem is: in our zeal to prove our point, we tortured the data until some statistic did what we wanted. A related tactic is **hypothesis switching** or **HARKing** – hypothesizing after the results are known: we have a dataset, maybe we have invested a lot of time and money in assembling it, so we need results. We come up with lots of different null hypotheses and test statistics, test them, and iterate, until we can report something.

These tactics violate the rules of hypothesis testing, as described in Section 6.3, where we laid out one sequential procedure of choosing the hypothesis and the test, and then collecting the data. But as we saw in Chapter 2, such tactics can be tempting in reality. With biological data, we tend to have so many different choices for "normalizing" the data, transforming the data, correcting for apparent batch effects, removing outliers, and so forth. The topic is complex and open-ended. Wasserstein and Lazar (2016) give a readable short summary of the problems with the ways p-values are used in science and some of the misconceptions. They also highlight how p-values can be fruitfully used. The essential message is: be completely transparent about your data, what analyses were tried, and how they were done. Provide the analysis code. Only with such contextual information can a p-value be useful.

Avoid fallacy.   Keep in mind that our statistical test is never attempting to prove that our null hypothesis is true – we are simply using it to assess whether or not there is evidence that the null hypothesis is false. If a high p-value *were* indicative of the truth of the null hypothesis, we could formulate a completely crazy null hypothesis, do an utterly irrelevant experiment, collect a small amount of inconclusive data, find a p-value that would just be a random number between 0 and 1 (and so with some high probability above our threshold α) and, whoosh, our hypothesis would be demonstrated!

6.7   Multiple testing

▶ Question **6.13** Look up *xkcd cartoon 882*. Why didn't the newspaper report the results for the other colors?   ◀

The quandary illustrated in the cartoon occurs with high-throughput data in biology. And with force! You will be dealing not only with 20 colors of jellybeans, but with, say, 20,000 genes that were tested for differential expression between two conditions, or

[16] http://fivethirtyeight.com/features/science-isnt-broken.

Test vs. reality	Null hypothesis is true	...is false	Total
Rejected	V	S	R
Not rejected	U	T	$m - R$
Total	m_0	$m - m_0$	m

Table 6.2: Types of errors in multiple testing. The letters designate the number of times each type of error occurs.

m: total number of hypotheses

m_0: number of null hypotheses

V: number of false positives (a measure of type I error)

T: number of false negatives (a measure of type II error)

S, U: number of true positives and true negatives

R: number of rejections

with 3 billion positions in the genome where a DNA mutation might have happened. So how do we deal with this? Let's look again at our table relating statistical test results with reality (Table 6.1), this time framing everything in terms of many hypotheses.

In the rest of this chapter, we look at different ways of taking care of the type I and II errors.

6.8   The family-wise error rate

The **family-wise error rate** (FWER) is the probability that $V > 0$, i.e., that we make one or more false positive errors. We can compute it as the complement of making no false positive errors at all:[17]

[17] Assuming independence.

$$P(V > 0) = 1 - P(\text{no rejection of any of } m_0 \text{ nulls}) = 1 - (1 - \alpha)^{m_0} \rightarrow 1$$
$$\text{as } m_0 \rightarrow \infty. \quad (6.4)$$

For any fixed α, this probability is appreciable as soon as m_0 is in the order of $1/\alpha$, and it tends toward 1 as m_0 becomes larger. This relationship can have serious consequences for experiments like DNA matching, where a large database of potential matches is searched. For example, if there is a one in a million chance that the DNA profiles of two people match by random error, and your DNA is tested against a database of 800,000 profiles, then the probability of a random hit with the database (i.e., without you being in it) is

```
1 - (1 - 1/1e6)^8e5
## [1] 0.5506712
```

That's pretty high. And once the database contains a few million profiles more, a false hit is virtually unavoidable.

▶ Question **6.14** Prove that probability (6.4) does indeed become very close to 1 when m_0 is large. ◀

6.8.1   Bonferroni correction

How are we to choose the per-hypothesis α if we want FWER control? The above computations suggest that the product of α with m_0 may be a reasonable ballpark estimate. Usually we don't know m_0, but we know m, which is an upper limit for m_0, since $m_0 \leqslant m$. The Bonferroni correction is simply that if we want FWER control at level α_{FWER}, we should choose the per-hypothesis threshold $\alpha = \alpha_{\text{FWER}}/m$. Let's check this on an example.

```
m = 10000
ggplot(tibble(
  alpha = seq(0, 7e-6, length.out = 100),
  p     = 1 - (1 - alpha)^m),
  aes(x = alpha, y = p)) + geom_line() +
  xlab(expression(alpha)) +
  ylab("Prob( no false rejection )") +
  geom_hline(yintercept = 0.05, col = "red")
```

In Figure 6.8, the black line intersects the red line (which corresponds to a value of 0.05) at $\alpha = 5.13 \times 10^{-6}$, which is just a little bit more than the value of $0.05/m$ implied by the Bonferroni correction.

▶ Question **6.15** Why are the two values not exactly the same? ◀

A potential drawback of this method, however, is that if m_0 is large, the rejection threshold is very small. This means that the individual tests need to be very powerful if we want to have any chance of detecting something. Often this is not possible, or would not be an effective use of our time and money. We'll see that there are more nuanced methods of controlling our type I error.

6.9   The false discovery rate

Let's look at some real data. We load up the RNA-Seq dataset `airway`, which contains gene expression measurements (gene-level counts) of four primary human airway smooth muscle cell lines with and without treatment with dexamethasone, a synthetic glucocorticoid. We'll use the *DESeq2* method, which we'll discuss in more detail in Chapter 8. For now it suffices to say that it performs a test for differential expression for each gene. Conceptually, the tested null hypothesis is very similar to the t-test, although the details are slightly more involved since we are dealing with count data.

```
library("DESeq2")
library("airway")
data("airway")
aw   = DESeqDataSet(se = airway, design = ~ cell + dex)
aw   = DESeq(aw)
awde = as.data.frame(results(aw)) %>% filter(!is.na(pvalue))
```

▶ Task Have a look at the content of `awde`. ◀

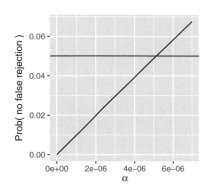

Figure 6.8: Bonferroni correction. The plot shows the graph of (6.4) for $m = 10^4$ as a function of α.

▶ Task   (Optional) Consult the *DESeq2* vignette and/or Chapter 8 for more information on what the above code chunk does.   ◀

6.9.1   The p-value histogram

The **p-value histogram** is an important sanity check for any analysis that involves multiple tests. It is a mixture composed of two components:

0: the p-values resulting from the tests for which the null hypothesis is true and
1: the p-values resulting from the tests for which the null hypothesis is not true.

The relative size of these two components depends on the fraction of true nulls and true alternatives, and can often be visually estimated from the histogram. If our analysis has high statistical power, then component 1 consists all of small p-values, i.e., appears as a peak near 0 in the histogram; if the power is not high for some of the alternatives, we expect that this peak extends toward the right, i.e., has a "shoulder". For component 0, we expect (by definition of the p-value for continuous data and test statistics) a uniform distribution in [0, 1]. Let's plot the histogram of p-values for the airway data.

```
ggplot(awde, aes(x = pvalue)) +
  geom_histogram(binwidth = 0.025, boundary = 0)
```

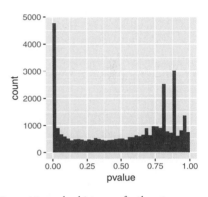

Figure 6.9: p-value histogram for the `airway` data.

In Figure 6.9 we see the expected mixture. We also see that the null component is not exactly flat (uniform): this is because the data are **counts**. While these appear quasi-continuous when high, for the tests with low counts, the discreteness of the data and the resulting p-values shows up in the spikes toward the right of the histogram.

Now suppose we reject all tests with a p-value less than α. We can visually determine an estimate of the false discovery proportion with a plot such as in Figure 6.10, generated by the following code.

```
alpha = binw = 0.025
pi0 = 2 * mean(awde$pvalue > 0.5)
ggplot(awde,
  aes(x = pvalue)) + geom_histogram(binwidth = binw, boundary = 0) +
  geom_hline(yintercept = pi0 * binw * nrow(awde), col = "blue") +
  geom_vline(xintercept = alpha, col = "red")
```

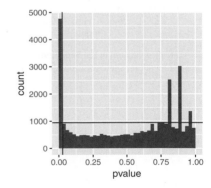

Figure 6.10: Visual estimation of the FDR with the p-value histogram.

We see that there are 4771 p-values in the first bin $[0, \alpha]$, among which we expect around 945 to be nulls (as indicated by the blue line). Thus we can estimate the fraction of false rejections as

```
pi0 * alpha / mean(awde$pvalue <= alpha)
## [1] 0.1980507
```

The **false discovery rate** (FDR) is defined as

$$\text{FDR} = E\left[\frac{V}{\max(R, 1)}\right], \tag{6.5}$$

where R and V are as in Table 6.2 and $E[\ ]$ stands for the **expected value**. The expression in the denominator makes sure that the FDR is well defined even if $R = 0$ (in that case, $V = 0$ by implication). Note that the FDR becomes identical to the FWER if all null hypotheses are true, i.e., if $V = R$. That means that the FDR is not a quantity associated with a specific outcome of V and R for one particular experiment. Rather, given our choice of tests and associated rejection rules for them, it is the average[18] proportion of type I errors out of the rejections made, where the average is taken (at least conceptually) over many replicate instances of the experiment.

[18] Since the FDR is an expectation value, it does not provide worst-case control: in any single experiment, the so-called false discovery proportion (FDP) – that is, the realized value v/r (without the $E[\ ]$) – could be much higher or lower.

6.9.2   The Benjamini–Hochberg algorithm for controlling the FDR

There is a more elegant alternative to the "visual FDR" method of the last section. The procedure, introduced by Benjamini and Hochberg (1995), has these steps:

- First, order the p-values in increasing order, $p_{(1)}, \ldots, p_{(m)}$.
- Then, for some choice of φ (our target FDR), find the largest value of k that satisfies $p_{(k)} \leqslant \varphi k/m$.
- Finally, reject the hypotheses $1, \ldots, k$.

We can see how this procedure works when applied to our RNA-Seq p-values through a simple graphical illustration.

```
phi  = 0.10
awde = mutate(awde, rank = rank(pvalue))
m    = nrow(awde)


ggplot(filter(awde, rank <= 7000), aes(x = rank, y = pvalue)) +
  geom_line() + geom_abline(slope = phi / m, col = "red")
```

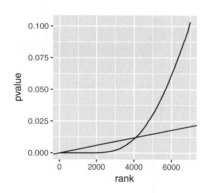

Figure 6.11: Visualization of the Benjamini–Hochberg procedure. Shown is a zoom-in to the 7000 lowest p-values.

The method finds the rightmost point where the black lines (our p-values) and red lines (slope φ/m) intersect. Then it rejects all tests to the left.

```
kmax = with(arrange(awde, rank),
         last(which(pvalue <= phi * rank / m)))
kmax

## [1] 4099
```

▶ Question **6.16** Compare the value of `kmax` with the number 4771 from above (Figure 6.10). Why are they different? ◀

▶ Question **6.17** Look at the code associated with the option `method="BH"` of the `p.adjust` function that comes with R. How does it compare to what we did above? ◀

6.10   The local FDR

While the xkcd cartoon in the chapter's opening figure ends with a rather sinister intepretation of the multiple testing problem as a way to accumulate errors, Figure 6.12 highlights the multiple testing opportunity: when we do many tests, we can use the multiplicity to increase our understanding beyond what's possible with a single test.

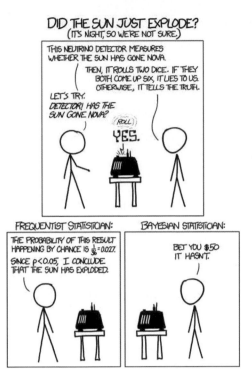

Figure 6.12: While the frequentist only has the currently available data, the Bayesian can draw on her understanding of the world or on previous experience. As a Bayesian, she would know enough about physics to understand that our sun's mass is too small to become a nova. Even if she does not know physics, she might be an *empirical Bayesian* and draw her prior from myriad previous days when the sun did not go nova. From http://xkcd.com/1132.

Let's get back to the histogram in Figure 6.10. Conceptually, we can think of it in terms of the so-called two-groups model (Efron, 2010):

$$f(p) = \pi_0 + (1 - \pi_0)f_{\text{alt}}(p). \tag{6.6}$$

Here, $f(p)$ is the density of the distribution (what the histogram would look like with an infinite amount of data and infinitely small bins), π_0 is a number between 0 and 1 that represents the size of the uniform component, and f_{alt} is the alternative component. This is a mixture model, as we already saw in Chapter 4. The mixture densities and the marginal density $f(p)$ are visualized in the top panel of Figure 6.13: the blue areas together correspond to the graph of $f_{\text{alt}}(p)$, the gray areas to that of $f_{\text{null}}(p) = \pi_0$. If we now consider one particular cutoff p (say, $p = 0.1$ as in Figure 6.13), then we can compute the probability that a hypothesis that we reject at this cutoff is a false positive, as follows. We decompose the value of f at the cutoff (red line) into the contribution from the nulls (light red, π_0) and from the alternatives (darker red, $(1 - \pi_0)f_{\text{alt}}(p)$). The **local false discovery rate** is then

$$\text{fdr}(p) = \frac{\pi_0}{f(p)}. \tag{6.7}$$

By definition, this quantity is between 0 and 1. Note how the fdr in Figure 6.13 is a monotonically increasing function of p, and this goes with our intuition that the fdr should be lowest for the smallest p and then gradually get larger, until it reaches 1 at the very right end. We can make a similar decomposition not only for the red line, but also for the area under the curve. This is

$$F(p) = \int_0^p f(t)\,dt, \tag{6.8}$$

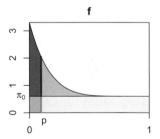

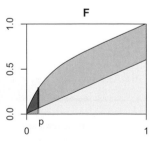

Figure 6.13: Local false discovery rate and the two-group model, with some choice of $f_{\text{alt}}(p)$ and $\pi_0 = 0.6$. Top: Densities. Bottom: Distribution functions.

fdr, Fdr, FDR

The convention is to use the lowercase abbreviation fdr for the local and the abbreviation Fdr for the tail-area false discovery rate in the context of the two-groups model (6.6). The abbreviation FDR is used for the original definition (6.5), which is a bit more general.

and the ratio of the dark gray area (that is, π_0 times p) to the overall area $F(p)$ is the *tail-area false discovery rate* (FDR):

$$\mathrm{Fdr}(p) = \frac{\pi_0\, p}{F(p)}. \tag{6.9}$$

We'll use the data version of F for diagnostics in Figure 6.17.

The packages *qvalue* and *fdrtool* offer facilities to fit these models to data.

```
library("fdrtool")
ft = fdrtool(awde$pvalue, statistic = "pvalue")
```

In *fdrtool*, what we called π_0 above is called eta0.

```
ft$param[,"eta0"]
##      eta0
## 0.8823238
```

▶ **Question 6.18** What do the plots produced by the above call to `fdrtool` show? ◀

▶ **Task** Explore the other elements of the *list* ft. ◀

▶ **Question 6.19** What does the *empirical* in empirical Bayes method stand for? ◀

6.10.1 Local versus total

The FDR (or the Fdr) is a set property – it is a single number that applies to a whole set of rejections made in the course of a multiple testing analysis. In contrast, the fdr is a local property – it applies to an individual additional hypothesis. Recall Figure 6.13, where the fdr was computed for each point along the x-axis of the density plot, whereas the Fdr depends on the areas to the left of the red line.

▶ **Question 6.20** Check out the concepts of *total cost* and *marginal cost* in economics. Can you see an analogy with Fdr and fdr? ◀

6.11 Independent filtering and hypothesis weighting

The Benjamini–Hochberg method and the two-groups model, as we have seen them so far, implicitly assume *exchangeability* indexexchangeability of the hypotheses: all we use are the p-values. Beyond these, we do not take into account any additional information. This is not always optimal, and here we'll study ways to improve on this.

Let's look at an example. Intuitively, the signal-to-noise ratio for genes with larger numbers of reads mapped to them should be better than for genes with few reads, and that should affect the power of our tests. We look at the mean of normalized counts across observations. In the *DESeq2* package this quantity is called the baseMean.

```
awde$baseMean[1]
## [1] 708.6022
cts = counts(aw, normalized = TRUE)[1, ]
cts
```

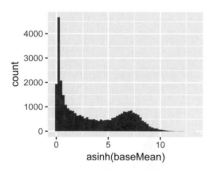

Figure 6.14: Histogram of `baseMean`. We see that it covers a large dynamic range, from close to 0 to around 3.3×10^5.

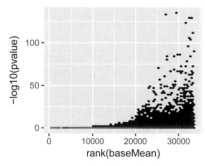

Figure 6.15: Scatterplot of the rank of `baseMean` versus the negative logarithm of the p-value. For small values of `baseMean`, no small p-values occur. Only for genes whose read counts across all observations have a certain size does the test for differential expression have power to come out with a small p-value.

```
## SRR1039508 SRR1039509 SRR1039512 SRR1039513 SRR1039516
##    663.3142    499.9070    740.1528    608.9063    966.3137
## SRR1039517 SRR1039520 SRR1039521
##    748.3722    836.2487    605.6024
mean(cts)
## [1] 708.6022
```

Next we produce the histogram of this quantity across genes, and plot it against the p-values (Figures 6.14 and 6.15).

```
ggplot(awde, aes(x = asinh(baseMean))) +
  geom_histogram(bins = 60)
ggplot(awde, aes(x = rank(baseMean), y = -log10(pvalue))) +
  geom_hex(bins = 60) +
  theme(legend.position = "none")
```

▶ Question **6.21** Why did we use the asinh transformation for the histogram? What does it look like with no transformation, the logarithm, the shifted logarithm, i.e., $\log(x + const.)$?   ◀

▶ Question **6.22** In the scatterplot, why did we use $-\log_{10}$ for the p-values? Why the rank transformation for the `baseMean`?   ◀

For convenience, we discretize `baseMean` into a factor variable `group`, which corresponds to six equal-sized groups.

```
awde = mutate(awde, stratum = cut(baseMean, include.lowest = TRUE,
    breaks = quantile(baseMean, probs = seq(0, 1, length.out = 7))))
```

In Figures 6.16 and 6.17 we see the histograms of p-values and the ECDFs stratified by `stratum`.

```
ggplot(awde, aes(x = pvalue)) + facet_wrap( ~ stratum, nrow = 4) +
  geom_histogram(binwidth = 0.025, boundary = 0)

ggplot(awde, aes(x = pvalue, col = stratum)) +
  stat_ecdf(geom = "step") + theme(legend.position = "bottom")
```

If we were to fit the two-group model to these strata separately, we would get quite different estimates for π_0 and f_{alt}. For the most lowly expressed genes, the power of the *DESeq2* test is low and the p-values essentially all come from the null component. As we go higher in average expression, the height of the small-p-values peak in the histogram increases, reflecting the increasing power of the test.

Can we use that for a better multiple testing correction? It turns out that this is possible. We can use either **independent filtering** (Bourgon et al., 2010) or **independent hypothesis weighting**, IHW (Ignatiadis et al., 2016).

```
library("IHW")
ihw_res = ihw(awde$pvalue, awde$baseMean, alpha = 0.1)
rejections(ihw_res)
## [1] 4896
```

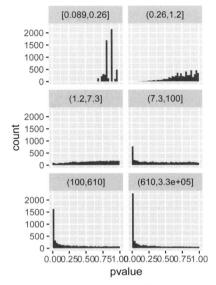

Figure 6.16: p-value histograms of the `airway` data, stratified into equally sized groups defined by increasing value of `baseMean`.

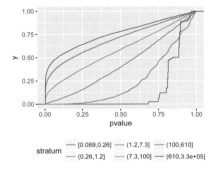

Figure 6.17: Same data as in Figure 6.16, shown with ECDFs.

Let's compare this to what we get from the ordinary (unweighted) Benjamini–Hochberg method.

```
padj_BH = p.adjust(awde$pvalue, method = "BH")
sum(padj_BH < 0.1)
## [1] 4099
```

With hypothesis weighting, we get more rejections. For these data, the difference is notable though not spectacular; this is because their signal-to-noise ratio is already quite high. In other situations, where there is less power to begin with (e.g., where there are fewer replicates, the data are more noisy, or the effect of the treatment is less drastic), the difference from using IHW can be more pronounced.

We can have a look at the weights determined by the `ihw` function (Figure 6.18).

```
plot(ihw_res)
```

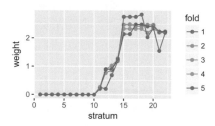

Figure 6.18: Hypothesis weights determined by the `ihw` function. Here the function's default settings chose 22 strata, while in our manual exploration above (Figures 6.16, 6.17) we used 6; in practice, this is a minor detail.

Intuitively, what happens here is that IHW chooses to put more weight on the hypothesis strata with higher `baseMean`, and low weight on those with very low counts. The Benjamini–Hochberg method has a certain type I error budget, and rather than spreading it equally among all hypotheses, here we take it away from those strata that have little change of small fdr anyway and "invest" it in strata where many hypotheses can be rejected at small fdr.

▶ **Question 6.23** Why does Figure 6.18 show five curves rather than only one?   ◀

Such possibilities for stratification by an additional summary statistic besides the p-value – in our case, the `baseMean` – exist in many multiple testing situations. Informally, we need these so-called *co-data* to be

- statistically independent from our p-values under the null, but
- informative of the prior probability π_0 and/or the power of the test (the shape of the alternative density, f_{alt}) in the two-groups model.

These requirements can be assessed through diagnostic plots as in Figures 6.14–6.17.

6.12   Summary of this chapter

We explored the concepts behind *single hypothesis testing* and then moved on to *multiple testing*. We have seen how some of the limitations of interpreting a single p-value from a single test can be overcome once we are able to consider a whole distribution of outcomes from many tests. We have also seen that there are often additional summary statistics of our data, besides the p-values. We called them *co-data* and saw how we can use them to weigh the p-values and overall get more (or better) discoveries.

The use of hypothesis testing in the *multiple testing* scenario is quite different from that in the *single test* case: for the latter, the hypothesis test might literally be the final result, the culmination of a long and expensive data acquisition campaign (ideally, with a prespecified hypothesis and data analysis plan). In the multiple testing case, its outcome will often just be an intermediate step: a subset of most worthwhile hypotheses selected by screening a large initial set. This subset is then followed up by more careful analyses.

We have seen the concept of the *false discovery rate* (FDR). It is important to keep in mind that this is an average property for the subset of hypotheses that were selected. Like other averages, it does not say anything about the individual hypotheses. Then there is the concept of the *local false discovery rate* (fdr), which indeed does apply to an individual hypothesis. The local false discovery rate is, however, quite unrelated to the p-value, as the two-group model showed us. Much of the confusion and frustration about p-values seems to come from the fact that people would like to use them for purposes that the fdr is made for. It is perhaps a historical aberration that so much of applied science focuses on p-values and not local false discovery rates. On the other hand, there are also practical reasons, since a p-value is readily computed, whereas a fdr is difficult to estimate or control from data without making strong modeling assumptions.

We saw the importance of diagnostic plots, in particular, that you should always look at the p-value histograms when encountering a multiple testing analysis.

6.13 Further reading

- A comprehensive textbook treatment of multiple testing is Efron (2010).
- For outcome switching in clinical trials, visit `http://compare-trials.org`.
- For hypothesis weighting, see the *IHW* vignette, the IHW paper (Ignatiadis et al., 2016) and the references therein.

6.14 Exercises

▶ Exercise **6.1** Identify an application from your scientific field of expertise that relies on multiple testing. Find an exemplary dataset and plot the histogram of p-values. Are the hypotheses all exchangeable, or are there informative co-data? Plot the stratified histograms. ◀

▶ Exercise **6.2** Why do mathematical statisticians focus so much on the null hypothesis of a test, compared to the alternative hypothesis? ◀

▶ Exercise **6.3** How can we ever prove that the null hypothesis is true? Or that the alternative is true? ◀

▶ Exercise **6.4** Make a less extreme example of correlated test statistics than the data duplication at the end of Section 6.5. Simulate data with true null hypotheses only, and let the data morph from having completely independent replicates (columns) to highly correlated as a function of some continuous-valued control parameter. Check type I error control (e.g., with the p-value histogram) as a function of this control parameter. ◀

▶ Exercise **6.5** Find an example in the published literature that looks as if p-value hacking, outcome switching or HARKing played a role. ◀

7.1 Goals for this chapter

In this chapter we will:

- See examples of matrices that come up in the study of biological data.
- Perform dimension reduction to understand correlations between variables.
- Preprocess, rescale and center data before starting a multivariate analysis.
- Build new variables, called principal components (PCs), that are more useful than the original measurements.
- See what is "under the hood" of PCA: the singular value decomposition of a matrix.
- Visualize what SVD achieves and learn how to choose the number of principal components.
- Run through a complete PCA analysis from start to finish.
- Project factor covariates onto the PCA map for a more useful interpretation of results.

7.2 What are the data? Matrices and their motivation

First, let's look at a set of examples of rectangular **matrices** used to represent tables of measurements. In each matrix, the rows and columns represent specific entities.

Turtles A very simple dataset that will help us understand the basic principles is a matrix of three dimensions of biometric measurements on painted turtles.

```
turtles = read.table("../data/PaintedTurtles.txt", header = TRUE)
turtles[1:4,]
```

```
##   sex length width height
## 1   f     98    81     38
## 2   f    103    84     38
## 3   f    103    86     42
## 4   f    105    86     40
```

The last three columns are length measurements (in millimeters), whereas the first column is a factor variable that tells us the sex of each animal.

Athletes This matrix is an interesting example from the sports world. It reports the performances of 33 athletes in the 10 disciplines of the decathlon: m100, m400 and m1500 are times in seconds for the 100, 400 and 1500 meters, respectively; m110 is the time to finish the 110 meter hurdles; pole is the polevault height, and highj and long are the results of the high and long jumps, all in meters; weight, disc and javel are the lengths in meters that the athletes were able to throw the weight, discus and javelin. Here are the variables for the first three athletes.

```
load("../data/athletes.RData")
athletes[1:3,]
```

```
##    m100 long weight highj  m400  m110  disc pole javel  m1500
## 1 11.25 7.43  15.48  2.27 48.90 15.13 49.28  4.7 61.32 268.95
## 2 10.87 7.45  14.97  1.97 47.71 14.46 44.36  5.1 61.76 273.02
## 3 11.18 7.44  14.20  1.97 48.29 14.81 43.66  5.2 64.16 263.20
```

Cell types Holmes et al. (2005) studied gene expression profiles of sorted T-cell populations from different subjects. The columns are a subset of gene expression measurements and correspond to 156 genes that show differential expression between cell types.

```
load("../data/Msig3transp.RData")
round(Msig3transp,2)[1:5, 1:6]

##              X3968 X14831 X13492 X5108 X16348  X585
## HEA26_EFFE_1 -2.61  -1.19  -0.06 -0.15   0.52 -0.02
## HEA26_MEM_1  -2.26  -0.47   0.28  0.54  -0.37  0.11
## HEA26_NAI_1  -0.27   0.82   0.81  0.72  -0.90  0.75
## MEL36_EFFE_1 -2.24  -1.08  -0.24 -0.18   0.64  0.01
## MEL36_MEM_1  -2.68  -0.15   0.25  0.95  -0.20  0.17
```

Bacterial species abundances Matrices of counts are used in microbial ecology studies (as we saw in Chapter 5). Here the columns represent different species (or operational taxonomic units, OTUs) of bacteria, which are identified by numerical tags. The rows are labeled according to the samples in which they were measured, and the (integer) numbers represent the number of times each OTU was observed in each of the samples.

```
data("GlobalPatterns", package = "phyloseq")
GPOTUs = as.matrix(t(phyloseq::otu_table(GlobalPatterns)))
GPOTUs[1:4, 6:13]

## OTU Table:          [8 taxa and 4 samples]
##                  taxa are columns
##       246140 143239 244960 255340 144887 141782 215972 31759
## CL3        0      7      0    153      3      9      0      0
## CC1        0      1      0    194      5     35      3      1
## SV1        0      0      0      0      0      0      0      0
## M31Fcsw    0      0      0      0      0      0      0      0
```

Notice the propensity of the matrix entries to be zero; we call such data **sparse**.

mRNA reads RNA-Seq transcriptome data report the number of sequence reads matching each gene[2] in each of several biological samples. We will study this type of data in detail in Chapter 8.

[2] Or sub-gene structures, such as exons.

```
library("SummarizedExperiment")
data("airway", package = "airway")
assay(airway)[1:3, 1:4]

##                 SRR1039508 SRR1039509 SRR1039512 SRR1039513
## ENSG00000000003        679        448        873        408
## ENSG00000000005          0          0          0          0
## ENSG00000000419        467        515        621        365
```

It is customary in the RNA-Seq field – and so it is for the `airway` data above – to report genes in rows and samples in columns. Compared with the other matrices we look at here, this is *transposed*: rows and columns are swapped. Such different conventions easily lead to errors, so they are worthwhile paying attention to.[3]

[3] The Bioconductor project tries to help users and developers to avoid such ambiguities by defining data containers in which such conventions are explicitly fixed. In Chapter 8, we will see the example of the *SummarizedExperiment* class.

Proteomic profiles Here the columns are aligned **mass spectroscopy** peaks or molecules identified through their *m/z* ratios; the entries in the matrix are the measured intensities.[4]

[4] More details can be found on Wikipedia.

```
metab = t(as.matrix(read.csv("../data/metabolites.csv",
        row.names = 1)))
metab[1:4, 1:4]

##            146.0985388 148.7053275 310.1505057 132.4512963
## KOGCHUM1     29932.36    17055.70     1132.82      785.5129
## KOGCHUM2     94067.61    74631.69    28240.85     5232.0499
## KOGCHUM3    146411.33   147788.71    64950.49    10283.0037
## WTGCHUM1    229912.57   384932.56   220730.39    26115.2007
```

In many of the matrices we see here, important information is stored in the row or column names. However, this far from the best place to store all available information on the subjects (columns) and features (rows). A much better approach is the Bioconductor *SummarizedExperiment* class.

▶ **Task** When a peak was not detected for a particular m/z score in the mass spectrometry run, a zero was recorded in `metab`. Similarly, zeros in `GPOTUs` or in the `airway` object occur when there are no matching sequence reads detected. Tabulate the frequencies of zeros in these data matrices.   ◀

▶ **Question 7.1**

(a) What are the columns of these data matrices usually called?

(b) In each of these examples, what are the rows of the matrix?

(c) What does a cell in a matrix represent?

(d) If the data matrix is called `athletes` and you want to see the value of the third variable for the fifth athlete, what do you type into R?   ◀

7.2.1   Low-dimensional data summaries and preparation

[5] The third column of a matrix X is denoted mathematically by $x_{\bullet 3}$ or accessed in R using `X[, 3]`.

If we are studying only one variable, e.g., just the third column of the turtles matrix,[5] we say we are looking at one-dimensional data. Such a vector, say all the turtle weights, can be visualized by plots such as those that we saw in Section 3.6, e.g., a histogram. If we compute a one-number summary, say mean or median, we have made a zero-dimensional summary of our one-dimensional data. This is already an example of dimension reduction.

In Chapter 3 we studied two-dimensional scatterplots. We saw that if there are too many observations, it can be beneficial to group the data into (hexagonal) bins: these are *two-dimensional* histograms. When considering two variables (x and y) measured together on a set of observations, the **correlation coefficient** measures how the variables co-vary. This is a single-number summary of two-dimensional data. Its formula involves

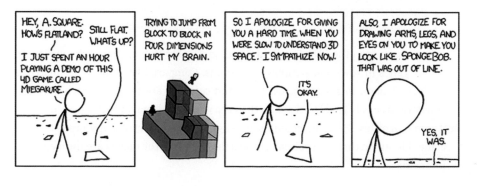

Figure 7.1: What do we mean by low-dimensional? We live in three dimensions, or four if you count time, a plane has two dimensions and a line has one dimension. A point is said to be zero-dimensional. The amusing novel alluded to in the cartoon is Abbott (1884). Image credit: xkcd.com.

the summaries $\bar{x}$ and $\bar{y}$:

$$\hat{\rho} = \frac{\sum_{i=1}^{n}(x_i - \bar{x})(y_i - \bar{y})}{\sqrt{\sum_{i=1}^{n}(x_i - \bar{x})^2}\sqrt{\sum_{j=1}^{n}(y_j - \bar{y})^2}}. \tag{7.1}$$

In R, we use the `cor` function to calculate its value. Applied to a matrix, this function computes all the two-way correlations between continuous variables. In Chapter 9 we will see how to analyze multivariate categorical data.

▶ **Question 7.2** Compute the matrix of all correlations between the measurements from the turtles data. What do you notice?   ◀

▶ **Solution 7.2**   We take out the categorical variable and compute the matrix.

```
cor(turtles[, -1])
##           length      width    height
## length 1.0000000 0.9783116 0.9646946
## width  0.9783116 1.0000000 0.9605705
## height 0.9646946 0.9605705 1.0000000
```

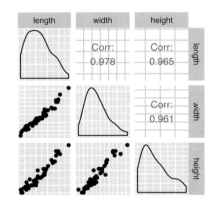

Figure 7.2: All pairs of bivariate scatterplots for the three biometric measurements on painted turtles.

We see that this square matrix is symmetric and the values are all close to 1. The diagonal values are always 1.   □

It is always beneficial to start a multidimensional analysis by checking these simple one-dimensional and two-dimensional summary statistics and making visual displays such as those in Figures 7.2 and 7.3.

▶ **Question 7.3**   (a) Produce all pairwise scatterplots, as well as the one-dimensional histograms on the diagonal, for the turtles data. The result should look something like Figure 7.2. Use the package *GGally*.
(b) Guess the underlying or "true" dimension of these data.   ◀

▶ **Solution 7.3**

```
library("ggplot2")
library("dplyr")
library("GGally")
ggpairs(turtles[, -1], axisLabels = "none")
```

It seems that all three of the variables mostly reflect the same "underlying" variable, which we might interpret as the *size* of the turtle.   □

▶ **Question 7.4** Make a pairs plot of the `athletes` data. What do you notice?   ◀

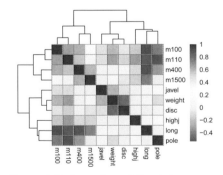

Figure 7.3: Heatmap of correlations between variables in the `athletes` data. Higher values are color coded red–orange. The hierarchical clustering shows the grouping of the related disciplines.

▶ **Solution 7.4**   We can confirm some of the structure apparent in the correlations by a call to the `pheatmap` function as shown in Figure 7.3.

```
library("pheatmap")
pheatmap(cor(athletes), cell.width = 10, cell.height = 10)
```

Figure 7.3 shows how the *hierarchical clustering* of the variables clusters them into three groups: running, throwing and jumping.   □

[6] Common measures of scale are the range and the standard deviation. For instance, the times for the 110 meters vary between 14.18 and 16.2, with a standard deviation of 0.51, whereas the times to complete the 1500 meters vary between 256.64 and 303.17, with a standard deviation of 13.66, more than an order of magnitude larger. Moreover, the `athletes` data also contain measurements in different units (seconds, meters), whose choice is arbitrary (lengths could also be recorded in centimeters or feet, times in milliseconds).

7.2.2   Preprocessing the data

In many cases, different variables are measured in different units, so they have different baselines and different scales.[6] These are not directly comparable in their original form.

For PCA and many other methods, we therefore need to transform the numeric values to some common scale in order to make comparisons meaningful. **Centering** means subtracting the mean, so that the mean of the centered data is at the origin. **Scaling** or **standardizing** then means dividing by the standard deviation, so that the new standard deviation is 1. In fact, we have already encountered these operations when computing the correlation coefficient (Equation 7.1): the **correlation coefficient** is simply the vector product of the centered and scaled variables. To perform these operations, there is the R function `scale`, whose default behavior when given a matrix or a dataframe is to make every column have a mean of 0 and a standard deviation of 1.

▶ Question **7.5** (a) Compute the means and standard deviations of the `turtle` data, then use the `scale` function to center and standardize the continuous variables. Call this `scaledTurtles`, then verify the new values for mean and standard deviation of `scaledTurtles`.

(b) Make a scatterplot of the scaled and centered width and height variables of the turtle data and color the points by their sex.   ◀

▶ **Solution 7.5**

```
apply(turtles[,-1], 2, sd)
##    length     width    height
## 20.481602 12.675838  8.392837
apply(turtles[,-1], 2, mean)
##    length     width    height
## 124.68750  95.43750  46.33333
scaledTurtles = scale(turtles[, -1])
apply(scaledTurtles, 2, mean)
##         length         width         height
## -1.432050e-18  1.940383e-17 -2.870967e-16
apply(scaledTurtles, 2, sd)
## length  width height
##      1      1      1
data.frame(scaledTurtles, sex = turtles[, 1]) %>%
  ggplot(aes(x = width, y = height, group = sex)) +
    geom_point(aes(color = sex)) + coord_fixed()
```

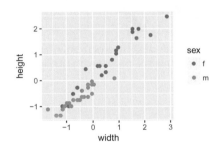

Figure 7.4: Turtles data projected onto the plane defined by the `width` and `height` variables, each point colored according to `sex`.

We have already encountered other data transformation choices in Chapters 4 and 5, where we used the `log` and `asinh` functions. The aim of these transformations is (usually) variance stabilization, i.e., to make the variances of replicate measurements of *one and the same variable* in different parts of its dynamic range more similar. In contrast, the standardizing transformation described above aims to make the scale (as measured by mean and standard deviation) of *different variables* the same.

Sometimes it is preferable to leave variables at different scales because they are truly of different importance. If their original scale is relevant, then we can (and should) leave the data alone. In other cases, the variables have different precisions known a priori. We will see in Chapter 9 that there are several ways of weighting such variables.

After preprocessing the data, we are ready to undertake **data simplification** through **dimension reduction**.

7.3   Dimension reduction

We will explain dimension reduction from several different perspectives. It was invented in 1901 by Karl Pearson (Pearson, 1901) as a way of reducing a two-variable scatterplot to a single coordinate. It was used by statisticians in the 1930s to summarize a battery of psychological tests run on the same subjects (Hotelling, 1933), thus providing overall scores that summarize many test variables at once. This idea of **principal** scores inspired the name principal component analysis (PCA). PCA is called an **unsupervised learning** technique because, as in clustering, it treats all variables as having the same **status**. We are not trying to predict or explain one particular variable's value from the others; rather, we are trying to find a mathematical model for an underlying structure for all the variables. PCA is primarily an exploratory technique that produces maps that show the relations between variables and between observations in a useful way.

We first provide a flavor of what this multivariate analysis does to the data. There is an elegant mathematical formulation of these methods through linear algebra, although here we will try to minimize its use and focus on visualization and data examples.

We use geometric **projections** that take points in higher-dimensional spaces and project them down onto lower dimensions. Figure 7.5 shows the projection of the point *A* onto the line generated by the vector $\boldsymbol{v}$.

PCA is a **linear** technique, meaning that we look for linear relations between variables and that we will use new variables that are linear functions of the original ones $(f(ax + by) = af(x) + b(y))$. The linearity constraint makes computations particularly easy. We will see nonlinear techniques in Chapter 9.

7.3.1   Lower-dimensional projections

Here we show one way of projecting two-dimensional data onto a line, using the `athletes` data. The code below provides the preprocessing and plotting steps that were used to generate Figure 7.6.

```
athletes = data.frame(scale(athletes))
ath_gg = ggplot(athletes, aes(x = weight, y = disc)) +
  geom_point(size = 2, shape = 21)
ath_gg + geom_point(aes(y = 0), colour = "red") +
  geom_segment(aes(xend = weight, yend = 0), linetype = "dashed")
```

Useful books with relevant chapters are Flury (1997) for an introductory account and Mardia et al. (1979) for a detailed mathematical approach.

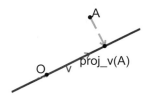

Figure 7.5: Point *A* is projected onto the red line generated by the vector $\boldsymbol{v}$. The dashed projection line is perpendicular (or *orthogonal*) to the red line. The intersection point of the projection line and the red line is called the orthogonal projection of *A* onto the red line generated by the vector $\boldsymbol{v}$.

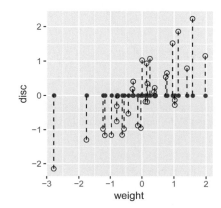

Figure 7.6: Scatterplot of two variables showing the projection on the horizontal *x*-axis (defined by $y = 0$) in red, and the lines of projection appear as dashed.

▶ Task (a) Calculate the variance of the red points in Figure 7.6.
(b) Make a plot showing projection lines onto the y-axis and projected points.
(c) Compute the variance of the points projected onto the vertical y-axis. ◀

7.3.2   How do we summarize two-dimensional data by a line?

In general, we lose information about the points when we project from two dimensions (a plane) onto one (a line). If we do it just by using the original coordinates, as we did on the `weight` variable in Figure 7.6, we lose all the information about the `disc` variable. Our goal is to keep as much information as we can about *both* variables. There are actually many ways of projecting a point cloud onto a line. One is to use what are known as **regression lines**. Let's look at these lines and how they are constructed in R.

Regressing one variable on the other

If you have seen linear regression, you already know how to compute lines that summarize scatterplots; **linear regression** is a **supervised** method that gives preference to minimizing the residual sum of squares in one direction: that of the response variable.

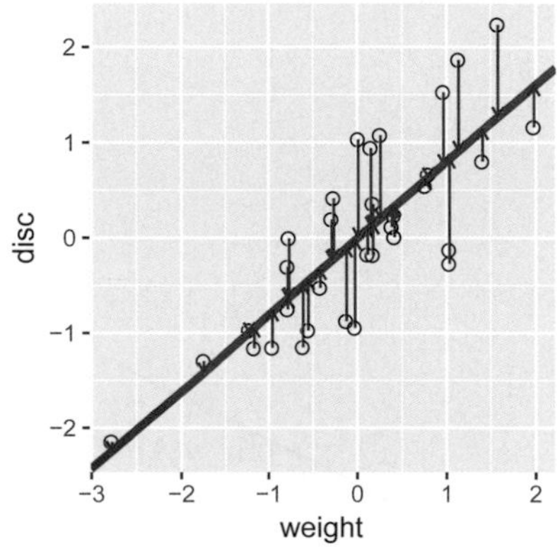

Regression of the `disc` variable on `weight`. In Figure 7.7, we use the `lm` (linear model) function to find the regression line. Its slope and intercept are given by the values in the `coefficients` slot of the resulting object `reg1`.

```
reg1 = lm(disc ~ weight, data = athletes)
a1 = reg1$coefficients[1] # intercept
b1 = reg1$coefficients[2] # slope
pline1 = ath_gg + geom_abline(intercept = a1, slope = b1,
    col = "blue", lwd = 1.5)
pline1 + geom_segment(aes(xend = weight, yend = reg1$fitted),
    colour = "red", arrow = arrow(length = unit(0.15, "cm")))
```

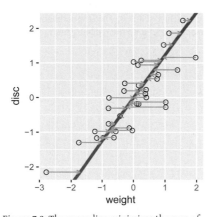

Figure 7.7: The blue line minimizes the sum of squares of the vertical residuals (in red).

Regression of `weight` on `disc`. Figure 7.8 shows the line produced when the roles of the two variables are reversed; `weight` becomes the response variable.

```
reg2 = lm(weight ~ disc, data = athletes)
a2 = reg2$coefficients[1] # intercept
b2 = reg2$coefficients[2] # slope
pline2 = ath_gg + geom_abline(intercept = -a2/b2, slope = 1/b2,
    col = "darkgreen", lwd = 1.5)
pline2 + geom_segment(aes(xend=reg2$fitted, yend=disc),
    colour = "orange", arrow = arrow(length = unit(0.15, "cm")))
```

Figure 7.8: The green line minimizes the sum of squares of the horizontal residuals (in orange).

Each of the regression lines in Figures 7.7 and 7.8 gives us an approximate linear relationship between `disc` and `weight`. However, the relationship differs depending on which variable we choose to be the **predictor** and which the **response**.

▶ Question **7.6** How large is the variance of the projected points that lie on the blue regression line of Figure 7.7? Compare this to the variance of the data when projected on the original axes, `weight` and `disc`. ◀

▶ **Solution 7.6** Pythagoras' theorem tells us that the square of the hypotenuse of a right-angled triangle is equal to the sum of the squares of the other two sides, which we apply as follows.

```
var(athletes$weight) + var(reg1$fitted)
## [1] 1.650204
```

The variances of the points along the original axes `weight` and `disc` are 1, since we scaled the variables.   □

A line that minimizes distances in both directions

Figure 7.9 shows the line chosen to minimize the sum of squares of the orthogonal (perpendicular) projections of data points onto it; we call this the **principal component** line. All of our three ways of fitting a line (Figures 7.7–7.9) together in one plot are shown in Figure 7.10.

```
xy = cbind(athletes$disc, athletes$weight)
svda = svd(xy)
pc = xy %*% svda$v[, 1] %*% t(svda$v[, 1])
bp = svda$v[2, 1] / svda$v[1, 1]
ap = mean(pc[, 2]) - bp * mean(pc[, 1])
ath_gg + geom_segment(xend = pc[, 1], yend = pc[, 2]) +
  geom_abline(intercept = ap, slope = bp, col = "purple", lwd = 1.5)
```

▶ **Question 7.7** (a) What is particular about the slope of the purple line?
(b) Redo the plots on the original (unscaled) variables. What happens?   ◀

▶ **Solution 7.7** The lines computed here depend on the choice of units. Because we have made the standard deviation equal to 1 for both variables, the PCA line is the diagonal that cuts exactly in the middle of both regression lines. Since the data were centered by subtracting their means, the line passes through the origin $(0, 0)$.   □

▶ **Question 7.8** Compute the variance of the points on the purple line.   ◀

▶ **Solution 7.8** We computed the coordinates of the points when we made the plot; these are in the `pc` vector.

```
apply(pc, 2, var)
## [1] 0.9031761 0.9031761
sum(apply(pc, 2, var))
## [1] 1.806352
```

We see that the variance along this axis is larger than the other variances we calculated in Question 7.6.   □

Pythagoras' theorem tells us two interesting things here:

• If we are minimizing in both horizontal and vertical directions, we are in fact minimizing the orthogonal projections onto the line from each point.

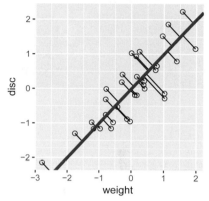

Figure 7.9: The purple **principal component** line minimizes the sums of squares of the orthogonal projections.

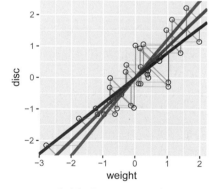

Figure 7.10: The blue line minimizes the sum of squares of the vertical residuals, the green line minimizes the horizontal residuals, the purple line, called the *principal component*, minimizes the orthogonal projections. Notice the ordering of the slopes of the three lines.

- The total variability of the points is measured by the sum of squares of the projection of the points onto the center of gravity, which is the origin (0,0) if the data are centered. This is called the *total variance* or the **inertia** of the point cloud. This inertia can be decomposed into the sum of the squares of the projections onto the line plus the variances along that line. For a fixed variance, minimizing the projection distances also maximizes the variance along that line. Often we define the first principal component as the line with maximum variance.

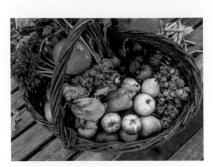

Image credit: Sara Holmes.

7.4   The new linear combinations

The PC line we found in the previous section could be written

$$PC = \frac{1}{2}\text{disc} + \frac{1}{2}\text{weight}. \tag{7.2}$$

Principal components are *linear combinations* of the variables that were originally measured: they provide a *new coordinate system*. To understand what a **linear combination** really is, we can take an analogy. When making a healthy juice mix, you will follow a recipe like

$$V = 2 \times \text{Beet} + 1 \times \text{Carrot} + \frac{1}{2}\text{Gala} + \frac{1}{2}\text{GrannySmith} + 0.02 \times \text{Ginger} + 0.25 \times \text{Lemon}.$$

This recipe is a linear combination of individual juice types (the original variables). The result is a new variable, V, and the coefficients $(2, 1, \frac{1}{2}, \frac{1}{2}, 0.02, 0.25)$ are called the **loadings**.

▶ Question **7.9** How would you compute the calories in a glass of juice?   ◀

7.4.1   Optimal lines

A linear combination of variables defines a line in higher dimensions in the same way we constructed lines in the scatterplot plane of two dimensions. As we saw in that case, there are many ways to choose lines onto which we project the data; there is, however, a "best" line for our purpose.

The total variance of all the points in all the variables can be decomposed. In PCA, we use the fact that the total sums of squares of the distances between the points and any line can be decomposed into the distance to the line and the variance along the line.

We saw that the principal component minimizes the distance to the line, and it also maximizes the variance of the projections along the line.

Why is maximizing the variance along a line a good idea? Let's look at another example of a projection from three dimensions onto two. In fact, human vision depends on such dimension reduction.

Figure 7.11: A mystery silhouette.

▶ Question **7.10** In Figure 7.11, there is a two-dimensional projection of a three-dimensional object. What is the object?   ◀

▶ Question **7.11** Which of the two projections, Figure 7.11 or 7.13, do you find more informative, and why?   ◀

▶ Solution **7.11** One can argue that the projection that maximizes the area of the shadow shows more "information".   □

7.5   The PCA workflow

PCA is based on the principle of finding the axis showing the largest inertia/variability, removing the variability in that direction, and then iterating to find the next best orthogonal axis, and so on. In fact, we do not have to run iterations: all the axes can be found in one operation called the **s**ingular **v**alue **d**ecomposition (we will delve more deeply into the details below).

In the diagram in Figure 7.12, we see that first the means and variances are computed and we have to choose whether or not to work with rescaled covariances – the correlation matrix. Then the next step is the choice of k, the number of components relevant to the data. We say that k is the rank of the approximation we choose; we give below a careful explanation of how we make that choice. Unlike clustering, it is impossible to choose the number of components before doing part of the analysis. The choice of k requires looking at a plot of the variances explained by the successive principal components *before* proceeding to the projections of the data.

The end results of the PCA workflow are useful maps of both the variables and the samples. Understanding how these maps are constructed will maximize the information we can gather from them.

7.6   The inner workings of PCA: rank reduction

This is a small section for those whose background in linear algebra is but a faint memory. It tries to give some intuition to the singular value decomposition method underlying PCA, without too much notation.

The singular value decomposition of a matrix finds horizontal and vertical vectors (called *singular vectors*) and normalizing values (called *singular values*). As before, we start by giving the forward-generative explanation before doing the actual reverse engineering that is used in creating the decomposition. To calibrate the meaning of each step, we will start with an artificial example before moving to the complexity of real data.

7.6.1   Rank-one matrices

A simple generative model demonstrates the meaning of the **rank of a matrix** and explains how we find it in practice. Suppose we have two vectors, $\boldsymbol{u}$ (a one-column matrix)

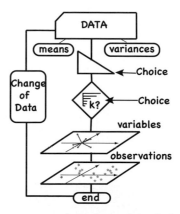

Figure 7.12: Many choices have to be made during PCA processing.

$\boldsymbol{u} = \begin{pmatrix} 1 \\ 2 \\ 3 \\ 4 \end{pmatrix}$ and $\boldsymbol{v} = \begin{pmatrix} 2 \\ 4 \\ 8 \end{pmatrix}$. The transpose of $\boldsymbol{v}$ is written $\boldsymbol{v}^{\mathrm{T}} = t(\boldsymbol{v}) = (2\ 4\ 8)$.

The $(2, 3)$ entry of the matrix X, written $x_{2,3}$, is obtained by multiplying $\boldsymbol{u}_2$ by $\boldsymbol{v}_3$. We can write this

$$X = \begin{pmatrix} 2 & 4 & 8 \\ 4 & 8 & 16 \\ 6 & 12 & 24 \\ 8 & 16 & 32 \end{pmatrix} = \boldsymbol{u} * t(\boldsymbol{v}) = \boldsymbol{u} * \boldsymbol{v}^{\mathrm{T}}.$$

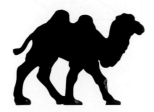

Figure 7.13: Another two-dimensional projection of the same object shown in Figure 7.11. Here, the perspective is more informative. Generally, choosing the perspective such that the spread (in other words, the variance) of the points is maximal provides most information. We want to see as much of the variation as possible: that's what PCA does. Exercise inspired by the cover of Fénelon (1981).

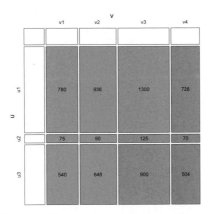

Figure 7.14: Some special matrices have numbers in them that make them easy to decompose. Each colored rectangle in this diagram has an area that corresponds to the number in it.

and $\boldsymbol{v}^{\mathrm{T}} = t(\boldsymbol{v})$ (a one-row matrix – the transpose of a one-column matrix $\boldsymbol{v}$). We multiply a copy of $\boldsymbol{u}$ by each of the elements of $\boldsymbol{v}^{\mathrm{T}}$ in turn as follows.

```
X | 2  4  8      X | 2  4  8      X | 2  4  8      X | 2  4  8
-----------      -----------      ------------     ------------
1 |              1 | 2            1 | 2  4         1 | 2  4  8
2 |              2 | 4            2 | 4  8         2 | 4  8 16
3 |              3 | 6            3 | 6 12         3 | 6 12 24
4 |              4 | 8            4 | 8 16         4 | 8 16 32
Step 0           Step 1          Step 2           Step 3
```

The matrix X we obtain here is said to be of rank 1, because both u and v have one column.

▶ Question 7.12 Why can we say that writing $X = \boldsymbol{u} * \boldsymbol{v}^{\mathrm{T}}$ is more economical than spelling out the full matrix X? ◀

▶ Solution 7.12 X has 12 elements, while in terms of $\boldsymbol{u}$ and $\boldsymbol{v}$ it can be expressed by only seven numbers. □

On the other hand, suppose that we want to reverse the process and simplify another matrix X given below with three rows and four columns (12 numbers). Can we always express it in a similar way as a product of vectors without loss of information? In the diagrams shown in Figures 7.14 and 7.15, the colored boxes have areas proportional to the numbers in the cells of the matrix (7.3).

▶ Question 7.13 Here is a matrix X we want to decompose:

X	$x_{.1}$	$x_{.2}$	$x_{.3}$	$x_{.4}$
$x_{1.}$	780	936	1300	728
$x_{2.}$	75	90	125	70
$x_{3.}$	540	648	900	504

(7.3)

We've redrawn X as a series of rectangles in Figure 7.14. What numbers could we put in the white $\boldsymbol{u}$ and $\boldsymbol{v}$ boxes there so that the values of the sides of the rectangle give the numbers as their product? ◀

A matrix with the special property of being perfectly "rectangular" like X is said to be of rank 1. We can represent the numbers in X by the areas of rectangles, where the sides of rectangles are given by the values in the side vectors ($\boldsymbol{u}$ and $\boldsymbol{v}$).

We see in Figure 7.15 that the decomposition of X is not unique: there are several candidate choices for the vectors $\boldsymbol{u}$ and $\boldsymbol{v}$. We will choose these marginal vectors so that each vector has its coordinates' sum of squares add to 1 (we say the vectors $\boldsymbol{v}$ and $\boldsymbol{u}$ have **norm** 1). Then we have to keep track of one extra number by which to multiply each of the products, which represents the "overall scale" of X. This is the value we have put in the upper left-hand corner. It is called the **singular value** s_1. In the R code below, we start by supposing we know the values in u, v and s1; later we will see a function that finds them for us. Let's check the multiplication and norm properties in R.

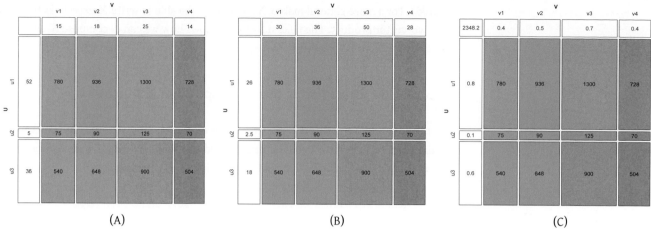

Figure 7.15: The numbers in the cells are equal to the product of the corresponding margins in (A), (B) and (C). We could make the cells from products in several ways. In (C) we force the margins to have norm 1.

```
X = matrix(c(780,    75,  540,
             936,    90,  648,
            1300,   125,  900,
             728,    70,  504), nrow = 3)
u = c(0.8196, 0.0788, 0.5674)
v = c(0.4053, 0.4863, 0.6754, 0.3782)
s1 = 2348.2
sum(u^2)
## [1] 1
sum(v^2)
## [1] 1
s1 * u %*% t(v)
##        [,1] [,2] [,3] [,4]
## [1,]   780  936 1300  728
## [2,]    75   90  125   70
## [3,]   540  648  900  504
X - s1 * u %*% t(v)
##            [,1]    [,2]   [,3]   [,4]
## [1,] -0.03419  0.0745 0.1355 0.1221
## [2,]  0.00403  0.0159 0.0252 0.0186
## [3,] -0.00903  0.0691 0.1182 0.0982
```

▶ Question **7.14** Try `svd(X)` in R. Look at the components of the output of the `svd` function carefully. Check the norm of the columns of the matrices that result from this call. Where did the above value of `s1` = 2348.2 come from?   ◀

▶ **Solution 7.14**

```
svd(X)$u[, 1]
svd(X)$v[, 1]
sum(svd(X)$u[, 1]^2)
sum(svd(X)$v[, 1]^2)
svd(X)$d
```

In fact, in this particular case we were lucky: we see that the second and third singular values are 0 (up to the numeric precision we care about). That is why we say that X is of

rank 1. For a more general matrix X, it is rare to be able to write X exactly as this type of two-vector product. The next subsection shows how we can decompose X when it is not of rank 1: we will just need more pieces.

7.6.2   How do we find such a decomposition in a unique way?

In the above decomposition, there were three elements: the horizontal and vertical singular vectors, and the diagonal corner, called the singular value. These can be found using the singular value decomposition function (svd). For instance:

```
Xtwo = matrix(c(12.5, 35.0, 25.0, 25, 9, 14, 26, 18, 16, 21, 49, 32,
       18, 28, 52, 36, 18, 10.5, 64.5, 36), ncol = 4, byrow = TRUE)
USV = svd(Xtwo)
```

▶ Question **7.15** Look at the USV object, the result of calling the svd function. What are its components?   ◀

▶ Solution **7.15**

```
names(USV)

## [1] "d" "u" "v"

USV$d

## [1] 1.350624e+02 2.805191e+01 3.103005e-15 1.849559e-15
```

So 135.1 is the first singular value USV$d[1].   □

▶ Question **7.16** Check how each successive pair of singular vectors improves our approximation to Xtwo. What do you notice about the third and fourth singular values?

◀

▶ Solution **7.16**

```
Xtwo - USV$d[1] * USV$u[, 1] %*% t(USV$v[, 1])
Xtwo - USV$d[1] * USV$u[, 1] %*% t(USV$v[, 1]) -
       USV$d[2] * USV$u[, 2] %*% t(USV$v[, 2])
```

The third and fourth singular values are so small that they do not improve the approximation, so we can conclude that Xtwo is of rank 2.   □

Again, there are many ways to write a rank-2 matrix such as Xtwo as a sum of rank-1 matrices; in order to ensure uniqueness, we impose yet another[7] condition on the singular vectors. The output vectors of the singular decomposition do not only have their norms equal to 1: each vector in the U matrix is orthogonal to all the previous ones. Ditto for the V matrix. The expression $u_{\bullet 1} \perp u_{\bullet 2}$ means that the sum of the products of the values in the same positions is 0: $\sum_i u_{i1} u_{i2} = 0$.

▶ Task Check the *orthonormality* by computing the crossproduct of the U and V matrices.

```
t(USV$u) %*% USV$u
t(USV$v) %*% USV$v
```
◀

Let's submit our rescaled turtles matrix to a singular value decomposition.

[7] Above, we chose the norm of the vectors to be 1.

```
turtles.svd = svd(scaledTurtles)
turtles.svd$d
## [1] 11.746475  1.419035  1.003329
turtles.svd$v
##              [,1]        [,2]         [,3]
## [1,] 0.5787981 -0.3250273 -0.74789704
## [2,] 0.5779840 -0.4834699  0.65741263
## [3,] 0.5752628  0.8127817  0.09197088
dim(turtles.svd$u)
## [1] 48  3
```

▶ Question **7.17** What can you conclude about the `turtles` matrix from the `svd` output?   ◀

▶ Solution **7.17** The first column of `turtles.svd$v` shows that the coefficients for the three variables are practically equal. Other noticeable "coincidences" include:

```
sum(turtles.svd$v[,1]^2)
## [1] 1
sum(turtles.svd$d^2) / 47
## [1] 3
```

We see that the coefficients are in fact $\sqrt{1/3}$ and the sum of squares of the singular values is equal to $(n - 1) \times p$.   □

7.6.3   Singular value decomposition

We decompose X additively into rank-1 pieces. Each of the u vectors is combined into the U matrix, and each of the v vectors into V. The *singular value decomposition* is

$$X = USV^{\mathrm{T}}, \qquad V^{\mathrm{T}}V = \mathbb{I}, \qquad U^{\mathrm{T}}U = \mathbb{I}, \tag{7.4}$$

where S is the diagonal matrix of singular values, V^{T} is the transpose of V and $\mathbb{I}$ is the identity matrix. Expression (7.4) can be written element-wise as

$$X_{ij} = u_{i1}s_1v_{1j} + u_{i2}s_2v_{2j} + u_{i3}s_3v_{3j} + \cdots + u_{ir}s_rv_{rj}.$$

We say U and V are **orthonormal**,[8] because their self-crossproducts are the identity matrix.

[8] Nothing to do with the normal distribution; it stands for orthogonal and having norm 1.

7.6.4   Principal components

The singular vectors from the singular value decomposition (provided by the `svd` function in R) contain the coefficients to put in front of the original variables to make the more informative ones we call the principal components. We write this as

$$Z_1 = c_1 X_{\bullet 1} + c_2 X_{\bullet 2} + c_3 X_{\bullet 3} + \cdots + c_p X_{\bullet p}.$$

If `usv = svd(X)`, then $(c_1, c_2, c_3, \ldots)$ will be given by the first column of `usv$v`. These new variables $Z_1, Z_2, Z_3, \ldots$ will have variances that decrease in size: $s_1^2 \geqslant s_2^2 \geqslant s_3^2 \geqslant \cdots$.

▶ Question **7.18** Compute the first principal component for the turtles data by multiplying by the first singular value `usv$d[1]` by `usv$u[,1]`.
What is another way of computing it?   ◀

▶ Solution **7.18** We show this using the code:

```
turtles.svd$d[1] %*% turtles.svd$u[,1]
scaledTurtles %*% turtles.svd$v[,1]
```

Matrix manipulations can also show that XV and US are the same: remember that V is orthogonal, so $V^\mathsf{T} V = \mathbb{I}$ and $XV = USV^\mathsf{T} V = US\mathbb{I}$.   □

Note. If you feel lost about which output matrices we are dealing with, remember the dimension of the principal components: each $C = (c_1, c_2, \ldots, c_p)$ is of length n, the number of observations, which is also the number of rows of each of the vectors $X_{\bullet 1}, X_{\bullet 2}, \ldots, X_{\bullet p}$.

Here are two useful facts, first in words, then with the mathematical shorthand.

The number of principal components k is always chosen to be less than the number of original variables or the number of observations. We are "lowering" the dimension of the problem:

$$k \leqslant \min(n, p).$$

The principal component transformation is defined so that the first principal component has the largest possible variance (that is, accounts for as much of the variability in the data as possible), and each successive component in turn has the highest variance possible under the constraint that it be orthogonal to the preceding components:

$$\max_{aX \perp bX} \mathrm{var}(\mathrm{Proj}_{aX}(X)), \qquad \text{where } bX = \text{previous components.}$$

7.7   Plotting the observations in the principal plane

We revisit our two-variable athletes data with the `disc` and `weight` variables. In Section 7.3.2, we computed the first principal component and represented it as the purple line in Figure 7.10. We showed that Z_1 was the linear combination given by the diagonal. As the coefficients have to have their sum of squares add to 1, we have that

```
Z1 = -0.707*athletes$disc -0.707*athletes$weight.
```

This is the same as if the two coordinates were $c_1 = 0.7071$ and $c_2 = 0.7071$.

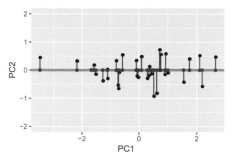 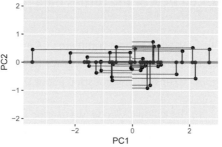

Figure 7.16: In the case where we only have two original variables, the PCA transformation is a simple rotation; the new coordinates are always chosen to be the horizontal and vertical axes.

▶ Question **7.19** What part of the output of the `svd` functions leads us to the first PC coefficients, also known as the PC **loadings**?   ◀

▶ Solution **7.19**

```
svda$v[,1]
## [1] -0.7071068 -0.7071068
```

We use `svda`, which is the svd applied to the two variables `disc` and `weight`.

If we rotate the `(disc,weight)` plane, making the purple line the horizontal *x*-axis, we obtain what is know as the first **principal plane**.

```
ppdf = tibble(PC1n = -svda$u[, 1] * svda$d[1],
              PC2n = svda$u[, 2] * svda$d[2])
ggplot(ppdf, aes(x = PC1n, y = PC2n)) + geom_point() + xlab("PC1 ")+
    ylab("PC2") + geom_point(aes(x=PC1n,y=0),color="red") +
    geom_segment(aes(xend = PC1n, yend = 0), color = "red") +
    geom_hline(yintercept = 0, color = "purple", lwd=1.5, alpha=0.5)+
    xlim(-3.5, 2.7) + ylim(-2,2) + coord_fixed()
```

▶ Question **7.20** (a) What is the mean of the sums of squares of the red segments in Figure 7.16 equal to?

(b) How does this compare to the variance of the red points?

(c) Compute the ratio of the standard deviation of the red segments to the blue segments in Figure 7.16. Compare this to the ratio of singular values 1 and 2.   ◀

▶ Solution **7.20** (a) The mean sum of squares of the red segments corresponds to the square of the second singular value.

```
svda$d[2]^2
## [1] 6.196729
```

(b) The variance of the red points is `var(ppdf$PC1n)`, which is larger than the number calculated in (a) by design of the first PC.

(c) We take the ratios of the standard deviations explained by the points on the vertical and horizontal axes by computing:

```
sd(ppdf$PC1n)/sd(ppdf$PC2n)
svda$d[1]/svda$d[2]
```

▶ Task Use `prcomp` to compute the PCA of the first two columns of the athletes data; look at the output. Compare to the singular value decomposition.   ◀

7.7.1   PCA of the turtles data

We now want to do a complete PCA analysis on the turtles data. Remember, we already looked at the summary statistics for the one- and two-dimensional data. Now we are going to answer the question about the "true" dimensionality of these rescaled data.

In the following code, we use the function `princomp`. Its return value is a list of all the important pieces of information needed to plot and interpret a PCA.

```
cor(scaledTurtles)
##          length     width    height
## length 1.0000000 0.9783116 0.9646946
## width  0.9783116 1.0000000 0.9605705
## height 0.9646946 0.9605705 1.0000000
pcaturtles = princomp(scaledTurtles)
pcaturtles
## Call:
## princomp(x = scaledTurtles)
##
## Standard deviations:
##    Comp.1    Comp.2    Comp.3
## 1.6954576 0.2048201 0.1448180
##
## 3  variables and  48 observations.
library("factoextra")
fviz_eig(pcaturtles, geom = "bar", bar_width = 0.4) + ggtitle("")
```

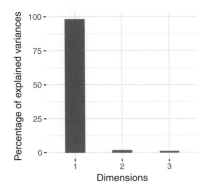

Figure 7.17: The screeplot shows the eigenvalues for the standardized turtles data (`scaledTurtles`): there are one large value and two small ones. The data are (almost) one-dimensional. We will see why this dimension is called an axis of size, a frequent phenomenon in biometric data (Jolicoeur et al., 1960).

> ▶ **Question 7.21** Many PCA functions have been created by different teams working in different areas at different times. This can lead to confusion, especially because they have different naming conventions. Let's compare three of them. Run the following lines of code and look at the resulting objects.

```
svd(scaledTurtles)$v[, 1]
prcomp(turtles[, -1])$rotation[, 1]
princomp(scaledTurtles)$loadings[, 1]
dudi.pca(turtles[, -1], nf = 2, scannf = FALSE)$c1[, 1]
```

What happens when you disable the scaling in the `prcomp` and `princomp` functions?   ◀

In fact, PCA is such a fundamental technique that there are many different implementations of it in various R packages. Unfortunately, the input arguments and the formatting and naming of their output is not standardized, and some even use different conventions for the *scaling* of their output. We will experiment with several different ones to familiarize ourselves with these choices.

Figure 7.18: A biplot of the first two dimensions showing both variables and observations. The arrows show the variables. The turtles are labeled by sex. The extended horizontal direction is due to the size of the first eigenvalue, which is much larger than the second.

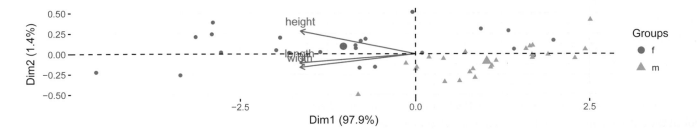

In what follows, we always suppose that the matrix X represents the centered and scaled matrix.

▶ Question **7.22** The coordinates of the observations in the new variables from the `prcomp` function (call it `res`) are in the `scores` slot of the result. Take a look at PC1 for `turtles` and compare it to `res$scores`. Compare the standard deviation `sd1` to that in the `res` object and to that of the scores.   ◀

▶ **Solution 7.22**

```
res = princomp(scaledTurtles)
PC1 = scaledTurtles %*% res$loadings[,1]
sd1 = sqrt(mean(res$scores[, 1]^2))                                    □
```

▶ Question **7.23** Check the orthogonality of the `res$scores` matrix. Why can't we say that it is orthonormal?   ◀

Now we are going to combine both the PC scores (US) and the loadings coefficients (V). The plots with both the samples and the variables represented are called **biplots**. This can be done in one line using the following *factoextra* package function.

```
fviz_pca_biplot(pcaturtles, label = "var", habillage = turtles[, 1]) +
   ggtitle("")
```

▶ Question **7.24** Is it possible to have a PCA plot with the PC1 as the horizontal axis whose height is longer than its width?   ◀

▶ **Solution 7.24** The variance of points in the PC1 direction is $\lambda_1 = s_1^2$, which is always larger than $\lambda_2 = s_2^2$, so the PCA plot will always be wider than high.   □

▶ Question **7.25** Looking at Figure 7.18: (a) Did the male or female turtles tend to be larger?
(b) What do the arrows tell us about the correlations?   ◀

▶ Question **7.26** Compare the variance of each new coordinate to the eigenvalues returned by the PCA `dudi.pca` function.   ◀

▶ **Solution 7.26**

```
pcadudit = dudi.pca(scaledTurtles, nf = 2, scannf = FALSE)
apply(pcadudit$li, 2, function(x) sum(x^2)/48)

##       Axis1        Axis2
## 2.93573765 0.04284387

pcadudit$eig

## [1] 2.93573765 0.04284387 0.02141848                                   □
```

Now we look at the relationships between the variables, both old and new, by drawing what is known as the correlation circle. The aspect ratio is 1 here and the variables are represented by arrows, as shown in Figure 7.19. The lengths of the arrows indicate the quality of the projections onto the first principal plane.

```
fviz_pca_var(pcaturtles, col.circle = "black") + ggtitle("") +
   xlim(c(-1.2, 1.2)) + ylim(c(-1.2, 1.2))
```

Beware the aspect ratio when plotting a PCA. It is rare to have two components with similar norm, so square-shaped plots will be the exception. More common are elongated plots, which show that the horizontal (first) principal component is more important than the second. This matters, e.g., for interpreting distances between points in the plots.

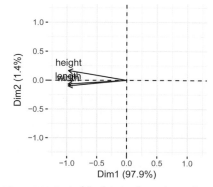

Figure 7.19: Part of the "circle of correlations" showing the original variables. Their *correlations* with each other and with the new principal components are given by the angles between the vectors and between the axes and the vectors.

The first column is just $c_1 = s_1 u_1$. Note that $||c_1||^2 = s_1^T u_1^T u_1 s_1 = s_1^2 u_1^T u_1 = s_1^2 = \lambda_1$.
Keep in mind: $X^T C = V S U^T U S = V S^2$.

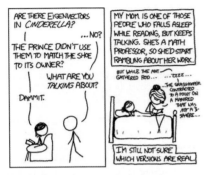

Figure 7.20: Another great xkcd take: this time eigenvectors. Image credit: xkcd.com.

eigen-decomposition
The crossproduct of X with itself satisfies

$$X^T X = V S U^T U S V^T = V S^2 V^T = V \Lambda V^T,$$

where V is called the eigenvector matrix of the symmetric matrix $X^T X$ and Λ is the diagonal matrix of eigenvalues of $X^T X$.

[9] This sum of the diagonal elements is called the **trace** of the matrix.

For help with the basics of linear algebra, a motivated student pressed for time may consult the Khan Academy. If you have more time and would like in-depth coverage, *Gil Strang's MIT course* is a classic and some of the book is available online (Strang, 2009).

▶ **Question 7.27** Explain the relationships between the number of rows of our turtles data matrix and the following numbers.

```
svd(scaledTurtles)$d/pcaturtles$sdev
sqrt(47)
```
◀

▶ **Solution 7.27** When computing the variance-covariance matrix, many implementations use $1/(n-1)$ as the denominator. Here, $n = 48$, so the sum of the variances is off by a factor of 48/47. □

These data are a good example of how sometimes almost all the variation in the data can be captured in a lower-dimensional space: here, three-dimensional data can be essentially replaced by a line. The **principal components** are the columns of the matrix $C = US$. The p columns of U (the matrix given as USV\$u in the output from the svd function above) are rescaled to have norms $(s_1^2, s_2^2, \ldots, s_p^2)$. Each column has a different variance it is responsible for explaining. Notice that these will be decreasing numbers.

If the matrix X comes from the study of n different samples or specimens, then the principal components provide new coordinates for these n points, as in Figure 7.16. These are sometimes called the scores in the results of PCA functions.

Before we go into more detailed examples, let's summarize what SVD and PCA provide:

- Each principal component has a variance measured by the corresponding eigenvalue, the square of the corresponding singular value.
- The new variables are made to be orthogonal. Since they are also centered, this means they are uncorrelated. In the case of normal distributed data, this also means they are independent.
- When the variables are rescaled, the sum of the variances of all the variables is the number of variables (i.e., p). The sum of the variances is computed by adding the diagonal of the crossproduct matrix.[9]
- The principal components are ordered by the size of their eigenvalues. We always check the screeplot before deciding how many components to retain. It is also best practice to do as we did in Figure 7.18 and annotate each PC axis with the proportion of variance it explains.

▶ **Task** Look up *eigenvalue* on Wikipedia.
Try to find a sentence that defines it without using a formula.
Why would eigenvectors come into use in Cinderella (at a stretch)?
(See the cartoon in Figure 7.20.) ◀

7.7.2 A complete analysis: the decathlon athletes

We looked briefly at part of this data earlier in the chapter; here we will follow, step by step, a complete multivariate analysis. First we take a second look at the rounded correlation matrix capturing the essentials of the bivariate associations. These correlations are represented with colors in Figure 7.3.

```
cor(athletes) %>% round(1)
##           m100 long weight highj m400 m110 disc pole javel m1500
## m100       1.0 -0.5   -0.2  -0.1  0.6  0.6  0.0 -0.4  -0.1   0.3
## long      -0.5  1.0    0.1   0.3 -0.5 -0.5  0.0  0.3   0.2  -0.4
## weight    -0.2  0.1    1.0   0.1  0.1 -0.3  0.8  0.5   0.6   0.3
## highj     -0.1  0.3    0.1   1.0 -0.1 -0.3  0.1  0.2   0.1  -0.1
## m400       0.6 -0.5    0.1  -0.1  1.0  0.5  0.1 -0.3   0.1   0.6
## m110       0.6 -0.5   -0.3  -0.3  0.5  1.0 -0.1 -0.5  -0.1   0.1
## disc       0.0  0.0    0.8   0.1  0.1 -0.1  1.0  0.3   0.4   0.4
## pole      -0.4  0.3    0.5   0.2 -0.3 -0.5  0.3  1.0   0.3   0.0
## javel     -0.1  0.2    0.6   0.1  0.1 -0.1  0.4  0.3   1.0   0.1
## m1500      0.3 -0.4    0.3  -0.1  0.6  0.1  0.4  0.0   0.1   1.0
```

Then we start looking at the screeplot, which will help us choose a rank k for these data.

```
pca.ath = dudi.pca(athletes, scannf = FALSE)
pca.ath$eig
##  [1] 3.4182381 2.6063931 0.9432964 0.8780212 0.5566267 0.4912275
##  [7] 0.4305952 0.3067981 0.2669494 0.1018542
fviz_eig(pca.ath, geom = "bar", bar_width = 0.3) + ggtitle("")
```

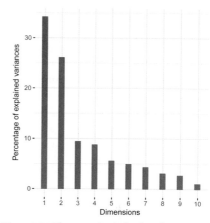

Figure 7.21: The screeplot is the first thing to consult. It tells us that it's satisfactory to use a two-dimensional plot.

Figure 7.21 shows that eigenvalues in the screeplot make a clear drop after the second eigenvalue. This indicates that a good approximation will be obtained at rank 2. Let's look at an interpretation of the first two axes by projecting the loadings of the original (old) variables as they project onto the two new ones.

```
fviz_pca_var(pca.ath, col.circle = "black") + ggtitle("")
```

The correlation circle in Figure 7.22 displays the projection of the original variables onto the two first new principal axes. The angles between vectors are interpreted as correlations. On the right-hand side of the plane, we have the track events (m110, m100, m400, m1500), and on the left, we have the throwing and jumping events. Maybe there is an opposition of skills as characterized in the correlation matrix. We did see that the correlations were negative between variables from these two groups. How can we interpret this?

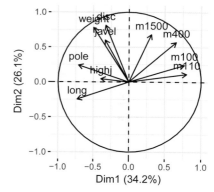

Figure 7.22: Correlation circle of the original variables.

It seems that those who throw the best have lower scores in the track competitions. In fact, if we look at the original measurements, we can see what is happening. The athletes who run faster times are the stronger ones, as are the athletes who throw or jump farther. We should probably change the scores of the track variables and redo the analysis.

▶ Question 7.28 What transformations of the variables induce the best athletic performances to vary in the same direction, i.e., be mostly positively correlated?   ◀

▶ Solution 7.28 If we change the signs on the running performances, almost all the variables will be positively correlated.

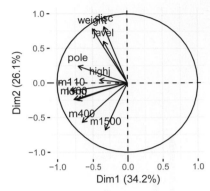

Figure 7.23: Correlation circle after changing the signs of the running variables.

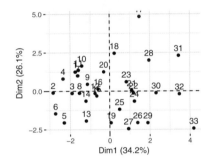

Figure 7.24: First principal plane showing the projections of the athletes. Do you notice something about the organization of the numbers?

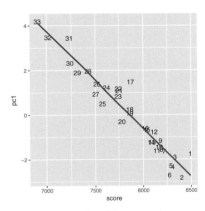

Figure 7.25: Scatterplot of the scores given as a supplementary variable and the first principal component. The points are labeled by their order in the dataset. We can see a very strong correlation between this supplementary score variable and the first principal coordinate – why is it not a perfectly linear fit?

```
athletes[, c(1, 5, 6, 10)] = -athletes[, c(1, 5, 6, 10)]
cor(athletes) %>% round(1)
##            m100 long weight highj m400 m110 disc pole javel m1500
## m100        1.0  0.5    0.2   0.1  0.6  0.6  0.0  0.4   0.1   0.3
## long        0.5  1.0    0.1   0.3  0.5  0.5  0.0  0.3   0.2   0.4
## weight      0.2  0.1    1.0   0.1 -0.1  0.3  0.8  0.5   0.6  -0.3
## highj       0.1  0.3    0.1   1.0  0.1  0.3  0.1  0.2   0.1   0.1
## m400        0.6  0.5   -0.1   0.1  1.0  0.5 -0.1  0.3  -0.1   0.6
## m110        0.6  0.5    0.3   0.3  0.5  1.0  0.1  0.5   0.1   0.1
## disc        0.0  0.0    0.8   0.1 -0.1  0.1  1.0  0.3   0.4  -0.4
## pole        0.4  0.3    0.5   0.2  0.3  0.5  0.3  1.0   0.3   0.0
## javel       0.1  0.2    0.6   0.1 -0.1  0.1  0.4  0.3   1.0  -0.1
## m1500       0.3  0.4   -0.3   0.1  0.6  0.1 -0.4  0.0  -0.1   1.0
pcan.ath = dudi.pca(athletes, nf = 2, scannf = FALSE)
pcan.ath$eig
##  [1] 3.4182381 2.6063931 0.9432964 0.8780212 0.5566267 0.4912275
##  [7] 0.4305952 0.3067981 0.2669494 0.1018542
fviz_pca_var(pcan.ath, col.circle="black") + ggtitle("")
```

Figure 7.23 shows the correlation circle of the transformed variables. We now see that we have an axis of **size**, and all the arrows are pointing in the same direction.

Now all the negative correlations are quite small. The screeplot will show no change, as the eigenvalues are unchanged. The signs in the coefficients of the PC loadings for the *m* variables are the only output that changes.

We now plot the athletes projected in the first principal plane using:

```
fviz_pca_ind(pcan.ath) + ggtitle("")
```

▶ Question **7.29** If we look at the athletes themselves as they are shown in Figure 7.24, we notice a slight ordering effect. Do you see a relation between the quality of the athletes and their number on the figure? ◀

▶ Solution **7.29** If you play join the dots following the order of the numbers, you will probably realize that you are spending more time on one side of the plot than you would be if the numbers were randomly assigned. □

It turns out that *supplementary information* is available on the olympic data. An extra variable called score is a vector of the final scores at the competition (men's decathlon at the 1988 Olympics).

```
data("olympic", package = "ade4")
olympic$score
##  [1] 8488 8399 8328 8306 8286 8272 8216 8189 8180 8167 8143 8114
## [13] 8093 8083 8036 8021 7869 7860 7859 7781 7753 7745 7743 7623
## [25] 7579 7517 7505 7422 7310 7237 7231 7016 6907
```

We now make the scatterplot comparing the first principal component score of the athletes to this score from the data. This is shown in Figure 7.25; we can see a strong correlation between the two variables. We notice that athlete number 1 (who in fact won the Olympic decathlon gold medal) has the highest score but not the highest value for the PC1 linear combination. Why do you think that is?

7.7.3 How to choose k, the number of dimensions?

We have seen in the examples that the first step in PCA is to make the screeplot of variances of the new variables (equal to the *eigenvalues*). We cannot decide how many dimensions are needed before seeing this plot. The reason is that there are situations when the principal components are ill defined: when two or three successive PCs have very similar variances, giving a screeplot as in Figure 7.26, the subspace corresponding to a group of similar eigenvalues exists. In this case it would be 3D space generated by u_2, u_3, u_4. The vectors are not meaningful individually and one cannot interpret their loadings. This is because a very slight change in one observation could give a completely different set of three vectors. These would generate the same 3D space, but could have very different loadings. We say the PCs are unstable.

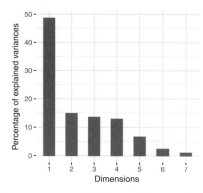

Figure 7.26: A screeplot showing "dangerously" similar variances. Choosing the cutoff at a hard threshold of 80% of the variance would give unstable PC plots. With no such cutoff, the axes corresponding to the 3D subspace of three similar eigenvalues are unstable and cannot be individually interpreted.

7.8 PCA as an exploratory tool: using extra information

We have seen that, unlike regression, PCA treats all variables equally (to the extent that they were preprocessed to have equivalent standard deviations). However, it is still possible to map other continuous variables or categorical factors onto the plots in order to help interpret the results. Often we have **supplementary information** on the samples, for example, diagnostic labels in the diabetes data or cell types in the T-cell gene expression data.

Here we see how we can use such extra variables to inform our interpretation. The best place to store such so-called **metadata** is in appropriate slots of the data object (such as in the Bioconductor *SummarizedExperiment* class); the second best is in additional columns of the data frame that also contains the numeric data. In practice, such information is often stored in a more or less cryptic manner in the row names of the matrix. Below, we need to face the latter scenario; we use `substr` gymnastics to extract the cell types and show the screeplot in Figure 7.27 and the PCA in Figure 7.28.

```
pcaMsig3 = dudi.pca(Msig3transp, center = TRUE, scale = TRUE,
                    scannf = FALSE, nf = 4)
fviz_screeplot(pcaMsig3) + ggtitle("")
```

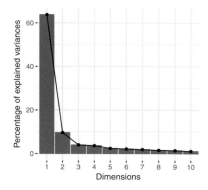

Figure 7.27: T-cell expression PCA screeplot.

```
ids = rownames(Msig3transp)
celltypes = factor(substr(ids, 7, 9))
status = factor(substr(ids, 1, 3))
table(celltypes)
## celltypes
## EFF MEM NAI
##  10   9  11
cbind(pcaMsig3$li, tibble(Cluster = celltypes, sample = ids)) %>%
ggplot(aes(x = Axis1, y = Axis2)) +
  geom_point(aes(color = Cluster), size = 5) +
  geom_hline(yintercept = 0, linetype = 2) +
  geom_vline(xintercept = 0, linetype = 2) +
  scale_color_discrete(name = "Cluster") + coord_fixed()
```

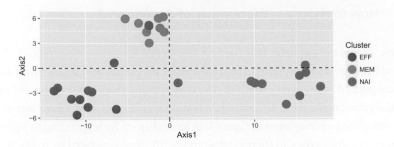

Figure 7.28: PCA of gene expression for a subset of 156 genes involved in specificities of each of the three T-cell types: effector, naive and memory. Again, we see that the plot is elongated along the the first axis, as that explains much of the variance. Notice that one of the T cells seems to be mislabeled.

7.8.1   Mass spectroscopy data analysis

These data require delicate preprocessing before we can obtain our desired matrix with the relevant features as columns and the samples as rows. Starting with the raw mass spectroscopy readings, the steps involve extracting peaks of relevant features, aligning them across multiple samples and estimating peak heights. We refer the reader to the vignette of the Bioconductor *xcms* package for gruesome details. We load a matrix of data generated in such a way from the file `mat1xcms.RData`. The output of the code below is shown in Figures 7.29 and 7.30.

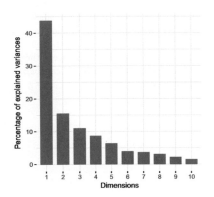

Figure 7.29: Screeplot showing the eigenvalues for the mice data.

```
load("../data/mat1xcms.RData")
dim(mat1)

## [1] 399  12

pcamat1 = dudi.pca(t(mat1), scannf = FALSE, nf = 3)
fviz_eig(pcamat1, geom = "bar", bar_width = 0.7) + ggtitle("")
```

```
dfmat1 = cbind(pcamat1$li, tibble(
    label = rownames(pcamat1$li),
    number = substr(label, 3, 4),
    type = factor(substr(label, 1, 2))))
pcsplot = ggplot(dfmat1,
  aes(x=Axis1, y=Axis2, label=label, group=number, colour=type)) +
  geom_text(size = 4, vjust = -0.5) + geom_point(size = 3)
pcsplot + geom_hline(yintercept = 0, linetype = 2) +
  geom_vline(xintercept = 0, linetype = 2)
```

▶ Question **7.30** Looking at Figure 7.30, do the samples seem to be randomly placed in the plane? Do you notice any structure explained by the labels?   ◀

▶ Solution **7.30** The answer becomes (even more) evident if you make this plot:

```
pcsplot + geom_line(colour = "red")
```

Knockouts are always below their paired wild-type samples. We will revisit this example when we look at supervised multivariate methods in the next chapter.   □

7.8.2   Biplots and scaling

In the mass spectroscopy example, the number of variables measured was too large to enable useful concurrent plotting of both variables and samples. In this example we plot the PCA biplot of a simple dataset where chemical measurements were made on

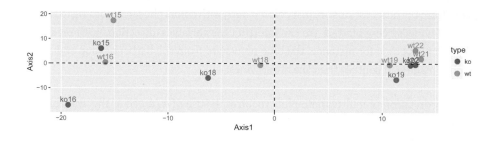

Figure 7.30: The first principal plane for the `mat1` data. It explains 59% of the variance.

different wines for which we also have a categorical `wine.class` variable. We start the analysis by looking at the two-dimensional correlations and a heatmap of the variables.

```
library("pheatmap")
load("../data/wine.RData")
load("../data/wineClass.RData")
wine[1:2, 1:7]

##   Alcohol MalicAcid  Ash AlcAsh  Mg Phenols Flav
## 1   14.23      1.71 2.43   15.6 127    2.80 3.06
## 2   13.20      1.78 2.14   11.2 100    2.65 2.76

pheatmap(1 - cor(wine), treeheight_row = 0.2)
```

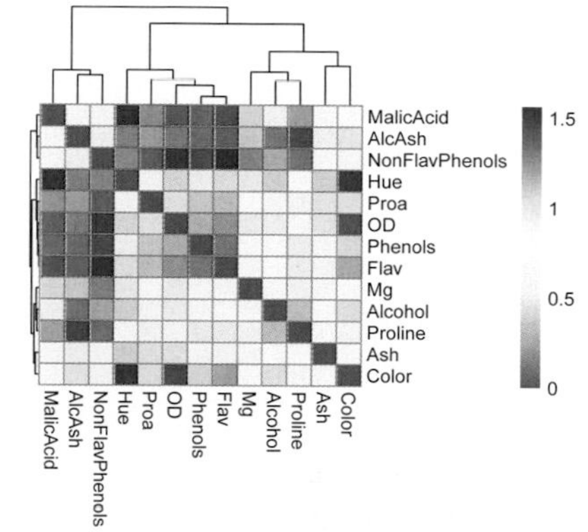

```
winePCAd = dudi.pca(wine, scannf=FALSE)
table(wine.class)

## wine.class
##    barolo grignolino    barbera
##        59         71         48

fviz_pca_biplot(winePCAd, geom = "point", habillage = wine.class,
  col.var = "violet", addEllipses = TRUE, ellipse.level = 0.69) +
  ggtitle("") + coord_fixed()
```

Figure 7.31: The difference between 1 and the correlation can be used as a *distance* between variables and is used to make a heatmap of the associations between the variables.

A **biplot** is a simultaneous representation of both the space of observations and the space of variables. In the case of a PCA biplot as in Figure 7.32, the arrows represent the directions of the old variables as they project onto the plane defined by the first two new

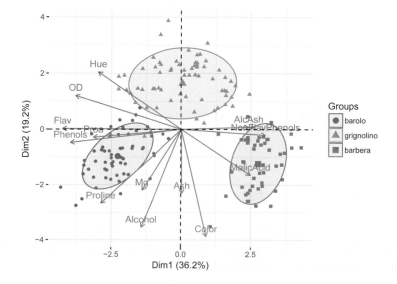

Figure 7.32: PCA biplot including ellipses for the three types of wine: barolo, grignolino and barbera. For each ellipsis, the axis lengths are given by one standard deviation. Small angles between the vectors `Phenols`, `Flav` and `Proa` indicate that they are strongly correlated, whereas `Hue` and `Alcohol` are uncorrelated.

axes. Here the observations are just colored dots, with colors chosen according to which type of wine is being plotted. We can interpret the variables' directions with regard to the sample points; for instance, the blue points are from the barbera group and show higher malic acid content than the other wines.

Interpretation of multivariate plots requires the use of as much of the available information as possible; here we used the samples and their groups as well as the variables to understand the main differences between the wines.

7.8.3   An example of weighted PCA

Sometimes we want to see variability between different groups of observations but want to weight them. This can be the case if, e.g., the groups have very different sizes. Let's re-examine the Hiiragi data we saw in Chapter 3 (Ohnishi et al., 2014). In the code below, we select the wild-type (WT) samples and the top 100 features with the highest overall variance.

```
data("x", package = "Hiiragi2013")
xwt = x[, x$genotype == "WT"]
sel = order(rowVars(exprs(xwt)), decreasing = TRUE)[1:100]
xwt = xwt[sel, ]
tab = table(xwt$sampleGroup)
tab

##
##     E3.25 E3.5 (EPI)  E3.5 (PE) E4.5 (EPI)  E4.5 (PE)
##        36         11         11          4          4
```

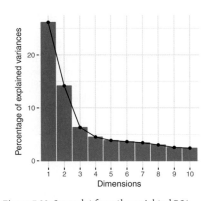

Figure 7.33: Screeplot from the weighted PCA of the Hiiragi data. The drop after the second eigenvalue suggests that a two-dimensional PCA is appropriate.

We see from `tab` that the groups are represented rather unequally. To account for this, we reweigh each sample by the inverse of its group size. The function `dudi.pca` in the *ade4* package has a `row.w` argument into which we can enter the weights. The output of the below code is shown in Figures 7.33 and 7.34.

```
xwt$weight = 1 / as.numeric(tab[xwt$sampleGroup])
pcaMouse = dudi.pca(as.data.frame(t(exprs(xwt))),
  row.w = xwt$weight,
  center = TRUE, scale = TRUE, nf = 2, scannf = FALSE)
fviz_eig(pcaMouse) + ggtitle("")
```

```
fviz_pca_ind(pcaMouse, geom = "point", col.ind = xwt$sampleGroup) +
  ggtitle("") + coord_fixed()
```

7.9   Summary of this chapter

Preprocessing matrices Multivariate data analyses require "conscious" preprocessing. After consulting all the means, variances and one-dimensional histograms, we saw how to rescale and recenter the data.

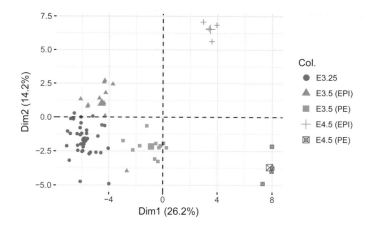

Figure 7.34: Output from weighted PCA on the Hiiragi data. The samples are colored according to their groups.

Projecting onto new variables We saw how we can make projections on lower dimensions (planes and 3D are the most frequently used) of very high-dimensional data without losing too much information. PCA searches for new "more informative" variables that are linear combinations of the original (old) ones.

Matrix decomposition PCA is based on finding a decomposition, called SVD, of the matrix X. This decomposition provides lower rank approximation and is equivalent to the eigenanalysis of $X^\mathsf{T}X$. The squares of the singular values are equal to the eigenvalues and to the variances of the new variables. We systematically plot these values before deciding how many axes are necessary to reproduce the signal in the data.

Two eigenvalues that are quite close can give rise to scores or PC scores which are highly unstable. It is always necessary to look at the screeplot of the eigenvalues and avoid separating the axes corresponding to these close eigenvalues. This may require using interactive three- or four-dimensional projections, which are available in several R packages.

Biplot representations The space of observations is naturally a p-dimensional space (the p original variables provide the coordinates). The space of variables is n-dimensional. Both decompositions we have studied (singular values/eigenvalues and singular vectors/eigenvectors) provide new coordinates for both of these spaces: sometimes we call one the dual of the other. We can plot the projections of both the observations and the variables onto the same eigenvectors. This provides a biplot that can be useful for interpreting the PCA output.

Projecting other group variables Interpretation of PCA can also be facilitated by redundant or contiguous data about the observations.

7.10 Further reading

The best way to deepen your understanding of singular value decomposition is to read Chapter 7 of Strang (2009). The whole book sets the foundation for the linear algebra necessary to understand the meaning of the rank of a matrix and the duality between row spaces and column spaces (Holmes, 2006).

Complete textbooks have been written on the subject of PCA and related methods.

Mardia et al. (1979) is a standard text that covers all multivariate methods in a classical way, with linear algebra and matrices. By making the parametric assumption that the data come from multivariate normal distributions, Mardia et al. (1979) also provide inferential tests for the number of components and limiting properties for principal components. Jolliffe (2002) is a book-length treatment of everything to do with PCA, with extensive examples.

We can incorporate supplementary information into weights for the observations and the variables. This technique was introduced in the 1970s by French data scientists; see Holmes (2006) for a review and Chapter 9 for further examples.

Improvements to the interpretation and stability of PCA can be obtained by adding a penalty that minimizes the number of non-zero coefficients that appear in the linear combinations. Zou et al. (2006) and Witten et al. (2009) have developed sparse versions of principal components, and their packages *elasticnet* and *PMA* provide implementations in R.

7.11   Exercises

▶ Exercise **7.1** Review the basics of SVD by reading Sections 1, 2 and 3 of the Wikipedia article on *singular value decomposition*. It will also be beneficial to read about the related eigenvalue decomposition by reading Sections 1, 2 and 2.1 of the Wikipedia article about *eigendecomposition of a matrix*. We know that we can decompose an n-row by p-column rank-1 matrix X as

$$X = \begin{pmatrix} x_{11} & x_{12} & \cdots & x_{1p} \\ x_{21} & x_{22} & \cdots & x_{2p} \\ \vdots & \vdots & \vdots & \vdots \\ x_{n1} & x_{n2} & \cdots & x_{np} \end{pmatrix} = \begin{pmatrix} u_{11} \\ u_{21} \\ \vdots \\ u_{n1} \end{pmatrix} \times \begin{pmatrix} v_{11} & v_{21} & \cdots & v_{p1} \end{pmatrix}.$$

a. If X has no rows and no columns that are all zeros, then is this decomposition unique?
b. Generate a rank-1 matrix. Start by taking a vector of length 15 with values from 2 to 30 in increments of 2, and a vector of length 4 with values 3, 6, 9, 12. Take their "product".

```
u = seq(2, 30, by = 2)
v = seq(3, 12, by = 3)
X1 = u %*% t(v)
```

Why do we have to take t(v)?
c. Now we add some noise in the form of a matrix we call Materr so we have an "approximately rank-1" matrix.

```
Materr = matrix(rnorm(60,1),nrow=15,ncol=4)
X = X1+Materr
```

Visualize X using ggplot.
d. Redo the same analysis with a rank-2 matrix.   ◀

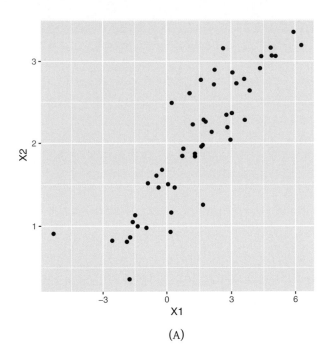

(A)

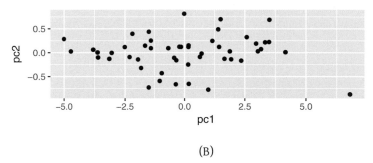

(B)

Figure 7.35: The original data shown in scatterplot (A) and the plot obtained using the principal component rotation (B).

► **Exercise 7.2**

a. Create a matrix of highly correlated bivariate data such as the data shown in Figure 7.35. Hint: use the function `mvrnorm`. Check the rank of the matrix by looking at its singular values.

b. Perform PCA and show the rotated principal component axes. ◄

► **Exercise 7.3** Panel (B) in Figure 7.35 shows a very elongated plotting region – why? What happens if you do not use the `coord_fixed()` option and have a square plotting zone? Why can this be misleading? ◄

► **Exercise 7.4** Let's revisit the Hiiragi data and compare the weighted and unweighted approaches.

a. Make a correlation circle for the unweighted Hiiragi data `xwt`. Which genes have the best projections on the first principal plane (best approximation)?

b. Make a biplot showing the labels of the extreme gene variables that explain most of the variance in the first plane. Add the sample points. ◄

CHAPTER 8

High-Throughput Count Data

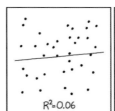 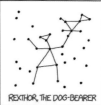

I DON'T TRUST LINEAR REGRESSIONS WHEN IT'S HARDER TO GUESS THE DIRECTION OF THE CORRELATION FROM THE SCATTER PLOT THAN TO FIND NEW CONSTELLATIONS ON IT.

Many measurement devices in biotechnology are based on massively parallel sampling and counting of molecules. One example is high-throughput DNA sequencing. Its applications fall broadly into two main classes of data output. In the first case, the outputs of interest are the sequences themselves, perhaps also their polymorphisms or differences from other sequences seen before. In the second case, the sequences themselves are more or less well understood (if, say, we have a well-assembled and annotated genome) and our interest is is the abundance of different sequence regions in our sample.

For instance, in **RNA-Seq** (Ozsolak and Milos, 2011), we sequence the RNA molecules found in a population of cells or in a tissue. In **ChIP-Seq**, we sequence DNA regions that are bound to particular DNA-binding proteins (selected by immuno-precipitation). In **CLIP-Seq**, we sequence RNA molecules or regions of them bound to a particular RNA-binding protein. In **DNA-Seq**, we sequence genomic DNA and are interested in the prevalence of genetic variants in heterogeneous populations of cells, for instance the clonal composition of a tumor. In high-throughput chromatin conformation capture (HiC) we aim to map the 3D spatial arrangement of DNA. In **genetic screens** (using, say, RNAi or CRISPR-Cas9 libraries for perturbation and high-throughput sequencing for readout), we're interested in the proliferation or survival of cells upon gene knockdown, knockout or modification. In microbiome analysis, we study the abundance of different microbial species in complex microbial habitats.

Ideally, we might want to sequence and count *all* molecules of interest in the sample. Generally this is not possible: the biochemical protocols are not 100% efficient, and some molecules or intermediates get lost along the way. Moreover, it's often also not even necessary. Instead, we sequence and count a *statistical sample*. The sample size will depend on the complexity of the sequence pool assayed; it can go from tens of thousands to billions. This *sampling* nature of the data is important when it comes to analyzing them. We hope that the sampling is sufficiently representative for us to identify interesting trends and patterns.

Strictly speaking, we don't sequence the RNA but rather the complementary DNA (cDNA) obtained from reverse transcription. The pool of all RNA might be reduced to a subset of interest (e.g., messenger RNA) by biochemical means, such as poly-A selection or ribosomal RNA depletion. Sensitive variants of RNA-Seq exist that enable assaying single cells, and large numbers of them.

8.1   Goals of this chapter

In this chapter, we will become familiar with count data in high-throughput sequencing applications such as RNA-Seq. We will understand and model the sampling processes that underlie the data in order to interpret them. Our main aim is to detect and quantify systematic changes between samples from different conditions, say *untreated* versus *treated*, where the task is to distinguish such systematic changes from sampling variations and experimental variability within the same conditions. In order to do this, we will also equip ourselves with a set of needed statistical concepts and tools:

- multifactorial designs, linear models and analysis of variance;
- generalized linear models;
- robustness and outlier detection; and
- shrinkage estimation.

In fact, these concepts have a much wider range of application: they can also be applied to other types of data where we want to detect differences in noisy data as a function of some experimental covariate. In particular, the framework of generalized linear models is quite abstract and generic, but this has the advantage that it can be adapted to many different data types so that we don't need to reinvent the wheel, but rather can immediately enjoy a wide range of associated tools and diagnostics.

As a bonus, we will also look at data transformations that make the data amenable to unsupervised methods such as those we saw in Chapters 5 and 7, and that make it easier to visualize the data.

8.2   Some core concepts

Before we start, let's settle some key terminology.

- A **sequencing library** is the collection of DNA molecules used as input for the sequencing machine.
- **Fragments** are the molecules being sequenced. Since the most widely used current technology[1] can only deal with molecules of length around 300–1000 nucleotides, these are obtained by fragmenting the (generally longer) DNA or cDNA molecules of interest.
- A **read** is the sequence obtained from a fragment. With the current technology, the read covers not the whole fragment, but only one or both ends of it, and the read length on either side is up to around 150 nucleotides.

Between sequencing and counting, there is an important *aggregation* or clustering step, which aggregates sequences that belong together: for instance, all reads belonging to the same gene (in RNA-Seq) or to the same binding region (ChIP-Seq). There are several approaches to this task and choices to be made, depending on the aim of the experiment.[2] The methods include explicit alignment or hash-based mapping to a reference sequence,[3] and reference-independent sequence–similarity-based clustering of the reads – especially if there is no obvious reference, such as in metagenomics and metatranscriptomics. We need to choose whether to consider different alleles or isoforms separately, or to merge them into an equivalence class. For simplicity, we'll use the term *gene* in this chapter for these operational aggregates, even though they can be various things depending on the particular application.

[1] We refer to https://www.illumina.com/techniques/sequencing.html, as of September 2018.

[2] For any particular application, it's best to check the recent literature on the most appropriate approaches and choices.

[3] For example, in the case of RNA-Seq, the genome together with an annotation of its transcripts.

8.3 Count data

Let us load an example dataset. It resides in the experiment data package *pasilla*.

```
fn = system.file("extdata", "pasilla_gene_counts.tsv",
                 package = "pasilla", mustWork = TRUE)
counts = as.matrix(read.csv(fn, sep = "\t", row.names = "gene_id"))
```

The data are stored as a rectangular table in a tab-delimited file, which we've read into the matrix counts.

```
dim(counts)
## [1] 14599      7

counts[ 2000+(0:3), ]
##             untreated1 untreated2 untreated3 untreated4
## FBgn0020369       3387       4295       1315       1853
## FBgn0020370       3186       4305       1824       2094
## FBgn0020371          1          0          1          1
## FBgn0020372         38         84         29         28
##             treated1 treated2 treated3
## FBgn0020369     4884     2133     2165
## FBgn0020370     3525     1973     2120
## FBgn0020371        1        0        0
## FBgn0020372       63       28       27
```

The matrix tallies the number of reads seen for each gene in each sample. We call it the **count table**. It has 14,599 rows, corresponding to the genes, and seven columns, corresponding to the samples. When loading data from a file, a good plausibility check is to print out some of the data, not only from the very beginning, but also from some random point in the middle, as we have done above.

The table is a matrix of integer values: the value in the ith row and jth column of the matrix indicates how many reads have been mapped to gene i in sample j. The statistical sampling models that we discuss in this chapter rely on the fact that the values are the direct "raw" counts of sequencing reads – not some derived quantity, such as normalized counts, counts of covered base pairs or the like, which would only lead to nonsensical results.

8.3.1 The challenges of count data

What are the challenges that we need to overcome with such count data?

- The data have a large **dynamic range**, starting from zero up to millions. The variance and, more generally, the distribution shape of the data in different parts of the dynamic range are very different. We need to take this phenomenon, called **heteroscedasticity**, into account.
- The data are non-negative integers, and their distribution is not symmetric – thus normal or log-normal distribution models may be a poor fit.
- We need to understand the systematic sampling biases and adjust for them. Confusingly, such adjustment is often called **normalization**. Examples are the total

There are important conceptual and practical differences between experiments and studies – see Chapter 13.

[4] Distributions can be parameterized in various ways: often the parameters correspond to some measure of location and some measure of dispersion; a familiar measure of location is the mean, and a familiar measure of dispersion is the variance (or standard deviation), but for some distributions other measures are also in use.

sequencing depth of an experiment (even if the true abundance of a gene in two libraries is the same, we expect different numbers of reads for it depending on the total number of reads sequenced) and differing sampling probabilities (even if the true abundance of two genes within a biological sample is the same, we expect different numbers of reads for them if they have differing biophysical properties, such as length, GC content, secondary structure, binding partners).

- We need to understand the stochastic properties of the sampling, as well as other sources of stochastic experimental variation. For studies with large numbers of biological samples, this is usually straightforward, and we can even fall back on resampling- or permutation-based methods. For designed experiments, however, sample sizes tend to be limited.

For instance, there are four replicates from the *untreated* and three from the *treated* condition in the pasilla data. This means that resampling- or permutation-based methods will not have enough power. To proceed, we need to make distributional assumptions. Essentially, what such assumptions do is let us compute the probabilities of **rare events** in the tails of the distribution – i.e., extraordinarily high or low counts – from a small number of distribution parameters.

- But even that is often not enough; in particular, the estimation of **dispersion** parameters[4] is difficult with small sample sizes. In that case, we need to make further assumptions, such as that genes with similar locations also have similar dispersions. This is called sharing of information across genes, and we'll come back to it in Section 8.10.1.

8.3.2   RNA-Seq: what about gene structures, splicing, isoforms?

Eukaryotic genes are complex: most of them consist of multiple exons, and mRNAs result from concatenation of exons through a process called splicing. Alternative splicing and multiple possible choices of start and stop sites enable the generation of multiple alternative isoforms from the same gene locus. It is possible to use high-throughput sequencing to detect the isoform structures of transcripts. From the fragments that are characteristic for specific isoforms, it is also possible to detect isoform-specific abundances. With current RNA-Seq data, which give us only relatively short fragments of the full-length isoforms, it tends to be difficult to assemble and deconvolute full-length isoform structures and abundances (Steijger et al., 2013). Because of that, procedures with the more modest aim of making only local statements (e.g., inclusion or exclusion of individual exons) have been formulated (Anders et al., 2012), and these can be more robust. We can expect that future technologies will sequence full-length transcripts.

8.4   Modeling count data

8.4.1   Dispersion

Consider a sequencing library that contains n_1 fragments corresponding to gene 1, n_2 fragments for gene 2, and so on, with a total library size of $n = n_1 + n_2 + \ldots$. We submit the library to sequencing and determine the identity of r randomly sampled fragments. A welcome simplification comes from looking at the orders of magnitude of these numbers:

- the number of genes is in the tens of thousands;
- the value of n depends on the amount of cells that were used to prepare, but for bulk RNA-Seq it will be in the billions or trillions; and
- the number of reads r is usually in the tens of millions, thus much smaller than n.

From this we can conclude that the probability that a given read maps to the ith gene is $p_i = n_i/n$, and that this is pretty much independent of the outcomes for all the other reads. So we can model the number of reads for gene i by a Poisson distribution, where the *rate* of the Poisson process is the product of p_i, the initial proportion of fragments for the ith gene, times r; that is, $\lambda_i = rp_i$.

In practice, we are usually not interested in modeling the read counts within a single library, but in comparing the counts between libraries. That is, we want to know whether any differences that we see between different biological conditions – say, the same cell line with and without drug treatment – are larger than would be expected "by chance", i.e., larger than what we might expect even between biological replicates. Empirically, it turns out that replicate experiments vary more than the Poisson distribution predicts. Intuitively, what happens is that p_i, and therefore also λ_i, varies even between biological replicates; perhaps the temperature at which the cells grew was slightly different, or the amount of drug added varied by a few percent, or the incubation time was slightly longer. To account for that variation, we need to add another layer of modeling on top. We encountered hierarchical models and mixtures in Chapter 4. It turns out that the **gamma–Poisson** (aka negative binomial) distribution suits our modeling needs. Instead of a single λ – which represents both mean and variance – this distribution has two parameters. In principle, these can be different for each gene, and we will come back to the question of how to estimate them from the data.

8.4.2 Normalization

Often, systematic **biases** affect the data generation and are worth taking into account. Unfortunately, the term **normalization** is commonly used for that aspect of the analysis, even though it is misleading: it has nothing to do with the normal distribution, nor does it involve a data transformation. Rather, what we aim to do is identify the nature and magnitude of systematic biases and take them into account in our model-based analysis of the data.

The most important systematic bias stems from variations in the total number of reads in each sample. If we have more reads for one library than for another, then we might assume that, everything else being equal, the counts are proportional to each other with some proportionality factor s. Naively, we could propose that a decent estimate of s for each sample is simply given by the sum of the counts of all genes. However, it turns out that we can do better. To understand this, a toy example helps.

Read counts from a single library can be modeled by a Poisson distribution.

In principle, we should consider **sampling without replacement** and the multinomial distribution here: the probability of sampling a read for the ith gene depends on how many times the same gene and other genes have already been sampled. However, these dependencies are so negligibly small that we'll ignore them. This is because n is so much larger than r, the number of genes is large, and each individual n_i is small compared to n.

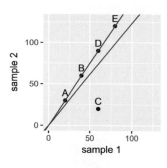

Figure 8.1: Size factor estimation. The points correspond to hypothetical genes whose counts in two samples are indicated by their x- and y-coordinates. The lines indicate the two different ways of estimating size factor explained in the text.

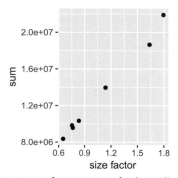

Figure 8.2: Size factors vs. sums for the pasilla data.

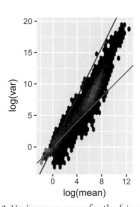

Figure 8.3: Variance vs. mean for the (size factor adjusted) counts data. The axes are logarithmic. Also shown are lines through the origin with slopes 1 (green) and 2 (red).

Consider a dataset with five genes and two samples, as displayed in Figure 8.1. If we estimate s for each of the two samples by its sum of counts, then the slope of the blue line represents their ratio. According to this, gene C is downregulated in sample 2 compared with sample 1, while the other genes are all somewhat upregulated. If we now instead estimate s such that their ratios correspond to the red line, then we will still conclude that gene C is downregulated, while the other genes are unchanged. The second version is more parsimonious and is often preferred by scientists. The slope of the red line can be obtained by robust regression. This is what the *DESeq2* method does.

▶ Question **8.1** For the example dataset `count` of Section 8.3, how does the output of *DESeq2*'s `estimateSizeFactorsForMatrix` compare with what you get by simply taking the column sums?   ◀

▶ Solution **8.1**   See Figure 8.2, produced by the code below. In this case there is not much difference; the results are nearly proportional.

```
library("tibble")
ggplot(tibble(
  `size factor` = estimateSizeFactorsForMatrix(counts),
  `sum` = colSums(counts)), aes(x = `size factor`, y = `sum`)) +
  geom_point()
```

▶ Task   Locate the R source for this book and look at the code that produces Figure 8.1.   ◀

▶ Question **8.2**   Plot the mean–variance relationship for the biological replicates in the pasilla dataset.   ◀

▶ Solution **8.2**   See Figure 8.3, produced by the following code.

```
library("ggplot2")
library("matrixStats")
sf = estimateSizeFactorsForMatrix(counts)
ncounts  = counts / matrix(sf,
   byrow = TRUE, ncol = ncol(counts), nrow = nrow(counts))
uncounts = ncounts[, grep("^untreated", colnames(ncounts)),
                    drop = FALSE]
ggplot(tibble(
        mean = rowMeans(uncounts),
        var  = rowVars( uncounts)),
     aes(x = log(mean), y = log(var))) +
  geom_hex() + coord_fixed() + theme(legend.position = "none") +
  geom_abline(slope = 1:2, color = c("forestgreen", "red"))
```

The green line (slope 1) is what we expect if the variance (v) equals the mean (m), as is the case for a Poisson-distributed random variable: $v = m$. We see that this approximately fits the data in the lower range. The red line (slope 2) corresponds to the quadratic mean–variance relationship $v = m^2$; lines parallel to it (not shown) would represent $v = cm^2$ for various values of c. We can see that in the upper range of the data, the quadratic relationship approximately fits the data, for some value of $c < 1$. □

8.5   A basic analysis

8.5.1   Example dataset: the pasilla data

Let's return to the *pasilla* data from Section 8.3. These data are from an experiment on *Drosophila melanogaster* cell cultures that investigated the effect of RNAi knockdown of the splicing factor *pasilla* (Brooks et al., 2011) on the cells' transcriptome. There were two experimental conditions, termed *untreated* and *treated* in the header of the count table that we loaded. They correspond to negative control and siRNA against *pasilla*. The experimental **metadata** of the seven samples in this dataset are provided in a spreadsheet-like table, which we load.

In the code shown here, we use the function `system.file` to locate a file that is shipped together with the *pasilla* package. When you work with your own data, prepare and load the corresponding file, or use some other way to generate a dataframe like `pasillaSampleAnno`.

```
annotationFile = system.file("extdata",
  "pasilla_sample_annotation.csv",
  package = "pasilla", mustWork = TRUE)
pasillaSampleAnno = readr::read_csv(annotationFile)
pasillaSampleAnno

## # A tibble: 7 x 6
##   file      condition type    `number of lane~ `total number of ~
##   <chr>     <chr>     <chr>            <int> <chr>
## 1 treate~   treated   single~              5 35158667
## 2 treate~   treated   paired~              2 12242535 (x2)
## 3 treate~   treated   paired~              2 12443664 (x2)
## 4 untrea~   untreated single~              2 17812866
## 5 untrea~   untreated single~              6 34284521
## 6 untrea~   untreated paired~              2 10542625 (x2)
## 7 untrea~   untreated paired~              2 12214974 (x2)
## # ... with 1 more variable: `exon counts` <int>
```

As we see here, the overall dataset was produced in two batches, the first consisting of three sequencing libraries that were subjected to single read sequencing, the second consisting of four libraries for which paired end sequencing was used. As so often, we need to do some data wrangling: we replace the hyphens in the `type` column with underscores, as arithmetic operators in factor levels are discouraged by *DESeq2*, and convert the `type` and `condition` columns into factors, explicitly specifying our preferred order of the levels (the default is alphabetical).

```
library("dplyr")
pasillaSampleAnno = mutate(pasillaSampleAnno,
condition = factor(condition, levels = c("untreated", "treated")),
type = factor(sub("-.*", "", type), levels = c("single", "paired")))
```

We note that the design is approximately **balanced** between the factor of interest, `condition`, and the "nuisance factor", `type`.

```
with(pasillaSampleAnno,
      table(condition, type))

##            type
## condition  single paired
##   untreated      2      2
##   treated        1      2
```

DESeq2 uses a specialized data container, called *DESeqDataSet*, to store the datasets it works with. Such use of specialized containers – or, in R terminology, *classes* – is a common principle of the Bioconductor project, as it helps users keep related data together. While this way of doing things requires users to invest a little more time up front to understand the classes, compared with just using basic R data types like *matrix* and *dataframe*, it helps in avoiding bugs due to loss of synchronization between related parts of the data. It also enables the abstraction and encapsulation of common operations that could be quite wordy if always expressed in basic terms.[5] *DESeqDataSet* is an extension of the class *SummarizedExperiment* in Bioconductor. The *SummarizedExperiment* class is also used by many other packages, so learning to work with it will enable you to use a large range of tools.

We use the constructor function `DESeqDataSetFromMatrix` to create a *DESeqDataSet* from the count data matrix `counts` and the sample annotation dataframe `pasillaSampleAnno`.[6]

```
mt = match(colnames(counts), sub("fb$", "", pasillaSampleAnno$file))
stopifnot(!any(is.na(mt)))


library("DESeq2")
pasilla = DESeqDataSetFromMatrix(
  countData = counts,
  colData   = pasillaSampleAnno[mt, ],
  design    = ~ condition)
class(pasilla)
## [1] "DESeqDataSet"
## attr(,"package")
## [1] "DESeq2"
is(pasilla, "SummarizedExperiment")
## [1] TRUE
```

The *SummarizedExperiment* class – and therefore *DESeqDataSet* – also contains facilities for storing annotations of the rows of the count matrix. For now, we are content with the gene identifiers from the row names of the `counts` table.

▶ Question **8.3** How can we access the row metadata of a *SummarizedExperiment* object, i.e., how can we read it out, and how can we change it? ◀

▶ Solution **8.3** Check the manual pages of the *SummarizedExperiment* class and the methods `rowData` and `rowData<-`. □

8.5.2 The *DESeq2* method

After these preparations, we are ready to jump straight into **differential expression analysis**. Our aim is to identify genes that are differentially abundant between the treated and the untreated cells. To this end, we will apply a test that is conceptually similar to the *t*-test, which we encountered in Section 6.5, although mathematically somewhat more involved. We postpone these details for now and return to them in Section 8.7. A choice of standard analysis steps are wrapped into a single function, `DESeq`.

[5] Another advantage is that classes can contain *validity* methods, which make sure that the data always fulfill certain expectations, for instance, that the counts are positive integers, or that the columns of the counts matrix align with the rows of the sample annotation dataframe.

[6] Note how, in the code below, we have to put in extra work to match the column names of the `counts` object with the `file` column of the `pasillaSampleAnno` dataframe; in particular, we need to remove the `"fb"` that happens to be used in the `file` column for some reason. Such data wrangling is very common. One of the reasons for storing the data in a *DESeqDataSet* object is that we then no longer have to worry about such things.

```
pasilla = DESeq(pasilla)
```

The `DESeq` function is simply a wrapper that calls, in order, the functions `estimateSizeFactors` (for normalization, as discussed in Section 8.4.2), `estimateDispersions` (dispersion estimation) and `nbinomWaldTest` (hypothesis tests for differential abundance). The test is between the two levels `untreated` and `treated` of the factor `condition`, since this is what we specified when we constructed the `pasilla` object through the argument `design = ~ condition`. You can always call each of these three functions individually if you want to modify their behavior or interject custom steps. Let's look at the results.

```
res = results(pasilla)
res[order(res$padj), ] %>% head
## log2 fold change (MLE): condition treated vs untreated
## Wald test p-value: condition treated vs untreated
## DataFrame with 6 rows and 6 columns
##              baseMean log2FoldChange       lfcSE        stat
##             <numeric>      <numeric>   <numeric>   <numeric>
## FBgn0039155  730.5958      -4.619006  0.16872512   -27.37593
## FBgn0025111 1501.4105       2.899863  0.12693550    22.84517
## FBgn0029167 3706.1165      -2.197001  0.09701773   -22.64535
## FBgn0003360 4343.0354      -3.179672  0.14352683   -22.15385
## FBgn0035085  638.2326      -2.560409  0.13731558   -18.64617
## FBgn0039827  261.9162      -4.162516  0.23258982   -17.89638
##                   pvalue          padj
##                <numeric>     <numeric>
## FBgn0039155 5.307308e-165 4.417272e-161
## FBgn0025111 1.632133e-115 6.792124e-112
## FBgn0029167 1.550286e-113 4.301011e-110
## FBgn0003360 9.577102e-109 1.992756e-105
## FBgn0035085  1.356647e-77  2.258274e-74
## FBgn0039827  1.258423e-71  1.745643e-68
```

8.5.3 Exploring the results

The first step after a differential expression analysis is to visualize the following three or four basic plots:

- the histogram of p-values (Figure 8.4),
- the MA plot (Figure 8.5), and
- an ordination plot (Figure 8.6).
- In addition, a heatmap (Figure 8.7) can be instructive.

These are essential data quality assessment measures – and the general advice on quality assessment and control given in Section 13.6 also applies here.

The p-value histogram is straightforward (Figure 8.4).

```
ggplot(as(res, "data.frame"), aes(x = pvalue)) +
  geom_histogram(binwidth = 0.01, fill = "Royalblue", boundary = 0)
```

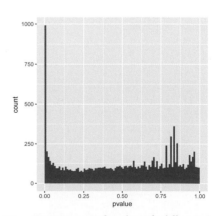

Figure 8.4: Histogram of p-values of a differential expression analysis.

[7] For the data shown here, the histogram also contains a few isolated peaks in the middle or toward the right; these stem from genes with small counts and reflect the discreteness of the data.

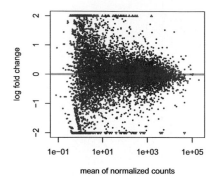

Figure 8.5: MA plot: fold change versus mean of size-factor normalized counts. Logarithmic scaling is used for both axes. By default, points are colored red if the adjusted p-value is less than 0.1. Points that fall out of the y-axis range are plotted as triangles.

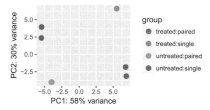

Figure 8.6: PCA plot. The seven samples are shown in the 2D plane spanned by their first two principal components.

The distribution displays two main components: a uniform background with values between 0 and 1, and a peak of small p-values at the left. The uniform background corresponds to the non-differentially expressed genes. Usually this is the majority of genes. The left-hand peak corresponds to differentially expressed genes.[7] As we saw in Chapter 6, the ratio of the level of the background to the height of the peak gives us a rough indication of the false discovery rate (FDR) that would be associated with calling the genes in the leftmost bin differentially expressed. In our case, the leftmost bin contains all p-values between 0 and 0.01, which correspond to 992 genes. The background level is at around 100, so the FDR associated with calling all genes in the leftmost bin would be around 10%.

A background distribution that is not uniform, but shows a tilted shape with an increase toward the right, tends to indicate batch effects, that is, underlying systematic variation that makes replicates look more different than expected.

▶ Question **8.4** If the histogram for your data suggests the presence of batch effects, what can you do?   ◀

To produce the MA plot, we can use the function `plotMA` in the *DESeq2* package (Figure 8.5).

```
plotMA(pasilla, ylim = c( -2, 2))
```

To produce PCA plots similar to those we saw in Chapter 7, we can use the *DESeq2* function `plotPCA` (Figure 8.6).

```
pas_rlog = rlogTransformation(pasilla)
plotPCA(pas_rlog, intgroup=c("condition", "type")) + coord_fixed()
```

As we saw in Chapter 7, this type of plot is useful for visualizing the overall effect of experimental covariates and/or detecting batch effects.

Here, the first principal axis, PC1, is mostly aligned with the experimental covariate of interest (untreated/treated), while the second axis is roughly aligned with the sequencing protocol (single/paired).

We used a data transformation, the **regularized logarithm** or **rlog**, which we will investigate more closely in Section 8.10.2.

▶ Question **8.5** Do the axes of a PCA plot always have to align with specific experimental covariates?   ◀

Heatmaps can be a powerful way to quickly get an overview of a matrix-like dataset, count tables included. Below, you see how to make a heatmap from the rlog-transformed data. For a matrix as large as `counts(pasilla)`, it is not practical to plot all of it, so we plot the subset of the 30 most variable genes.

```
library("pheatmap")
select = order(rowMeans(assay(pas_rlog)), decreasing = TRUE)[1:30]
pheatmap( assay(pas_rlog)[select, ],
    scale = "row",
    annotation_col = as.data.frame(
      colData(pas_rlog)[, c("condition", "type")] ))
```

By default, `pheatmap` arranges the rows and columns of the matrix by the dendrogram from (unsupervised) clustering. In Figure 8.7 we see that the clustering of the columns (samples) is dominated by the `type` factor. This highlights that our differential expression analysis above was probably too naive, and that we should adjust for this strong "nuisance" factor when we are interested in testing for differentially expressed genes between conditions; we'll do this in Section 8.9.

8.5.4 Exporting the results

An HTML report of the results with plots and sortable/filterable columns can be exported using the *ReportingTools* package on a *DESeqDataSet* object that has been processed by the `DESeq` function. For a code example, see the *RNA-Seq differential expression* vignette of the *ReportingTools* package or the manual page for the `publish` method for the *DESeqDataSet* class.

A CSV file of the results can be exported using `write.csv` (or its counterpart from the *readr* package).

```
write.csv(as.data.frame(res), file = "treated_vs_untreated.csv")
```

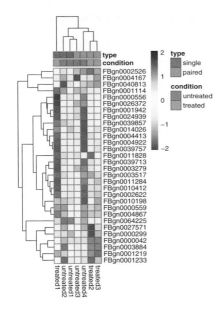

Figure 8.7: Heatmap of regularized log transformed data of the top 30 genes.

8.6 Critique of default choices and possible modifications

8.6.1 The few-changes assumption

Underlying the default normalization and the dispersion estimation in *DESeq2* (and many other differential expression methods) is the assumption that most genes are *not* differentially expressed. This assumption is often reasonable (well-designed experiments usually ask specific questions, so that not everything changes all at once), but what should we do if it does not hold? Instead of applying these operations on the data from all genes, we will then need to identify a subset of ("negative control") genes for which we believe the assumption is tenable, either because of prior biological knowledge or because we explicitly controlled their abundance as external "spiked in" features.

▶ Task Run the *DESeq2* workflow with size factors and dispersion parameters estimated from only a predefined subset of genes. ◀

8.6.2 Point-like null hypothesis

As a default, the `DESeq` function tests against the **null hypothesis** that each gene has the same abundance across conditions; this is a simple and pragmatic choice. Indeed, if the sample size is limited, what is statistically significant also tends to be strong enough to be biologically interesting. But as sample size increases, statistical significance in these tests may be present without much biological relevance. For instance, many genes may be slightly perturbed by downstream indirect effects. We can modify the test to use

For the normalization, though not for the dispersion estimation, one can slightly relax this assumption: it is still valid if many genes are changing, but in a way that is balanced between upward and downward directions.

a more permissive – harder to reject – interval-based null hypothesis;[8] we will further explore this in Section 8.10.4.

8.7   Multifactorial designs and linear models

8.7.1   What is a multifactorial design?

Let's assume that, in addition to the siRNA knockdown of the pasilla gene, we also want to test the effect of a certain drug. We could then envisage an experiment in which the experimenter treats the cells either with negative control, with the siRNA against pasilla, with the drug, or with both. To analyze this experiment, we can introduce the notation

$$y = \beta_0 + x_1\beta_1 + x_2\beta_2 + x_1x_2\beta_{12}. \tag{8.1}$$

Sometimes Equation (8.1) is written with an additional term x_0 that is multiplied with β_0, where it is understood that $x_0 = 1$ always. It turns out that this makes subsequent notation and bookkeeping easier, since then the intercept can be handled consistently together with the other βs instead of being a separate case.

This equation can be parsed as follows. The left-hand side, y, is the experimental measurement of interest, which in our case is the suitably transformed expression level of a gene (we'll discuss this in Section 8.8.3). Since in an RNA-Seq experiment there are lots of genes, we'll have as many copies of Equation (8.1), one for each. The coefficient β_0 is the base level of the measurement in the negative control; often it is called the **intercept**. The design factors x_1 and x_2 are binary indicator variables: x_1 takes the value 1 if the siRNA was transfected and 0 if not, and similarly, x_2 indicates whether the drug was administered. In the experiment where only the siRNA is used, $x_1 = 1$ and $x_2 = 0$, and the third and fourth terms of Equation (8.1) vanish. The equation then simplifies to $y = \beta_0 + \beta_1$. This means that β_1 represents the difference between treatment and control. If our measurements are on a logarithmic scale, then

$$\begin{aligned}
\beta_1 = y - \beta_0 &= \log_2(\text{expression}_{\text{treated}}) - \log_2(\text{expression}_{\text{untreated}}) \\
&= \log_2 \frac{\text{expression}_{\text{treated}}}{\text{expression}_{\text{untreated}}}
\end{aligned} \tag{8.2}$$

is the logarithmic fold change due to treatment with the siRNA. In exactly the same way, β_2 is the logarithmic fold change due to treatment with the drug. What happens if we treat the cells with both siRNA and drug? In that case, $x_1 = x_2 = 1$, and Equation (8.1) can be rewritten as

$$\beta_{12} = y - (\beta_0 + \beta_1 + \beta_2). \tag{8.3}$$

This means that β_{12} is the difference between the observed outcome, y, and the outcome expected from the individual treatments, obtained by adding to the baseline the effect of siRNA alone, β_1, and of drug alone, β_2.

The addition is on the logarithmic scale, which corresponds to multiplication on the original scale.

We call β_{12} the *interaction* effect of siRNA and drug. It has nothing to do with a physical interaction: the terminology indicates that the effects of these two different experimental factors do not simply add up, but combine in a more complicated fashion. For instance, if the target of the drug and of the siRNA were equivalent, leading to the same effect on the cells, then we would biologically expect that $\beta_1 = \beta_2$. We would also expect that their combination has no further effect, so that $\beta_{12} = -\beta_1$. If, on the other hand, the targets of the drug and of the siRNA are in parallel pathways that can buffer each other, we would expect that β_1 and β_2 are both relatively small, but the combined effect is synergistic, and β_{12} is large.

We don't always care about interactions. Many experiments are designed with multiple factors where we care most about each of their individual effects. In that case, the combinatorial treatment might not be present in the experimental design, and the model to use for the analysis is a version of Equation (8.1) with the rightmost term removed.

We can succinctly encode the design of the experiment in the **design matrix**. For instance, for the combinatorial experiment described above, the design matrix is

$$
\begin{array}{c|c|c}
x_0 & x_1 & x_2 \\
\hline
1 & 0 & 0 \\
1 & 1 & 0 \\
1 & 0 & 1 \\
1 & 1 & 1.
\end{array}
\tag{8.4}
$$

The columns of the design matrix correspond to the experimental factors, and its rows represent the different experimental conditions, four in our case. If, instead, the combinatorial treatment is not performed, then the design matrix is reduced to only the first three rows of (8.4).

8.7.2   What about noise and replicates?

Equation (8.1) provides a conceptual decomposition of the observed data into the effects caused by the different experimental variables. If our data (the ys) were absolutely precise, we could set up a linear system of equations, one equation for each of the four possible experimental conditions represented by the xs, and solve for the βs.

Of course, we usually wish to analyze real data that are affected by **noise**. We then need replicates to estimate the levels of noise and assess the uncertainty of our estimated βs. Only then can we empirically assess whether any of the observed changes between conditions are significantly larger than those occurring due just to experimental or natural variation. We need to slightly extend the equation:

$$
y_j = x_{j0}\,\beta_0 + x_{j1}\,\beta_1 + x_{j2}\,\beta_2 + x_{j1}\,x_{j2}\,\beta_{12} + \varepsilon_j.
\tag{8.5}
$$

We have added the index j and a new term ε_j. The index j now explicitly counts over our individual replicate experiments; for instance, if for each of the four conditions we perform three replicates, then j counts from 1 to 12. The design matrix now has 12 rows, and x_{jk} is the value of the matrix in its jth row and kth column. The additional terms ε_j, which we call the **residuals**, are there to absorb differences between replicates. However, one additional modeling component is needed: the system of 12 equations (8.5) would be underdetermined without further information, since it now has more variables (12 epsilons and four betas) than it has equations (12, one for each j). To fix this,

Remember that since β_0 is the intercept, $x_{j0} = 1$ for all j.

we require that the ε_j be small. One popular way – we'll encounter others – to overcome this is to minimize the sum of squared residuals,

$$\sum_j \varepsilon_j^2 \quad \rightarrow \quad \text{min.} \tag{8.6}$$

It turns out that with this requirement satisfied, the βs represent the *average* effects of each of the experimental factors, while the residuals ε_j reflect the experimental fluctuations around the mean between the replicates. This approach, which is called **least sum of squares fitting**, is mathematically convenient, since it can be achieved by straightforward matrix algebra. It is what the R function `lm` does.

▶ Question **8.6** An alternative way to write Equation (8.5) is

$$y_j = \sum_k x_{jk}\, \beta_k + \varepsilon_j. \tag{8.7}$$

How can this be mapped to Equation (8.5), i.e., where do we find the interaction term $x_{j1}\, x_{j2}\, \beta_{12}$? ◀

▶ Solution **8.6** This is really just a matter of notation: the sum extends over $k = 0, \ldots, 3$, where the terms for $k = 0, 1, 2$ are exactly as we know them already. We write β_3 instead of β_{12}, and define x_{j3} to be $x_{j1}x_{j2}$. The generic notation (8.7) is practical to use in computer software that implements linear models, and in mathematical proofs. It also highlights that the "scientific content" of a linear model is condensed in its design matrix. □

▶ Task Show that if we fit Equation (8.5) to data such that objective (8.6) holds, the fit residuals $\hat{\varepsilon}_j$ have an average of 0. ◀

8.7.3 Analysis of variance

A model that looks like (8.5) is called a **linear model**, and often it is implied that criterion (8.6) is used to fit it to data. This approach is elegant and powerful, but for novices it can take some time to appreciate all of its facets. What is the advantage over simply taking, for each distinct experimental condition, the average over replicates and comparing these values across conditions? In simple cases, the latter approach can be intuitive and effective. However, it reaches its limits when the replicate numbers are not all the same in the different groups, or when one or more of the x-variables is continuous valued. In these cases, we will invariably end up with something like fitting (8.5) to the data.

A useful way to think about (8.5) is encapsulated in the term **analysis of variance**, abbreviated ANOVA. In fact, what Equation (8.5) does is decompose the **variability** of y that we observed in the course of our experiments into elementary components: its baseline value, β_0; its variability caused by the effect of the first variable, β_1; its variability caused by the effect of the second variable, β_2; its variability caused by the effect of the interaction, β_{12}; and variability that is unaccounted for. The last of these we commonly call *noise*; the others, *systematic variability*.

The distinction between noise and systematic variability is in the eye of the beholder and depends on our model, not on reality.

8.7.4   Robustness

The sum (8.6) is sensitive to **outliers** in the data. A single measurement y_j with an outlying value can draw the β estimates far away from the values implied by the other replicates. This is the well-known fact that methods based on least sum of squares have a low **breakdown point**: if even a single data point is outlying, the whole statistical result can be strongly affected. For instance, the average of a set of n numbers has a breakdown point of $\frac{1}{n}$, meaning that it can be arbitrarily changed by changing only one of the numbers. On the other hand, the median has a much higher breakdown point. Changing a single number often has no effect at all, and when it does, the effect is limited to the range of data points in the middle of the ranking (i.e., those adjacent to rank $\frac{n}{2}$). To change the median by an arbitrarily large amount, you need to change half the observations. We call the median **robust**, and its breakdown point is $\frac{1}{2}$. Remember that the median of a set of numbers $y_1, y_2, \ldots$ minimizes the sum $\sum_j |y_j - \beta_0|$.

To achieve a higher degree of robustness against outliers, choices other than the sum of squares (8.6) can be used as the objective of minimization. Among these are

$$R = \sum_j |\varepsilon_j|, \qquad\qquad \text{Least absolute deviations} \qquad (8.8)$$

$$R = \sum_j \rho_s(\varepsilon_j), \qquad\qquad \text{M-estimation} \qquad (8.9)$$

$$R = Q_\theta\left(\{\varepsilon_1^2, \varepsilon_2^2, \ldots\}\right), \qquad\qquad \text{LTS, LQS} \qquad (8.10)$$

$$R = \sum_j w_j \varepsilon_j^2. \qquad\qquad \text{General weighted regression} \qquad (8.11)$$

Here, R is the quantity to be minimized.

Choice (8.8) is called **least absolute deviations** regression. It can be viewed as a generalization of the median. Although conceptually simple, and attractive on first sight, it is harder to minimize than the sum of squares, and it can be less stable and less efficient, especially if the data are limited or do not fit the model.[9]

Choice (8.9), called **M-estimation**, uses a penalization function ρ_s (least-squares regression is the special case with $\rho_s(\varepsilon) = \varepsilon^2$) that looks like a quadratic function for a limited range of ε, but has a smaller slope, flattens out, or even drops back to zero, for absolute values $|\varepsilon|$ that are larger than the scale parameter s. The intention behind this is to down-weight the effect of outliers, i.e., data points that have large residuals (Huber, 1964). A choice of s needs to be made, and it determines what is called an outlier. One can even drop the requirement that ρ_s is quadratic around 0 (as long as its second derivative is positive), and a variety of choices for the function ρ_s have been proposed in the literature. The aim is to give the estimator desirable statistical properties (say, bias and efficiency) when and where the data fit the model, but to limit or nullify the influence of those data points that do not fit, and to keep computations tractable.

▶ Question **8.7** Plot the graph of the function $\rho_s(\varepsilon)$ proposed by Huber (1964) for M-estimators. ◀

[9] The Wikipedia article on *least absolute deviations* gives an overview.

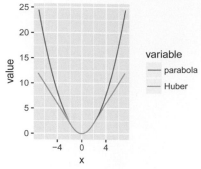

Figure 8.8: Graph of $\rho_s(\varepsilon)$ for the choice $s = 2$.

▶ **Solution 8.7**   Huber's paper defines, on page 75,

$$
\rho_s(\varepsilon) = \begin{cases} \frac{1}{2}\varepsilon^2, & \text{for } |\varepsilon| < s, \\ s|\varepsilon| - \frac{1}{2}s^2, & \text{for } |\varepsilon| \geqslant s. \end{cases}
$$

The graph produced by the code below is shown in Figure 8.8.

```r
rho = function(x, s)
  ifelse(abs(x) < s, x^2 / 2,  s * abs(x) - s^2 / 2)

df = tibble(
  x        = seq(-7, 7, length.out = 100),
  parabola = x ^ 2 / 2,
  Huber    = rho(x, s = 2))

ggplot(reshape2::melt(df, id.vars = "x"),
  aes(x = x, y = value, col = variable)) + geom_line()
```
□

Choice (8.10) generalizes the least sum of squares method in yet another way. In **least quantile of squares** (LQS) regression, the sum over the squared residuals is replaced with a quantile, for instance, Q_{50}, the median, or Q_{90}, the 90% quantile (Rousseeuw, 1987). In a variation, **least trimmed sum of squares** (LTS) regression, a sum of squared residuals is used; however, the sum extends not over all residuals, but only over the fraction $0 \leqslant \theta \leqslant 1$ of smallest residuals. The motivation in both cases is that outlying data points lead to large residuals, and as long as they are rare, they do not affect the quantile or the trimmed sum.

However, there is a price: while the least sum of squares optimization (8.6) can be performed through straightforward linear algebra, more complicated iterative optimization algorithms are needed for M-estimation, LQS and LTS regression.

Approach (8.11) represents an even more complex way of weighting down outliers. It assumes that we have some way of deciding what weight w_j we want to give to each observation, presumably down-weighting outliers. For instance, in Section 8.10.3, we will encounter the approach used by the *DESeq2* package, in which the leverage of each data point on the estimated βs is assessed using a measure called Cook's distance. For those data whose Cook's distance is deemed too large, the weight w_j is set to zero, whereas the other data points receive $w_j = 1$. In effect, this means that the outlying data points are discarded and ordinary regression is performed on the others. The extra computational effort of carrying the weights along is negligible, and the optimization is still straightforward linear algebra.

All these approaches to outlier robustness introduce a degree of subjectiveness and rely on sufficient replication. The subjectiveness is reflected by the parameter choices that need to be made: s in (8.9), θ in (8.10), the weights in (8.11). One scientist's outlier may be the Nobel Prize of another. On the other hand, outlier removal is no remedy for sloppy experiments and no justification for wishful thinking.

▶ **Task**   Search the documentation of R and CRAN packages for implementations of the above robust regression methods. A good place to start is the *CRAN task view on robust statistical methods*.   ◀

8.8 Generalized linear models

We need to explore two additional theoretical concepts before we can proceed to our next application example. Equations of the form (8.5) model the expected value of the outcome variable, y, as a linear function of the design matrix, and they are fitted to data according to the least sum of squares criterion (8.6) or a robust variant thereof. We now want to generalize these assumptions.

8.8.1 Modeling the data on a transformed scale

We have seen that it can be fruitful to consider data, not on the scale on which we obtained them, but after some transformation, for instance, the logarithm. This idea can be generalized since, depending on the context, other transformations are useful. For instance, the linear model (8.5) would not directly be useful for modeling outcomes that are bounded within an interval, say $[0, 1]$, as an indicator of disease risk. In a linear model, the values of y cover, in principle, the whole real axis. However, if we transform the expression on the right-hand side with a sigmoid function, for instance $f(y) = 1/(1 + e^{-y})$, then the range of this function[10] is bounded between 0 and 1 and can be used to model such an outcome.

[10] It is called the logistic function (Verhulst, 1845), and the associated regression model is called **logistic regression**.

8.8.2 Other error distributions

The other generalization concerns the minimization criterion (8.6). In fact, this criterion can be derived from a specific probabilistic model and the **maximum likelihood** principle (which we encountered in Chapter 2). To see this, consider the probabilistic model

$$p(\varepsilon_j) = \frac{1}{\sqrt{2\pi}\sigma} \exp \frac{\varepsilon_j^2}{2\sigma^2};$$

(8.12)

that is, we believe that the residuals follow a normal distribution with mean 0 and standard deviation σ. Then it is plausible to demand from a good model (i.e., a good set of βs) that these probabilities are large. Formally,

$$\prod_j p(\varepsilon_j) \quad \rightarrow \quad \max.$$

(8.13)

▶ Question **8.8** Show that maximizing the likelihood (8.13) is equivalent to minimizing the sum of squared residuals (8.6). ◀

▶ Solution **8.8** Insert (8.12) into (8.13) and take the logarithm. □

Let's review some core concepts. The left-hand side of Equation (8.13), i.e., the product of the probabilities of the residuals, is a function of both the model parameters $\beta_1, \beta_2, \ldots$ and the data $y_1, y_2, \ldots$; call it $f(\beta, y)$. If we think of the model parameters β as given and fixed, then the collapsed function $f(y)$ simply indicates the probability of the data. We could use it, for instance, to simulate data. If, on the other hand, we

It is good to remember that, while we can use the normal distribution as a convenient argument for motivating least sum of squares regression through the maximum likelihood principle, the data do not have to be distributed according to the normal for least sum of squares regression to provide a useful result. In fact, least sum of squares fitting often provides useful estimates for the βs even when the data are non-normal, although that depends on the specific circumstances.

consider the data as given, then $f(\beta)$ is a function of the model parameters, and it is called the *likelihood*. The second view is the one we take when we optimize (8.6) (and thus (8.13)), and hence the βs obtained this way are what are called *maximum likelihood estimates*.

The generalization that we can now make is to use a different probabilistic model. We can use the densities of distributions other than the normal instead of Equation (8.12). For instance, to be able to deal with count data, we will use the gamma–Poisson distribution.

8.8.3 A generalized linear model for count data

The differential expression analysis in *DESeq2* uses a generalized linear model of the form

$$K_{ij} \sim \mathrm{GP}(\mu_{ij}, \alpha_i), \tag{8.14}$$

$$\mu_{ij} = s_j \, q_{ij}, \tag{8.15}$$

$$\log_2(q_{ij}) = \sum_k x_{jk}\beta_{ik}. \tag{8.16}$$

Let's unpack this step by step. The counts K_{ij} for gene i, sample j are modeled using a gamma–Poisson (GP) distribution with two parameters, the mean μ_{ij} and the dispersion α_i. By default, the dispersion is different for each gene i, but the same across all samples; therefore it has no index j. Equation (8.15) states that the mean is composed of a sample-specific size factor[11] s_j and q_{ij}, which is proportional to the true expected concentration of fragments for gene i in sample j. The value of q_{ij} is given by the linear model in the third line via the *link function*, $\log_2$. The design matrix (x_{jk}) is the same for all genes (and therefore does not depend on i). Its rows j correspond to the samples, its columns k to the experimental factors. In the simplest case, for a pairwise comparison, the design matrix has only two columns, one of them everywhere filled with 1 (corresponding to β_0 of Section 8.7.1) and the other containing 0 or 1 depending on which group the sample belongs to. The coefficients β_{ik} give the $\log_2$-fold changes for gene i for each column of the design matrix X.

[11] The model can be generalized to use sample- *and* gene-dependent normalization factors s_{ij}. This is explained in the documentation of the *DESeq2* package.

8.9 Two-factor analysis of the pasilla data

Besides the treatment with siRNA, which we considered in Section 8.5, the *pasilla* data have another covariate, `type`, which indicates the type of sequencing that was performed.

We saw in the exploratory data analysis (EDA) plots in Section 8.5.3 that `type` had a considerable systematic effect on the data. Our basic analysis in Section 8.5 did not take this into account, but we will do so now. Introducing this second factor should help us get a more correct picture of which differences in the data are attributable to the treatment and which are confounded – or masked – by the sequencing type.

```
pasillaTwoFactor = pasilla
design(pasillaTwoFactor) = formula(~ type + condition)
pasillaTwoFactor = DESeq(pasillaTwoFactor)
```

Of the two variables `type` and `condition`, the one of primary interest is `condition`, and in *DESeq2*, the convention is to put it at the end of the formula. This convention has no effect on the model fitting, but it helps to simplify some of the subsequent results reporting. Again, we access the results using the `results` function, which returns a dataframe with the statistics of each gene.

```
res2 = results(pasillaTwoFactor)
head(res2, n = 3)
## log2 fold change (MLE): condition treated vs untreated
## Wald test p-value: condition treated vs untreated
## DataFrame with 3 rows and 6 columns
##                baseMean log2FoldChange      lfcSE        stat
##               <numeric>      <numeric>  <numeric>   <numeric>
## FBgn0000003  0.1715687     0.67455178  3.8710909   0.17425366
## FBgn0000008 95.1440790    -0.04067399  0.2222916  -0.18297586
## FBgn0000014  1.0565722    -0.08497708  2.1115384  -0.04024415
##                 pvalue       padj
##              <numeric>  <numeric>
## FBgn0000003  0.8616661         NA
## FBgn0000008  0.8548170  0.9520423
## FBgn0000014  0.9678985         NA
```

It is also possible to retrieve the $\log_2$-fold changes, p-values and adjusted p-values associated with the `type` variable. The function `results` takes an argument `contrast` that lets users specify the name of the variable, the level that corresponds to the numerator of the fold change and the level that corresponds to the denominator of the fold change.

```
resType = results(pasillaTwoFactor,
  contrast = c("type", "single", "paired"))
head(resType, n = 3)
## log2 fold change (MLE): type single vs paired
## Wald test p-value: type single vs paired
## DataFrame with 3 rows and 6 columns
##                baseMean log2FoldChange      lfcSE       stat
##               <numeric>      <numeric>  <numeric>  <numeric>
## FBgn0000003  0.1715687     -1.6115458  3.8710829 -0.4163036
## FBgn0000008 95.1440790     -0.2622592  0.2207626 -1.1879694
## FBgn0000014  1.0565722      3.2905815  2.0869727  1.5767247
##                 pvalue       padj
##              <numeric>  <numeric>
## FBgn0000003  0.6771878         NA
## FBgn0000008  0.2348455  0.5441805
## FBgn0000014  0.1148589         NA
```

So what did we gain from this analysis that took `type` into account as a nuisance factor (sometimes also called, more politely, a **blocking factor**), compared to the simple comparison between the two groups of Section 8.5? Let us plot the p-values from the two analyses against each other.

```
trsf = function(x) ifelse(is.na(x), 0, (-log10(x)) ^ (1/6))
ggplot(tibble(pOne = res$pvalue,
              pTwo = res2$pvalue),
    aes(x = trsf(pOne), y = trsf(pTwo))) +
    geom_hex(bins = 75) + coord_fixed() +
    xlab("Single factor analysis (condition)") +
    ylab("Two factor analysis (type + condition)") +
    geom_abline(col = "orange")
```

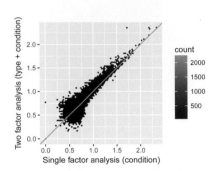

Figure 8.9: Comparison of p-values from the models with a single factor (condition) and with two factors (type + condition). The axes correspond to $(-\log_{10} p)^{1/6}$, an arbitrarily chosen monotonically decreasing transformation that compresses the dynamic range of the p-values for the purpose of visualization. We can see a trend for the joint distribution to lie above the bisector, indicating that the small p-values in the two-factor analysis are generally smaller than those in the one-factor analysis.

As we can see in Figure 8.9, the p-values in the two-factor analysis are similar to those in the one-factor analysis, but are generally smaller. The more sophisticated analysis has led to an, albeit modest, increase in power. We can also see this improvement by counting the number of genes that pass a certain significance threshold in each case:

```
compareRes = table(
    `simple analysis` = res$padj < 0.1,
    `two factor` = res2$padj < 0.1 )
addmargins( compareRes )
##                 two factor
## simple analysis FALSE TRUE  Sum
##           FALSE  6974  288 7262
##           TRUE     25 1036 1061
##           Sum    6999 1324 8323
```

The two-factor analysis found 1324 genes differentially expressed at an FDR threshold of 10%, while the one-factor analysis found 1061. The two-factor analysis has increased detection power. In general, the gain can be much larger, or also smaller, depending on the data. The proper choice of model requires informed adaptation to the experimental design and data quality.

▶ Question **8.9** Why do we detect fewer significant genes when we do not take into account the `type` variable? More generally, what does this mean about the benefit of taking into account (or not) blocking factors?   ◀

▶ Solution **8.9** When we don't model the blocking factor, the variability in the data that is associated with this factor has to be absorbed by the εs. This means that they are generally larger than in the model with the blocking factor. The higher level of noise leads to higher uncertainty in the β-estimates. On the other hand, the model with the blocking factor has more parameters that need to be estimated. In statistical parlance, the fit has fewer "degrees of freedom". These two effects counteract each other, and which of them prevails, and which of the modeling choices yields more or fewer significant results, depends on the data.   ☐

▶ Question **8.10** What is confounding? Can *not* taking into account a blocking factor also lead to the detection of *more* genes?   ◀

▶ **Solution 8.10** Yes. Imagine the variables `condition` and `type` were not as nicely balanced as they are, but partially or fully confounded. In that case, differences in the data due to `type` could be attributed to `condition` if a model is fitted that does not make it possible to absorb them in the `type` effect. Scientifically, such an experiment (and analysis) can be quite an embarrassment.   □

▶ Question **8.11** Consider a paired experimental design, say, 10 different cell lines, each with and without drug treatment. How should this be analyzed?   ◀

▶ **Solution 8.11** If we did just a simple two-group comparison (treated versus un-treated), many of the treatment effects would probably be swamped in the strong variation from cell line to cell line. However, we can set up a *paired* analysis simply by adding cell line identity as a blocking factor. (Cell line is then really an R *factor* with 10 different levels rather than just a 0/1 indicator variable, as with the variables that we have looked at so far. R's linear modeling facilities, and also *DESeq2*, have no problem dealing with that.)   □

▶ Question **8.12** What can you do if you suspect there are "hidden" factors affecting your data, but they are not documented? (Sometimes such undocumented covariates are also called **batch effects**.)   ◀

▶ **Solution 8.12** There are methods that try to identify blocking factors in an unsuper-vised fashion; see, e.g., Leek and Storey (2007) and Stegle et al. (2010).   □

8.10 Further statistical concepts

8.10.1 Sharing of dispersion information across genes

We saw an explanation of Bayesian (or empirical Bayes) analysis in Figure 6.12. The idea is to use additional information to improve our estimates, information that we either know a priori or have from analysis of other but similar data. This idea is particularly useful if the data per se are relatively noisy. *DESeq2* uses an empirical Bayes approach for the estimation of the dispersion parameters (the αs in Equation (8.16)) and, optionally, the logarithmic fold changes (the βs). The priors are, in both cases, taken from the dis-tributions of the maximum likelihood estimates (MLEs) across all genes. It turns out that both of these distributions are unimodal: in the case of the βs, with a peak at around 0, and in the case of the αs, at a particular value, the "typical" dispersion. The empirical Bayes machinery then "shrinks" each per-gene MLE toward that peak, by an amount that depends on the sharpness of the empirical prior distribution and the precision of the ML estimate (the better the latter, the less shrinkage will be done). The mathematics is explained in Love et al. (2014), and Figure 8.10 visualizes the approach for the βs.

▶ Task Advanced: check the source code that produces Figure 8.10. (It is a bit long, thus not shown here.)   ◀

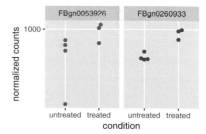

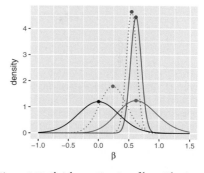

Figure 8.10: *Shrinkage estimation* of logarithmic fold change estimates by use of an empirical prior in *DESeq2*. Two genes with similar mean count and MLE logarithmic fold change are highlighted in green and blue. The normalized counts for these genes (upper panel) reveal low dispersion for the gene in blue and high dispersion for the gene in green. In the lower panel, density plots are shown of the normalized likelihoods (solid lines) and the posteriors (dashed lines) for the green and blue genes. In addition, the solid black line shows the prior estimated from the MLEs of all genes. Due to the higher dispersion of the green gene, its likelihood is wider and less sharp (indicating less information), and the prior has more influence on its posterior than in the case of the blue gene.

8.10.2   Count data transformations

When testing for differential expression, we operate on raw counts and use discrete distributions. For other downstream analyses – e.g., for visualization or clustering – it can be useful to work with transformed versions of the count data.

Maybe the most obvious choice of transformation is the logarithm. However, since count values for a gene can be zero, some analysts advocate the use of **pseudocounts**, i.e., transformations of the form

$$y = \log_2(n + 1) \quad \text{or more generally} \quad y = \log_2(n + n_0), \tag{8.17}$$

where n represents the count values and n_0 is a somehow chosen positive constant.

Let's look at two alternative approaches that offer more theoretical justification, and a rational way of choosing the parameter equivalent to n_0 above. One method incorporates priors on the sample differences, and the other uses the concept of variance-stabilizing transformations.

Variance-stabilizing transformation

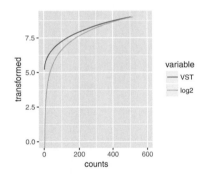

We explored **variance-stabilizing transformations** in Section 4.4.4. There we computed a piecewise linear transformation for a discrete set of random variables (Figure 4.25) and also saw how to use calculus to derive a smooth variance-stabilizing transformation for a gamma–Poisson mixture. These computations are implemented in the *DESeq2* package (Anders and Huber, 2010).

```
vsp = varianceStabilizingTransformation(pasilla)
```

Let us explore the effect of this transformation on the data, using the first sample as an example, and compare it to the $\log_2$ transformation; the plot is shown in Figure 8.11 and is made with the following code.

Figure 8.11: Graph of variance-stabilizing transformation for the data of one of the samples, and comparison with the $\log_2$ transformation. The variance-stabilizing transformation has finite values and finite slope even for counts close to zero, whereas the slope of $\log_2$ becomes very steep for small counts and is undefined for counts of zero. For large counts, the two transformations are essentially the same.

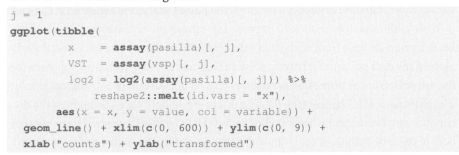

```
j = 1
ggplot(tibble(
        x    = assay(pasilla)[, j],
        VST  = assay(vsp)[, j],
        log2 = log2(assay(pasilla)[, j])) %>%
            reshape2::melt(id.vars = "x"),
      aes(x = x, y = value, col = variable)) +
  geom_line() + xlim(c(0, 600)) + ylim(c(0, 9)) +
  xlab("counts") + ylab("transformed")
```

Regularized logarithm (rlog) transformation

There is a second way to come up with a data transformation. It is conceptually distinct from variance stabilization. Instead, it builds upon the shrinkage estimation explored in Section 8.10.1. It works by transforming the original count data to a $\log_2$-like scale by fitting a "trivial" model with a separate term for each sample and a prior distribution

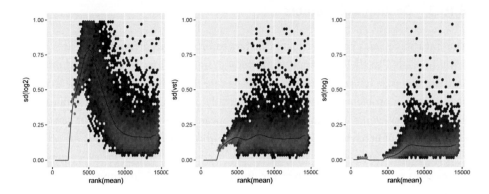

Figure 8.12: Per-gene standard deviation (sd, taken across samples) against the rank of the mean, for the shifted logarithm $\log_2(n + 1)$, the variance-stabilizing transformation (vst) and the rlog. Note that for the leftmost $\approx$2500 genes, the counts are all zero, and hence their standard deviation is zero. The mean-sd dependence becomes more interesting for genes with non-zero counts. Note also the high value of the standard deviation for genes that are weakly detected (but not with all zero counts) when the shifted logarithm is used, and compare to the relatively flat shape of the mean-sd relationship for the variance-stabilizing transformation.

on the coefficients that is estimated from the data. The fitting employs the same regularization as discussed in Section 8.10.1. The transformed data q_{ij} are defined by Equation (8.16), where the design matrix (x_{jk}) is of size $K \times (K + 1)$ – here K is the number of samples – and has the form

$$X = \begin{pmatrix} 1 & 1 & 0 & 0 & \cdot \\ 1 & 0 & 1 & 0 & \cdot \\ 1 & 0 & 0 & 1 & \cdot \\ \cdot & \cdot & \cdot & \cdot & \cdot \end{pmatrix}. \qquad (8.18)$$

Without priors, this design matrix would lead to a non-unique solution; however, the addition of a prior on non-intercept βs allows a unique solution to be found.

In *DESeq2*, this functionality is implemented in the function `rlogTransformation`. It turns out in practice that the rlog transformation is also approximately variance stabilizing, but in contrast to the variance-stabilizing transformation of Section 8.10.2, it deals better with data in which the size factors of the different samples are very distinct.

▶ Question **8.13** Plot mean against standard deviation between replicates for the shifted logarithm (8.17), the regularized log transformation and the variance-stabilizing transformation. ◀

▶ Solution **8.13** See Figure 8.12.

```
library("vsn")
rlp = rlogTransformation(pasilla)

msd = function(x)
  meanSdPlot(x, plot = FALSE)$gg + ylim(c(0, 1)) +
    theme(legend.position = "none")

gridExtra::grid.arrange(
  msd(log2(counts(pasilla, normalized = TRUE) + 1)) +
    ylab("sd(log2)"),
  msd(assay(vsp)) + ylab("sd(vst)"),
  msd(assay(rlp)) + ylab("sd(rlog)"),
  ncol = 3
)
```
□

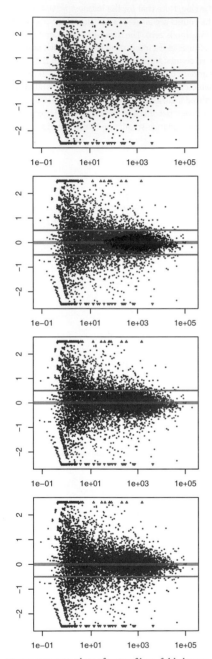

Figure 8.13: MA plots of tests of $\log_2$-fold change with respect to a threshold value. From top to bottom, the tests are for `altHypothesis = "greaterAbs"`, `"lessAbs"`, `"greater"` and `"less"`.

8.10.3 Dealing with outliers

The data sometimes contain isolated instances of very large counts that are apparently unrelated to the experimental or study design and may be considered outliers. Outliers can arise for many reasons, including rare technical or experimental artifacts, read mapping problems in the case of genetically differing samples, and genuine but rare biological events. In many cases, users appear primarily interested in genes that show consistent behavior, and this is the reason why, by default, genes that are affected by such outliers are set aside by `DESeq`. The function calculates, for every gene and for every sample, a diagnostic test for outliers called **Cook's distance** (Cook, 1977). Cook's distance is a measure of how much a single sample is influencing the fitted coefficients for a gene, and a large value of Cook's distance is intended to indicate an outlier count. *DESeq2* automatically flags genes with Cook's distance above a cutoff and sets their p-values and adjusted p-values to `NA`.

The default cutoff depends on the sample size and number of parameters to be estimated; *DESeq2* uses the 99% quantile of the $F(p, m - p)$ distribution (with p the number of parameters including the intercept and m the number of samples).

▶ Question **8.14** Check the documentation for *DESeq2* to see how the default cutoff can be changed, and how the outlier removal functionality can be disabled altogether. How can the computed Cook's distances be accessed? ◀

With many degrees of freedom – i.e., many more samples than number of parameters to be estimated – it might be undesirable to remove entire genes from the analysis just because their data include a single count outlier. An alternative strategy is to replace the outlier counts with the trimmed mean over all samples, adjusted by the size factor for that sample. This approach is **conservative**: it will not lead to false positives, as it replaces the outlier value with the value predicted by the null hypothesis.

8.10.4 Tests of $\log_2$-fold change above or below a threshold

Let's come back to the point we raised in Section 8.6: how to build into tests our scientific goal of detecting effects that have a strong enough size, as opposed to effects that are statistically significant but very small. Two arguments to the `results` function allow for threshold-based Wald tests: `lfcThreshold`, which takes a numeric of a non-negative threshold value, and `altHypothesis`, which specifies the kind of test. For the kind of test, we have the following four options, where β is the $\log_2$-fold change specified by the `name` argument and θ represents `lfcThreshold`:

- `greater`: $\beta > \theta$,
- `less`: $\beta < (-\theta)$,
- `greaterAbs`: $|\beta| > \theta$ (two-tailed test), and
- `lessAbs`: $|\beta| < \theta$ (p-values are the maximum of the upper and lower tests).

These tests are demonstrated in the following code and visually by MA plots in Figure 8.13. (Note that the `plotMA` method, which is defined in the *DESeq2* package, uses base graphics.)

```
par(mfrow = c(4, 1), mar = c(2, 2, 1, 1))
myMA = function(h, v, theta = 0.5) {
  plotMA(pasilla, lfcThreshold = theta, altHypothesis = h,
         ylim = c(-2.5, 2.5))
  abline(h = v * theta, col = "dodgerblue", lwd = 2)
}
myMA("greaterAbs", c(-1, 1))
myMA("lessAbs",    c(-1, 1))
myMA("greater",         1)
myMA("less",       -1    )
```

To produce results tables instead of MA plots, the same arguments as for `plotMA` (except `ylim`) would be provided to the `results` function.

8.11   Summary of this chapter

We have seen how to analyze count tables from high-throughput sequencing (and analogous data types) for differential abundance. We built upon the powerful and elegant framework of linear models. In this framework, we can analyze a basic two-groups comparison as well as more complex multifactorial designs, or experiments with covariates that have more than two levels or are continuous. In ordinary linear models, the sampling distribution of the data around the expected value is assumed to be independent and normal, with zero mean and the same variances. For count data, the distributions are discrete and tend to be skewed (asymmetric) with highly different variances across the dynamic range. We therefore employed a generalization of ordinary linear models, called generalized linear models (GLMs), and in particular considered gamma–Poisson distributed data with dispersion parameters that we needed to estimate from the data.

Since the *sampling depth* is typically different for different sequencing runs (replicates), we need to estimate the effect of this variable parameter and take it into account in our model. We did this through the size factors s_j. Often this part of the analysis is called *normalization* (the term is not particularly descriptive, but unfortunately it is now well established in the literature).

For designed experiments, the number of replicates is (and should be) usually too small to estimate the dispersion parameter (and perhaps even the model coefficients) from the data for each gene alone. Therefore we use shrinkage or empirical Bayes techniques, which promise large gains in precision for relatively small costs of bias.

While GLMs let us model the data on their original scale, sometimes it is useful to transform the data to a scale where they are more homoscedastic and fill out the range more uniformly – for instance, for plotting the data or subjecting them to general purpose clustering, dimension reduction or learning methods. To this end, we have the variance-stabilizing transformation.

A major, and quite valid, critique of differential expression testing as exercised here is that the null hypothesis – the effect size is exactly zero – is almost never true, and therefore our approach does not provide consistent estimates of what the differentially expressed genes are. In practice, this objection may be overcome by considering effect size as well as statistical significance. Moreover, we saw how to use interval-based null hypotheses.

8.12   Further reading

- The *DESeq2* method is explained in the paper by Love et al. (2014), and practical aspects of the software in the package vignette. See also the *edgeR* package and paper (Robinson et al., 2009) for a related approach.
- A classic textbook on robust regression and outlier detection is the book by Rousseeuw and Leroy (1987). For more recent developments, the *CRAN task view on robust statistical methods* is a good starting point.
- The Bioconductor RNA-Seq workflow at `https://www.bioconductor.org/help/workflows/rnaseqGene` (Love et al., 2015) covers a number of issues related specifically to RNA-Seq that we have sidestepped here.
- An extension of the generalized linear model to detecting alternative exon usage from RNA-Seq data is presented in the *DEXSeq* paper (Anders et al., 2012), and applications of these ideas to biological discovery are described by Reyes et al. (2013) and Reyes and Huber (2017).
- For some sequencing-based assays, such as RIP-Seq and CLIP-Seq, the biological analysis goal boils down to testing whether the ratio of *input* and *immunoprecipitate* (IP) has changed between conditions. Mike Love's post on the Bioconductor forum provides a clear and quick how-to: `https://support.bioconductor.org/p/61509`.

8.13   Exercises

▶ Exercise **8.1 edgeR.** Do the analyses of Section 8.5 with the *edgeR* package and compare the results: make a scatterplot of the $\log_{10}$ p-values, pick some genes where there are large differences, and visualize the raw data to see what is going on. Based on this, can you explain the differences? ◀

▶ Exercise **8.2 Robustness.** Write a *shiny* app that performs linear regression on an example (x, y) dataset (for instance, from the `mtcars` data) and displays the data as well as the fitted line. Add a widget that lets you move one of the points in the x- and/or y-direction in a wide range (extending a few times outside the original data range). Add a radio button widget that lets you choose between `lm`, `rlm` and `lqs` with its different choices of `method` (the latter two are in the *MASS* package). Bonus: add functions from the *robustbase* package. ◀

CHAPTER 9

Multivariate Methods for Heterogeneous Data

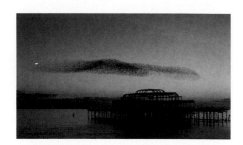

Real situations often involve graphs, point clouds, attraction points, noise and different spatial milieux, a little like this picture where we have a rigid skeleton, waves, sun, and starlings.

In Chapter 7, we saw how to summarize rectangular matrices whose columns were continuous variables. The maps we made used unsupervised dimension reduction techniques, such as principal component analysis, aimed at isolating the most important *signal* component in a matrix X when all the columns have meaningful variances.

Here we extend these ideas to more complex heterogeneous data, where continuous and categorical data are combined, and even to data where individual variables are not available. Indeed, sometimes our observations cannot be easily described by features – but it is possible to determine distances or (dis)similarities between them, or to put them into a graph or a tree. Examples include species in a species tree and biological sequences. Outside of biology, there are text documents and sound files, where we may have a reasonable method to determine (dis)similarity between objects, but no absolute "coordinate system" of features.

This chapter contains more advanced techniques for which we have omitted many technical details. We hope that hands-on experience with examples supplemented with extensive references will enable readers who have come this far to understand some of the more "cutting edge" techniques in nonlinear multivariate analysis.

9.1 Goals for this chapter

In this chapter we will:

- Extend linear dimension reduction methods to cases where the distances between observations are available. The method we use is known as **multid**imensional **s**caling (MDS) or principal coordinates analysis.
- Find modifications of MDS that are nonlinear and robust to outliers.
- Encode combinations of categorical data and continuous data as well as so-called supplementary information. We will see that this enables us to remove *batch effects*.

- Use chi-squared distances and **c**orrespondence **a**nalysis (CA) to see where categorical data (contingency tables) contain notable dependencies.
- Generalize clustering to methods that can uncover latent variables that are not categorical. This will allow us to detect gradients, "pseudotime" and hidden nonlinear effects in our data.
- Generalize the notion of variance and covariance to the study of tables of data from multiple different data domains.

9.2   Multidimensional scaling and ordination

Sometimes data are *not* represented as points in a feature space. This can occur when we are provided with (dis)similarity matrices between objects such as drugs, images, trees or other complex objects, which have no obvious coordinates in $\mathbb{R}^n$.

In Chapter 5 we saw how to produce **clusters** from distances. Here our goal is to visualize the data in maps in low-dimensional spaces (e.g., 2D planes), reminiscent of the representations we make from the first few principal axes in PCA.

We start with an example showing what we can do with simple geographic data. Figure 9.1 shows a heatmap and clustering based on the approximate road distances between some European cities.

```
library("pheatmap")
load("../data/distEuroN.RData")
seteuro = as.matrix(distEuroN)[1:12, 1:12]
pheatmap(seteuro, cluster_rows = TRUE,
    treeheight_row = 0.0001, treeheight_col = 0.8,
    fontsize_col = 8, cellwidth = 13, cellheight = 13)
```

Given these distances between cities, **multidimensional scaling** (MDS) provides a "map" of their relative locations. Of course, in this case the distances were originally measured as road distances (except for ferries), so we actually expect to find a two-dimensional map that represents the data well. With biological data, our maps are likely to be less clear-cut. We call the function with

```
MDSEuro = cmdscale(distEuroN, eig = TRUE)
```

We define a function `plotbar` that we can reuse to make an MDS screeplot from the result of a call to the `cmdscale` function.

```
library("tibble")
plotbar = function(res, m = 9) {
  tibble(eig = res$eig[seq_len(m)], k = seq(along = eig)) %>%
  ggplot(aes(x = k, y = eig)) +
    scale_x_discrete("k", limits = seq_len(m)) + theme_minimal() +
    geom_bar(stat="identity", width=0.5, color="orange", fill="pink")
}
plotbar(MDSEuro, m = 5)
```

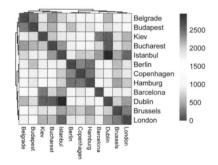

Figure 9.1: A heatmap of distances between European cities. The function has rearranged the order of the cities, grouping the closest ones.

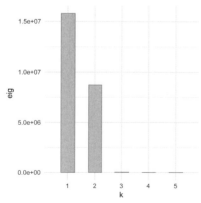

Figure 9.2: Screeplot of the first five eigenvalues. The drop after the first two eigenvalues is very visible.

▶ Question **9.1** Make a barplot of *all* the eigenvalues output by the `cmdscale` function. What do you notice?   ◀

▶ **Solution 9.1** Execute the following code.

```
plotbar(MDSEuro, m = length(MDSEuro$eig))
```

You will note that, unlike in PCA, there *are* negative eigenvalues; these occur because the data do not come from a Euclidean space.   □

To position the points on the map, we project them onto the new coordinates created from the distances (we will discuss how the algorithm works in the next section). Note that while relative positions in Figure 9.3 are correct, the orientation of the map is unconventional; e.g., Istanbul, which is in the southeast of Europe, is at the top left.

```
MDSeur = tibble(
  PCo1 = MDSEuro$points[, 1],
  PCo2 = MDSEuro$points[, 2],
  labs = rownames(MDSEuro$points))
g = ggplot(MDSeur, aes(x = PCo1, y = PCo2, label = labs)) +
  geom_point(color = "red") + xlim(-1950, 2000) + ylim(-1150, 1150) +
  coord_fixed() + geom_text(size = 4, hjust = 0.3, vjust = -0.5)
g
```

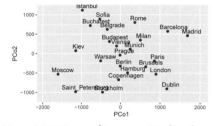

Figure 9.3: MDS map of European cities based on their distances.

We reverse the signs of the principal coordinates and redraw the map. We also read in the true longitudes and latitudes for the cities and plot these alongside for comparison (Figure 9.4).

```
g %+% mutate(MDSeur, PCo1 = -PCo1, PCo2 = -PCo2)
Eurodf = readRDS("../data/Eurodf.rds")
ggplot(Eurodf, aes(x = Long, y = Lat, label = rownames(Eurodf))) +
  geom_point(color = "blue") + geom_text(hjust = 0.5, vjust = -0.5)
```

▶ **Question 9.2** Which cities seem to have the worst representation on the map in the left-hand panel of Figure 9.4?   ◀

▶ **Solution 9.2** It seems that the cities at the extreme west – Dublin, Madrid and Barcelona – have worse projections than the central cities, perhaps because the data are more sparse in these areas and it is harder for the method to "triangulate" the outer cities. □

▶ **Question 9.3** We drew the longitudes and latitudes in the right-hand panel of Figure 9.4 without much attention to aspect ratio. What is the correct aspect ratio for this plot?   ◀

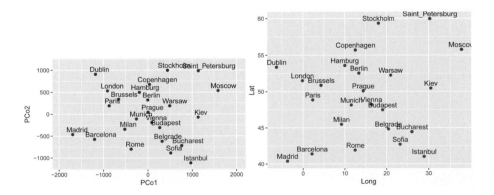

Figure 9.4: Left: Same as Figure 9.3, but with axes flipped. Right: True latitudes and longitudes.

▶ **Solution 9.3** There is no simple relationship between the distances that correspond to one degree change in longitude and one degree change in latitude, so the choice is difficult to make. Even under the simpliyfing assumption that our Earth is spherical and has a radius of 6371 km, it's complicated: one degree in latitude always corresponds to a distance of 111 km ($6371 \times 2\pi/360$), as does one degree of longitude at the equator. However, at the latitude of Barcelona (41.4 degrees), one degree of longitude is 83 km, and at that of Saint Petersburg (60 degrees), 56 km. Pragmatically, we could choose a value for the aspect ratio that's somewhere in between, say, the cosine for 50 degrees. Check out the internet for information on the Haversine formula.   □

Note. MDS creates output similar to PCA. However, there is only one "dimension" to the data (the sample points). There is no "dual" dimension, and biplots are unavailable. This is a drawback when trying to interpret the maps. Interpretation can be facilitated by carefully examining extreme points and their differences.

9.2.1   How does the method work?

Let's look at what would happen if we really started with points whose coordinates are known.[1] We put these coordinates into the two columns of a matrix X with 24 rows. Now we compute the distances between points based on these coordinates. In general, to go from coordinates X to distances, we write

$$d_{i,j}^2 = (x_{i1} - x_{j1})^2 + \cdots + (x_{ip} - x_{jp})^2.$$

[1] Here we commit a slight "abuse" by taking the latitude and longitude of our cities as the underlying cooordinates.

(In our example, p is 2.) We call the matrix of these squared distances DdotD in R and $D \cdot D$ in the text. To make a faithful "map", we want to find points such that the squares of their distances are as close as possible to the $D \cdot D$ observed.

D^2 would mean D multiplied by itself, which is different from $D \cdot D$.

```
Eurodf = readRDS("../data/Eurodf.rds")
X = as.matrix(Eurodf)
DdotD = as.matrix(dist(X)^2)
```

The relative distances do not depend on the point of origin of the data. We center the data using a matrix H, the centering matrix defined as $H = \mathbb{I} - \frac{1}{n}\mathbb{1}\mathbb{1}^{\mathsf{T}}$. Let's check the **centering** property of H.

$\mathbb{I}$ is the identity matrix, and $\mathbb{1}$ is the column vector of ones.

```
n = nrow(X)
H = diag(rep(1,n))-(1/n) * matrix(1, nrow = n, ncol = n)
Xc = sweep(X,2,apply(X,2,mean))
Xc[1:2, ]

##                       Lat      Long
## Saint_Petersburg 10.78194 15.543056
## Stockholm        10.16528  3.309722

HX = H %*% X
HX[1:2, ]

##           Lat      Long
## [1,] 10.78194 15.543056
## [2,] 10.16528  3.309722
```

```
apply(HX, 2, mean)
##           Lat         Long
## 7.901629e-15 2.266633e-15
```

▶ Question **9.4** Give the name `B0` to the matrix obtained by applying the centering matrix to both the right and left of `DdotD`. Consider the points centered at the origin given by the HX matrix and compute its crossproduct: we'll call this `B2`. What do you have to do to `B0` to make it equal to `B2`?   ◀

▶ **Solution 9.4**

```
B0 = H  %*% DdotD %*% H
B2 = HX %*% t(HX)
B2[1:3, 1:3] / B0[1:3, 1:3]

##      [,1] [,2] [,3]
## [1,] -0.5 -0.5 -0.5
## [2,] -0.5 -0.5 -0.5
## [3,] -0.5 -0.5 -0.5

max(abs(-0.5 * B0 - B2))
```
□
```
## [1] 3.694822e-13
```

Therefore, given the squared distances between rows $(D \cdot D)$ and the crossproduct of the centered matrix $B = (HX)(HX)^T$, we have shown that

$$-\frac{1}{2}H(D \cdot D)H = B. \tag{9.1}$$

This is always true, and we use it to reverse-engineer an X that satisfies Equation (9.1) when we are given $D \cdot D$ at the start.

From $D \cdot D$ to X using singular vectors.   We can go backward from a matrix $D \cdot D$ to X by taking the eigen-decomposition of B as defined in Equation (9.1). This also enables us to choose how many coordinates, or columns, we want for the X matrix. This is very similar to how PCA provides the best rank-r approximation.

Note.   As in PCA, we can write this using the singular value decomposition of HX (or the eigen-decomposition of $(HX)(HX)^T$):

$$HX^{(r)} = US^{(r)}V^T \text{ with } S^{(r)} \text{ the diagonal matrix of the first } r \text{ singular values.}$$

$$S^{(r)} = \begin{pmatrix} s_1 & 0 & 0 & 0 & \cdots \\ 0 & s_2 & 0 & 0 & \cdots \\ 0 & 0 & \cdots & \cdots & \cdots \\ 0 & 0 & \cdots & s_r & \cdots \\ \cdots & \cdots & \cdots & 0 & 0 \end{pmatrix}$$

This provides the best approximate representation in a Euclidean space of dimension r. The algorithm gives us the coordinates of points that have approximately the same distances as those provided by the D matrix.

This method is often called **principal coordinates analysis**, or PCoA, which stresses the connection to PCA.

Classical MDS algorithm.   In summary, given an $n \times n$ matrix of squared interpoint distances $D \cdot D$, we can find points and their coordinates $\widetilde{X}$ by the following operations:

1. Double centering the interpoint distance squared and multiplying it by $-\frac{1}{2}$:
   $B = -\frac{1}{2}HD \cdot DH$.
2. Diagonalizing B: $B = U\Lambda U^T s$.
3. Extracting $\widetilde{X}$: $\widetilde{X} = U\Lambda^{1/2}$.

Finding the right underlying dimensionality.   As an example, let's take objects for which we have similarities (surrogates for distances) but for which there is no natural underlying Euclidean space.

In a psychology experiment from the 1950s, Ekman (1954) asked 31 subjects to rank the similarities of 14 different colors. His goal was to understand the underlying dimensionality of color perception. The similarity or confusion matrix was scaled to have values between 0 and 1. The colors that were often confused had similarities close to 1. We transform the data into dissimilarities by subtracting the values from 1.

```
ekm = read.table("../data/ekman.txt", header=TRUE)
rownames(ekm) = colnames(ekm)
disekm = 1 - ekm - diag(1, ncol(ekm))
disekm[1:5, 1:5]

##       w434 w445 w465 w472 w490
## w434 0.00 0.14 0.58 0.58 0.82
## w445 0.14 0.00 0.50 0.56 0.78
## w465 0.58 0.50 0.00 0.19 0.53
## w472 0.58 0.56 0.19 0.00 0.46
## w490 0.82 0.78 0.53 0.46 0.00

disekm = as.dist(disekm)
```

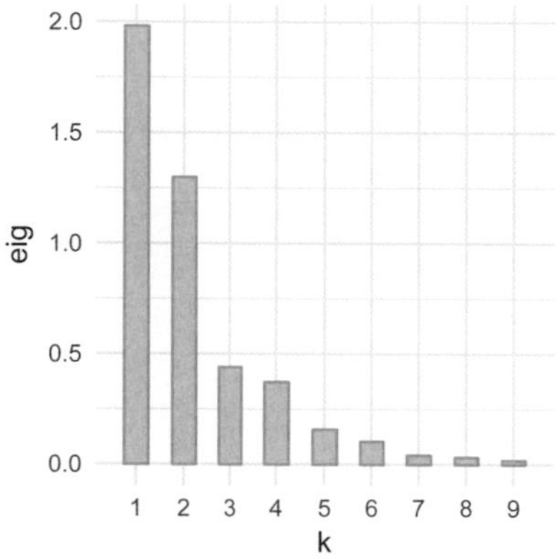

We compute the MDS coordinates and eigenvalues. We combine the eigenvalues in the screeplot shown in Figure 9.5.

```
mdsekm = cmdscale(disekm, eig = TRUE)
plotbar(mdsekm)
```

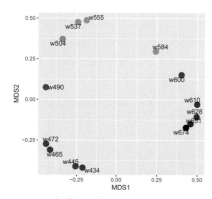

Figure 9.5: The screeplot shows us that the phenomenon is two-dimensional, giving a clean answer to Ekman's question.

We plot the different colors using the first two principal coordinates.

```
dfekm = as_tibble(mdsekm$points[,1:2])%>%
          setNames(paste0("MDS", 1:2))
dfekm$col  = rev(rainbow(nrow(dfekm)))
dfekm$name = rownames(ekm)
library("ggrepel")
ggplot(dfekm, aes(MDS1, MDS2)) +
  geom_point(aes(col = col), size=4) + guides(color = FALSE) +
  geom_text_repel(aes(label = name)) + coord_fixed()
```

Figure 9.6 shows the Ekman data in the new coordinates. There is a striking pattern that calls for a scientific explanation. This kind of horseshoe or arch structure in the points is often a good indicator of a latent ordering or gradient in the data (Diaconis et al., 2007a). We will revisit this idea in Section 9.5.

Figure 9.6: The form of the scatterpoints in the first two dimensions shows a horseshoe shape. The label orderings show that this arch or gradient can be explained by the wavelengths.

9.2.2   Robust versions of MDS

Multidimensional scaling aims to minimize the difference between the squared distances as given by $D \cdot D$ and the squared distances between the points with their new coordinates. Unfortunately, squared distances tend to be sensitive to outliers, and one single large value can skew the whole analysis. We might need procedures that are less dependent on the actual values of the distances but still take into account the relative rankings of the distances – with the most dissimilar objects represented as the farthest apart, the most similar represented as the closest together, and so forth. These rank-based methods are **robust**: their sensitivity to **outliers** is reduced.

We will use the Ekman data to show how useful robust methods are when we are not quite sure about the "scale" of our measurements. Robust ordination, called **non-metric multidimensional scaling** (NMDS for short), attempts only to embed the points in a new space such that the *order* of the reconstructed distances in the new map is the same as the ordering of the original distance matrix.

Non-metric MDS looks for a transformation f of the given dissimilarities in the matrix d and a set of coordinates in a low-dimensional space (the *map*) such that the distance in this new map is $\tilde{d}$ and $f(d) \approx \tilde{d}$. The quality of the approximation can be measured by the standardized residual sum of squares (STRESS) function:

$$\text{STRESS}^2 = \frac{\sum (f(d) - \tilde{d})^2}{\sum d^2}.$$

Non-metric MDS is not sequential in the sense that we have to specify the underlying dimensionality at the outset and the optimization is run to maximize the reconstruction of the distances in that dimension. There is no notion of percentage of variation explained by individual axes, as provided in PCA. However, we can make a ersatz screeplot by running the program for each of successive values of dimension k (i.e., $k = 1, 2, 3, \ldots$) and looking at how much the STRESS drops.

Here is an example of looking at these successive approximations and their goodness of fit. As in the case of diagnostics for clustering, we will take the number of axes *after* the STRESS has a steep drop.

Because each calculation of an NMDS result requires a new optimization that is both random and dependent on the k value, we use a procedure similar to that for clustering in Chapter 4. We execute the `metaMDS` function, say, 100 times for each of the four possible values of k and record the STRESS values.

```
library("vegan")
nmds.stress = function(x, sim = 100, kmax = 4) {
  sapply(seq_len(kmax), function(k)
    replicate(sim, metaMDS(x, k = k, autotransform = FALSE)$stress))
}
stress = nmds.stress(disekm, sim = 100)
dim(stress)
```

Let's look at the boxplots of results, which can be a useful diagnostic plot for choosing k (see Figure 9.7).

```
dfstr = reshape2::melt(stress, varnames = c("replicate","dimensions"))
ggplot(dfstr, aes(y = value, x = dimensions, group = dimensions)) +
  geom_boxplot()
```

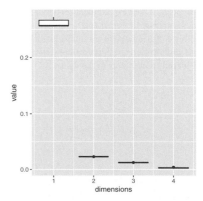

Figure 9.7: Several replicates at each dimension were run to evaluate the stability of the STRESS. We see that the STRESS drops dramatically with two or more dimensions, thus indicating that a two-dimensional solution is appropriate here.

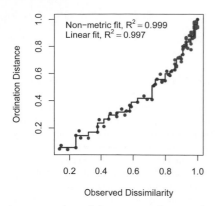

Figure 9.8: A Shepard plot compares the original distances or dissimilarities (along the horizontal axis) to the reconstructed distances (vertical axis), in this case for $k = 2$. The clustering of points near the diagonal means that $k = 2$ is a good choice.

We can also compare the distances and their approximations using what is known as a Shepard plot, computed for $k = 2$ for instance.

```
nmdsk2 = metaMDS(disekm, k = 2, autotransform = FALSE)
stressplot(nmdsk2, pch = 20)
```

Both the Shepard plot in Figure 9.8 and the screeplot in Figure 9.7 point to a two-dimensional solution for Ekman's color confusion study.

```
dfnmdsk2 = as_tibble(nmdsk2$points[,1:2]) %>%
            setNames(paste0("NmMDS", 1:2)) %>%
            bind_cols(select(dfekm, col, name))
ggplot(dfnmdsk2, aes(x = NmMDS1, y = NmMDS2)) +
  geom_point(aes(col = col), size = 4) + guides(color=FALSE) +
  geom_text_repel(aes(label = name))
```

Let's compare the output of the two different MDS programs: the classical metric least squares approximation and the non-metric rank approximation method. The right-hand panel of Figure 9.9 shows the result from the non-metric rank approximation; the left-hand panel is the same as Figure 9.6. The two projections are almost identical. For these data, it makes little difference whether we use a Euclidean or non-metric multi-dimensional scaling method.

9.3   Contiguous or supplementary information

In Chapter 3 we introduced the R *data.frame* class, which allows us to combine heterogeneous data types: categorical factors and continuous measurements. Each row of the dataframe corresponds to an object, or a record, and the columns are the different variables, or features.

Extra information about sample batches, dates of measurement and different protocols is often *misnamed* metadata. This information is actually *real* data that needs to be integrated into analyses.

metadata

Many programs and workflows in biological sequence analysis or assays separate the environmental and contextual information they call **metadata** from the assays or sequence read numbers; we discourage this practice, as the exact connections between the samples and covariates are important. The lost connection between the assays and covariates makes later analyses impossible. Covariates such as clinical history, time, batch and location are important and should be considered components of the *data*.

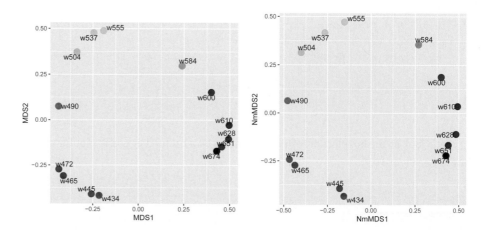

Figure 9.9: Comparison of the output from classical multidimensional scaling on the left (same as Figure 9.6), and the non-metric version on the right.

9.3.1 Known batches in data

Here we show an example of an analysis that was done by Holmes et al. (2011) on bacterial abundance data from *Phylochip* microarrays (Brodie et al., 2006). The experiment was designed to detect differences between a group of healthy rats and a group that had irritable bowel disease (Nelson et al., 2011). This example shows how nuisance **batch effects** can become apparent in the analysis of experimental data. It illustrates why best practices in data analysis are sequential and why it is better to analyze data as they are collected – to adjust for severe problems in the experimental design *as they occur* – instead of trying to deal with deficiencies *post mortem*.[2]

[2] Fisher's terminology – see Chapter 13.

When data collection started on this project, data for days 1 and 2 were delivered and we made the plot that appears in Figure 9.11. This shows a definite *day* effect. When investigating the source of this effect, we found that both the protocol and the array were different on days 1 and 2. This leads to uncertainty about the source of variation; we call this **confounding** of effects. We load the data and the libraries that we use for this section.

```
IBDchip = readRDS("../data/vsn28Exprd.rds")
library("ade4")
library("factoextra")
library("sva")
```

▶ Question 9.5 What class is IBDchip? Look at the last row of the matrix. What do you notice?   ◀

▶ Solution 9.5

```
class(IBDchip)
## [1] "matrix"
dim(IBDchip)
## [1] 8635   28
tail(IBDchip[,1:3])
##                             20CF     20DF     20MF
## bm-026.1.sig_st          7.299308 7.275802 7.383103
## bm-125.1.sig_st          8.538857 8.998562 9.296096
## bru.tab.d.HIII.Con32.sig_st  6.802736 6.777566 6.859950
## bru.tab.d.HIII.Con323.sig_st 6.463604 6.501139 6.611851
## bru.tab.d.HIII.Con5.sig_st   5.739235 5.666060 5.831079
## day                      2.000000 2.000000 2.000000
summary(IBDchip[nrow(IBDchip),])
##    Min. 1st Qu.  Median    Mean 3rd Qu.    Max.
##   1.000   1.000   2.000   1.857   2.000   3.000
```

The data are normalized abundance measurements of 8634 taxa measured on 28 samples. We use a rank-threshold transformation, giving the top 3000 most abundant taxa scores from 3000 to 1 and letting the 5634 least abundant all have a score of 1. We separate out the assay data from the day variable, which should be considered a factor.

```
assayIBD = IBDchip[-nrow(IBDchip), ]
day = factor(IBDchip[nrow(IBDchip), ])
```

Bioconductor container
The data provide an example of an awkward way of combining batch information from the actual data. The day information has been combined with the array data and encoded as a number and could be confused with a continuous variable. We will see in the next section a better practice for storing and manipulating heterogeneous data using a Bioconductor container called *SummarizedExperiment*.

Instead of using the continuous normalized data, we perform a robust analysis replacing the values by their ranks. The lower values are considered ties encoded as a threshold chosen to reflect the number of taxa expected to be present.

```
rankthreshPCA = function(x, threshold = 3000) {
  ranksM = apply(x, 2, rank)
  ranksM[ranksM < threshold] = threshold
  ranksM = threshold - ranksM
  dudi.pca(t(ranksM), scannf = FALSE, nf = 2)
}
pcaDay12 = rankthreshPCA(assayIBD[,day!=3])
day12 = day[day!=3]
fviz(pcaDay12, element="ind", axes=c(1,2), geom=c("point","text"),
  habillage = day12, repel = TRUE, palette = "Dark2",
  addEllipses = TRUE, ellipse.type = "convex") + ggtitle("") +
  coord_fixed()
```

▶ **Question 9.6** Why do we use a threshold for the ranks?   ◀

▶ **Solution 9.6** Low abundances, at noise level, occur for species that are not really present, which can be said of more than half. A large jump in rank for these observations would be meaningless and could easily occur without any meaningful effect. Thus we create a large number of ties at zero.   □

Figure 9.11 shows that the samples arrange themselves naturally into two different groups according to the day of the samples. After discovering this effect, we delved into the differences that could explain these distinct clusters. There were two different protocols used (protocol 1 on day 1, protocol 2 on day 2) *and*, unfortunately, two different provenances for the arrays used on those two days (array 1 on day 1, array 2 on day 2).

A third dataset of four samples had to be collected to deconvolve the confounded effects. Array 2 was used with protocol 2 on day 3; Figure 9.12 shows the new PCA plot with all the samples, created by the following code.

```
pcaDay123 = rankthreshPCA(assayIBD)
fviz(pcaDay123, element="ind", axes=c(1,2), geom=c("point","text"),
  habillage = day, repel=TRUE, palette = "Dark2",
  addEllipses = TRUE, ellipse.type = "convex") + ggtitle("") +
  coord_fixed()
```

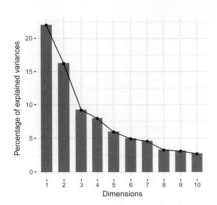

Figure 9.10: The screeplot shows us that the phenomenon can be usefully represented in two dimensions.

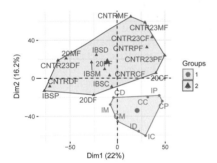

Figure 9.11: We use colors to identify the different days and keep the sample labels as well. We also add convex hulls for each day. The group mean is identified as the point with the larger symbol (circle, triangle or square).

Figure 9.12: When comparing the three-day analysis to that of the first two days, we notice an inversion of signs in the coordinates on the second axis; this has no biological relevance. The important finding is that group 3 overlaps heavily with group 1, indicating that it was the protocol change on day 2 that created the variability.

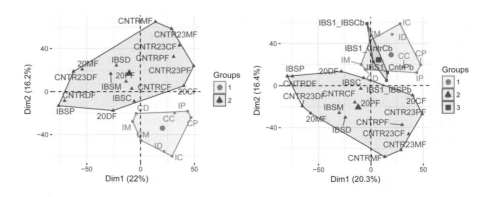

▶ **Question 9.7** In which situation would it be preferable to make confidence ellipses around the group means using the following code?

```
fviz_pca_ind(pcaDay123, habillage = day, labelsize = 3,
  palette = "Dark2", addEllipses = TRUE, ellipse.level = 0.69)      ◀
```

Through the visualization in Figure 9.12, we were able to uncover a flaw in the original experimental design. The first two batches, shown in green and brown, were both balanced with regard to IBS and healthy rats. They do show very different levels of variability and overall multivariate coordinates. In fact, there are two **confounded** effects. Both the arrays and protocols were different on those two days. We had to run a third batch of experiments on day 3, represented in purple; this used the protocol from day 1 and the arrays from day 2. The third group faithfully overlaps with batch 1, telling us that the change in protocol was responsible for the variability.

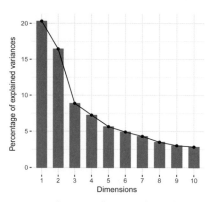

Figure 9.13: The eigenvalue screeplot in the case of three groups is extremely similar to that with two groups shown in Figure 9.10.

9.3.2   Removing batch effects

Through the combination of the continuous measurements from `assayIBD` and the **supplementary** batch number as a factor, the PCA map has provided an invaluable investigation tool. This is a good example of the use of **supplementary points**.[3] The mean barycenter points are created by using the group means of points in each of the three groups and serve as extra markers on the plot.

[3] This is called a supplementary point because the new observation point is not used in the matrix decomposition.

We can decide to realign the three groups by subtracting the group means so that all the batches are centered at the origin. A slightly more effective way is to use the `ComBat` function available in the *sva* package. This function uses a similar but slightly more sophisticated method (an empirical Bayes mixture approach; Leek et al., 2010). We can see its effect on the data by redoing our robust PCA.

```
model0 = model.matrix(~1,day)
combatIBD = ComBat(dat=assayIBD, batch=day, mod=model0)
## Standardizing Data across genes
pcaDayBatRM = rankthreshPCA(combatIBD)
fviz(pcaDayBatRM, element = "ind", geom = c("point", "text"),
  habillage = day, repel=TRUE, palette = "Dark2", addEllipses = TRUE,
  ellipse.type = "convex", axes =c(1,2)) + coord_fixed() + ggtitle("")
```

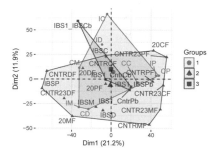

Figure 9.14: The modified data with batch effects removed now show three batch-groups heavily overlapping and centered almost at the origin.

9.3.3   Hybrid data and Bioconductor containers

A more rational way of combining the batch and treatment information into compartments of a composite object is to use *SummarizedExperiment* classes. These include special *slots* for the assay(s) where rows represent features of interest (e.g., genes, transcripts, exons, etc.) and columns represent samples. Supplementary information about the features can be stored in a *DataFrame* object, accessible using the function `rowData`. Each row of the *DataFrame* provides information on the feature in the corresponding row of the *SummarizedExperiment* object.

A confusing notational similarity occurs here; in the *SummarizedExperiment* framework, a `DataFrame` is not the same as a *data.frame*.

Here we insert the two covariates day and treatment in the `colData` object and combine it with assay data in a new *SummarizedExperiment* object.

```
library("SummarizedExperiment")
sampletypes = c("IBS","CTL")
status = c(1, 1, 1, 1, 2, 2, 2, 2, 2, 2, 2, 2, 2, 2,
           2, 2, 2, 2, 1, 1, 1, 1, 1, 1, 1, 1, 1, 1)
colData = DataFrame(day=day, treatment=factor(sampletypes[status]))
chipse = SummarizedExperiment(assays=list(abund = assayIBD),
                    colData=colData)
```

You can explore composite objects using the `Environment` pane in RStudio; you will see that some of the slots are empty.

This is the best way to keep all the relevant data together. It will also enable you to quickly filter the data while keeping all the information aligned properly.

▶ Question **9.8** Make a new *SummarizedExperiment* object by choosing the subset of the samples that were created on day 2.   ◀

▶ Solution **9.8**

```
chipse[,day==2]

## class: SummarizedExperiment
## dim: 8634 16
## metadata(0):
## assays(1): abund
## rownames(8634): 01010101000000.2104_gPM_GC
##    01010101000000.2141_gPM_GC ...
##    bru.tab.d.HIII.Con323.sig_st
##    bru.tab.d.HIII.Con5.sig_st
## rowData names(0):
## colnames(16): 20CF 20DF ... IBSM IBSP
## colData names(2): day treatment
```
□

Columns of the *DataFrame* represent different attributes of the features of interest, e.g., gene or transcript IDs. This is an example of a hybrid data container from a single-cell experiment (see Bioconductor workflow in Perraudeau et al. 2017, for more details). After the preprocessing and normalization steps prescribed in the workflow, we retain the 1000 most variable genes measured on 747 cells.

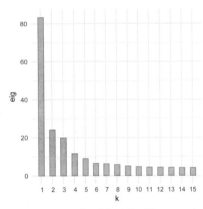

Figure 9.15: Screeplot of the PCA of the normalized data.

```
corese = readRDS("../data/normse.rds")
norm = assays(corese)$normalizedValues
```

▶ Question **9.9** How many different batches do the cells belong to?   ◀

▶ Solution **9.9**

```
length(unique(colData(corese)$Batch))

## [1] 18
```
□

We can look at a PCA of the normalized values and check graphically that the batch effect has been removed.

```
respca=dudi.pca(t(norm), nf=3, scannf=FALSE)
plotbar(respca, 15)
PCS = respca$li[,1:3]
```

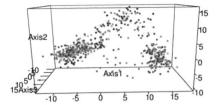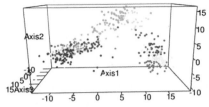

Figure 9.16: Three-dimensional plots: on the left the points are colored according to batch numbers, and on the right according to the original clustering. We can see that the batch effect has been effectively removed and the cells show the original clustering.

Since the screeplot in Figure 9.15 shows us that we must not dissociate axes 2 and 3, we will make a three-dimensional plot with the *rgl* package. We use the following interactive code.

```
library("rgl")
batch = colData(corese)$Batch
plot3d(PCS, aspect=sqrt(c(84,24,20)), col=col_batch[batch])
plot3d(PCS, aspect=sqrt(c(84,24,20)),
col = col_clus[as.character(publishedClusters)])
```

We have set up colors for the clusters as in the workflow (the code is not shown here).

Note. Of course, the book medium is limiting here, as we are showing two static projections that do not do justice to the depth available when looking at the **interactive** dynamic plots as they appear using the `plot3d` function. We encourage the reader to experiment extensively with these and other interactive packages, as they provide a much more intuitive experience of the data.

9.4 Correspondence analysis for contingency tables

9.4.1 Cross-tabulation and contingency tables

Categorical data abound in biological settings: sequence status (CpG/non-CpG), phenotypes and taxa are often coded as factors, as we saw in Chapter 2. Cross-tabulation of two such variables gives us a **contingency table**, the result of counting the co-occurrence of two phenotypes (sex and color blindness was such an example in Chapter 2). We saw that the first step is to look at the independence of the two categorical variables; the standard statistical measure of independence uses the **chi-squared distance**. This quantity will replace the variance we used for continuous measurements.

We're not in a supervised or regression-type setting, so we won't see a subject/variable divide; as a consequence, the rows and columns will have the same status and we will "center" both the rows and the columns. This symmetry will also appear in our use of **biplots**, where both dimensions appear on the same plot.

Transforming the data to tabular form. If the data are collected as long lists with each subject (or sample) associated to its levels of the categorical variables, we may want to transform them into a contingency table. For example, in Table 9.1 HIV mutations are tabulated as indicator (0/1) binary variables. These data are then transformed into the **mutation co-occurrence matrix** shown in Table 9.2. Some of these mutations tend to co-occur.

Table 9.1: Sample-by-mutation matrix from the HIV database (Rhee et al., 2003).

Patient	Mut1	Mut2	Mut3	...
AHX112	0	0	0	
AHX717	1	0	1	
AHX543	1	0	0	

Table 9.2: Cross-tabulation of the HIV mutations showing two-way co-occurrences.

	Mut1	Mut2	Mut3	...
Mut1	853	29	10	
Mut2	29	853	52	
Mut3	10	52	853	

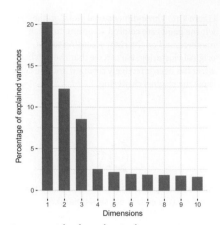

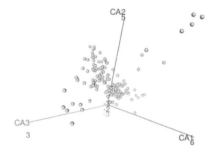

Figure 9.17: The dependencies between HIV mutations is clearly a three-dimensional phenomenon. The three first eigenvalues show a clear signal in the data.

Figure 9.18: A screenshot of the output from an interactive 3D plotting function (scatter3d).

▶ Question **9.10** What information is lost in this cross-tabulation? When will this matter? ◀

▶ Question **9.11** Test the hypothesis of independence of the mutations. ◀

Before explaining the details of how correspondence analysis works, let's look at the output of one of many correspondence analysis functions. We use dudi.coa from the *ade4* package to plot the mutations in a lower-dimensional projection; the procedure follows what we did for PCA.

```
cooc=read.delim2('../data/coccurHIV.txt',header=T,sep=',')
cooc[1:4,1:11]

##       X4S X6D X6K X11R X20R X21I X35I X35L X35M X35T X39A
## 4S      0  28   8    0   99    0   22    5   15    3   45
## 6D     26   0   0   34  131    0  108    4   30   13   84
## 6K      7   0   0    6   45    0    5   13   38   35   12
## 11R     0  35   7    0  127   12   60   17   15    6   42

HIVca=dudi.coa(cooc,nf=4,scannf=FALSE)
fviz_eig(HIVca,geom="bar",bar_width=0.6)+ggtitle("")
```

Looking at the screeplot in Figure 9.17, we see that the underlying variation is definitely three-dimensional, so we plot these three dimensions. Ideally this would be done with an interactive three-dimensional plotting function such as that provided by the package *rgl*, as shown in Figure 9.18.

▶ Question **9.12** Using the *car* and *rgl* packages, make a 3D scatterplot similar to Figure 9.18. Compare it to the plot obtained using aspect=FALSE with the plot3d function from *rgl*. What structure do you notice by rotating the cloud of points? ◀

▶ **Solution 9.12**

```
CA1=HIVca$li[,1];CA2=HIVca$li[,2];CA3=HIVca$li[,3]
scatter3d(CA1,CA2,CA3,surface=FALSE)
plot3d(CA1,CA2,CA3,aspect=FALSE,col="purple")

fviz_ca_row(HIVca,axes = c(1, 2),geom="text", col.row="purple",
  labelsize=3)+ggtitle("") + xlim(-0.55, 1.7) + ylim(-0.53,1.1) +
  theme_bw() + coord_fixed()
```
□

▶ Question **9.13** Show the code for plotting the plane defined by axes 1 and 3 of the correspondence analysis respecting the scaling of the vertical axis, as shown in the right-hand panel of Figure 9.19. ◀

▶ **Solution 9.13**

```
fviz_ca_row(HIVca,axes = c(1, 3), geom="text", col.row="purple",
    labelsize=3)+ ggtitle("")+ theme_minimal() +
    coord_fixed()
```
□

This first example shows how to map all the different levels of one categorical variable (mutations) in a way similar to how PCA projects continuous variables. We will now explore how this can be extended to two or more categorical variables.

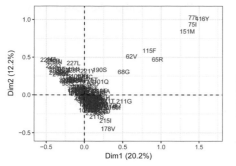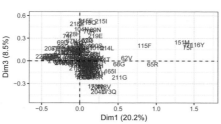

Figure 9.19: Two planar maps of the mutations defined with the horizontal axis corresponding to the first eigenvector of the CA, the vertical axis being the second axis on the left and the third on the right; notice the difference in height.

9.4.2   Hair color, eye color and phenotype co-occurrence

We will consider a small table so we can follow the analysis in detail. The data are a contingency table of hair color and eye color phenotypic co-occurrence among students, as shown in Table 9.3. In Chapter 2 we used a chi-squared test of independence that uncovered the existence of possible dependencies.

```
HairColor = HairEyeColor[,,2]
chisq.test(HairColor)

##
##   Pearson's Chi-squared test
##
## data:  HairColor
## X-squared = 106.66, df = 9, p-value < 2.2e-16
```

However, stating *non-independence* between hair and eye color is not enough. We need a more detailed explanation of where the dependencies occur: which hair color occurs more often with green eyes? Are some of the variable levels independent? In fact, we can study the departure from independence using a special weighted version of SVD. This method can be understood as a simple extension of PCA and MDS to contingency tables.

Table 9.3: Cross-tabulation of student hair and eye color.

	Brown	Blue	Hazel	Green
Black	36	9	5	2
Brown	66	34	29	14
Red	16	7	7	7
Blond	4	64	5	8

Independence: computationally and visually.   We start by computing the row and column sums and use them to build the table that would be expected if the two phenotypes were independent. We call this expected table `HCexp`.

```
rowsums=as.matrix(apply(HairColor,1,sum))
rowsums

##          [,1]
## Black    52
## Brown    143
## Red      37
## Blond    81

colsums=as.matrix(apply(HairColor,2,sum))
t(colsums)

##       Brown Blue Hazel Green
## [1,]    122  114    46    31

HCexp=rowsums%*%t(colsums)/sum(colsums)
```

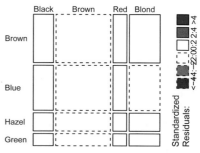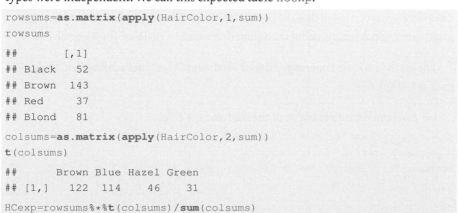

Figure 9.20: Here is a schematic representation of the expected table `HCexp`. We see that it has the "rectangular" property characteristic of the rank-1 matrices we saw in Chapter 7. The boxes are all white.

Now we compute the chi-squared statistic, which is the sum of the scaled residuals for each of the cells of the table.

```
sum((HairColor  - HCexp)^2/HCexp)
## [1] 106.6637
```

We can study these residuals from the expected table, first numerically, and then visually in Figure 9.21.

```
round(t(HairColor-HCexp))
##         Hair
## Eye      Black Brown Red Blond
##   Brown     16    10   2   -28
##   Blue     -10   -18  -6    34
##   Hazel     -3     8   2    -7
##   Green     -3     0   3     0
library("vcd")
mosaicplot(HairColor,shade=TRUE,las=1,type="pearson",
    cex.axis=0.7,main="")
```

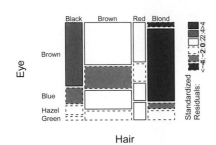

Figure 9.21: Visualization of the departure from independence. The boxes are now proportional in size to the actual observed counts, and we no longer have a "rectangular" property. The departure from independence is measured in chi-squared distance for each of the boxes and colored according to whether the residuals are large and positive. Dark blue indicates a positive association, for instance, between blue eyes and blond hair; red indicates a negative association, as in the case of blond hair and brown eyes.

$\mathbb{1}_I$ and $\mathbb{1}_J$ are I and J dimensional vectors of ones, respectively.

Mathematical formulation.   Here are the computations we just did in R in mathematical form. For a general contingency table N with I rows and J columns and a total sample size of $n = \sum_{i=1}^{I} \sum_{j=1}^{J} n_{ij} = n_{..}$, if the two categorical variables are independent, each cell frequency is approximately equal to

$$n_{ij} = \frac{n_{i.}}{n} \frac{n_{.j}}{n} \times n,$$

which can also be written as

$$N = cr \times n, \qquad \text{where } c = \frac{1}{n}N\mathbb{1}_I \text{ and } r^{\mathsf{T}} = \frac{1}{n}N^{\mathsf{T}}\mathbb{1}_J.$$

The departure from independence is measured by the **chi-squared statistic**:

$$\mathcal{X}^2 = \sum_{i,j} \left[\frac{(n_{ij} - \frac{n_{i.}}{n}\frac{n_{.j}}{n}n)^2}{\frac{n_{i.}n_{.j}}{n^2}n} \right].$$

Correspondence analysis functions include CCA in *vegan*, CA in *FactoMineR*, ordinate in *phyloseq* and dudi.coa in *ade4*.

Once we have ascertained that the two variables are not independent, we use a weighted multidimensional scaling using chi-squared distance to visualize the associations.

The method is called **correspondence analysis** (CA) or **dual scaling**, and multiple R packages implement it.

Here we make a simple biplot of the hair and eye colors.

```
HC=as.data.frame.matrix(HairColor)
coaHC=dudi.coa(HC,scannf=FALSE,nf=2)
round(coaHC$eig[1:3]/sum(coaHC$eig)*100)
## [1] 89 10  2
fviz_ca_biplot(coaHC,repel=TRUE)+ggtitle("")+ylim(c(-0.5,0.5))
```

▶ Question **9.14** What percentage of the chi-squared statistic is explained by the first two axes of the correspondence analysis?   ◀

▶ Question **9.15** Compare the results with those obtained by using CCA in the *vegan* package with the appropriate value for the scaling parameter.   ◀

▶ **Solution 9.15**

```
library("vegan")
res.ca=vegan::cca(HairColor)
plot(res.ca,scaling=3)
```    □

Interpreting the biplots

Correspondence analysis has a special barycentric property: the biplot scaling is chosen so that the row points are placed at the center of gravity of the column levels with their respective weights. For instance, the blue-eyes column point is at the center gravity of (black, brown, red, blond) with weights proportional to (9,34,7,64). The blond row point is very heavily weighted. This is why Figure 9.22 shows blond and blue quite close together.

9.5   Finding time ... and other important gradients

All the methods we have studied so far in this chapter are commonly known as **ordination** methods. In the same way that **clustering** allows us to detect and interpret a hidden factor/categorical variable, ordination enables us to detect and interpret a hidden ordering, gradient or latent variable in the data.

Ecologists have a long history of interpreting the arches formed by observation points in correspondence analysis and principal components as ecological gradients (Prentice, 1977). Let's illustrate this, first, with a very simple dataset on which we perform a correspondence analysis.

```
load("../data/lakes.RData")
lakelike[1:3,1:8]
##      plant1 plant2 plant3 plant4 plant5 plant6 plant7 plant8
## loc1      6      4      0      3      0      0      0      0
## loc2      4      5      5      3      4      2      0      0
## loc3      3      4      7      4      5      2      1      1
reslake=dudi.coa(lakelike,scannf=FALSE,nf=2)
round(reslake$eig[1:8]/sum(reslake$eig),2)
## [1] 0.56 0.25 0.09 0.03 0.03 0.02 0.01 0.00
fviz_ca_row(reslake,repel=TRUE)+ggtitle("")+ylim(c(-0.55,1.7))
```

We plot the location points on the left-hand side of Figure 9.23 and the biplot of both location and plant species on the right-hand side.

```
fviz_ca_biplot(reslake,repel=TRUE)+ggtitle("")+ylim(c(-0.55,1.7))
```

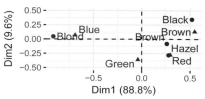

Figure 9.22: The CA plot gives a representation of a large proportion of the chi-squared distance between the data and the values expected under independence. The first axis shows a contrast between black- and blond-haired students, mirrored by the brown eye, blue eye opposition. In CA the two categories play symmetric roles and we can interpret the proximity of blue eyes and blond hair to mean that there is strong co-occurrence of these categories.

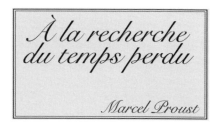

The first example of seriation or chronology detection was that of archaeological artifacts by Kendall (1969), who used the presence or absence of features on pottery to date them. These so-called seriation methods are still relevant today, for example as we follow developmental trajectories in single-cell data.

Figure 9.23: The locations near the lake are ordered along an arch, as shown on the left. In the biplot on the right, we can see which plants are most frequent at which locations by looking at the red triangles closest to the blue points.

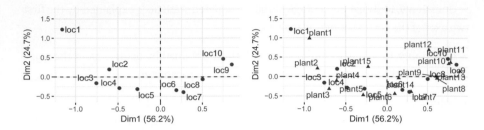

▶ **Question 9.16** Looking back at the raw matrix `lakes` as it appears, do you see a pattern in its entries? What would happen if the plants had been ordered by actual taxa names, for instance?   ◀

9.5.1 Dynamics of cell development

We will now analyze a more interesting dataset that was published by Moignard et al. (2015). That paper describes the dynamics of blood cell development. The data are single-cell gene expression measurements of 3934 cells with blood and endothelial potential from five populations between embryonic days E7.0 and E8.25.

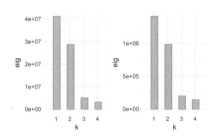

Figure 9.24: The four cell populations studied here are representative of three sequential states (PS, NP, HF) and two possible final branches (4SG and 4SFG⁻).

Remember from Chapter 4 that several different distances are available for comparing our cells. Here, we start by computing both the L_2 distance and the L_1 distance between the 3934 cells – the Euclidean and Manhattan distances.

```
Moignard = readRDS("../data/Moignard.rds")
cellt = rowData(Moignard)$celltypes
colsn = c("red", "purple", "orange", "green", "blue")
blom = assay(Moignard)
dist2n.euclid=dist(blom)
dist1n.l1=dist(blom,"manhattan")
```

We carry out classical multidimensional scaling on these two distance matrices.

```
ce1Mds=cmdscale(dist1n.l1,k=20,eig=TRUE)
ce2Mds=cmdscale(dist2n.euclid,k=20,eig=TRUE)
perc1=round(100*sum(ce1Mds$eig[1:2])/sum(ce1Mds$eig))
perc2=round(100*sum(ce2Mds$eig[1:2])/sum(ce2Mds$eig))
```

We look at the underlying dimension and see in Figure 9.25 that two dimensions can provide a substantial percentage of the variance.

```
plotbar(ce1Mds,m=4)
plotbar(ce2Mds,m=4)
```

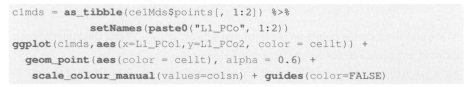

Figure 9.25: Screeplots from MDS on L_1 (left) and L_2 (right) distances. We see that the eigenvalues are extremely similar and both point to a two-dimensional phenomenon.

The first two coordinates account for 78% of the variability when the L_1 distance is used between cells, and 57% when the L_2 distance is used. Figure 9.26A plots the first two coordinates created by applying MDS to the L_1 distances between cells.

```
c1mds = as_tibble(ce1Mds$points[, 1:2]) %>%
            setNames(paste0("L1_PCo", 1:2))
ggplot(c1mds, aes(x=L1_PCo1,y=L1_PCo2, color = cellt)) +
  geom_point(aes(color = cellt), alpha = 0.6) +
    scale_colour_manual(values=colsn) + guides(color=FALSE)
```

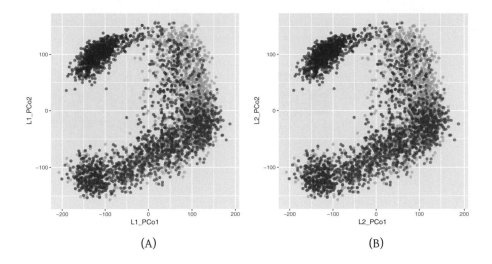

(A)   (B)

Figure 9.26: Moignard cell data colored according to cell type (blue: PS, green: NP, yellow: HF, red: 4SG, purple: 4SFG⁻) in the two-dimensional MDS plots created, on the left (A) using L_1 distances and on the right (B) using L_2 distances.

cell type
● 4SG
● 4SGF−
● HF
● NP
● PS

Figure 9.26B is created in the same way for MDS applied to the L_2 distances.

```
c2mds = as_tibble(celMds$points[, 1:2]) %>%
            setNames(paste0("L2_PCo", 1:2))
ggplot(c2mds, aes(x=L2_PCo1, y=L2_PCo2, color = cellt)) +
  geom_point(aes(color = cellt), alpha = 0.6) +
    scale_colour_manual(values = colsn) + guides(color = FALSE)
```

Figure 9.26 shows that both distances (L_1 and L_2) give the same first plane for the MDS, with very similar representations of the underlying gradient followed by the cells.

We can see from Figure 9.26 that the cells are not distributed uniformly in the lower dimensions we have been considering: there is definite organization of the points. All the cells of type 4SG, represented in red, form an elongated cluster in which they are much less mixed with the other cell types.

9.5.2   Local nonlinear methods

Multidimensional scaling and non-metric multidimensional scaling aim to represent *all* distances as precisely as possible, and the large distances between far-apart points skew the representations. It can be beneficial when looking for gradients or low-dimensional manifolds to restrict ourselves to approximations of points that are close together. This idea calls for methods that try to represent local (small) distances well and do not try to approximate distances between widely separated points with too much accuracy.

There has been substantial progress on such methods in recent years. The use of **kernels** computed using the calculated interpoint distances allows us to decrease the importance of points that are far apart. A radial basis kernel is of the form

$$1 - \exp\{-\frac{d(x,y)^2}{\sigma^2}\}, \text{ where } \sigma^2 \text{ is fixed.} \tag{9.2}$$

It has the effect of heavily discounting large distances. This can be very useful, as the

This is an advanced topic.

Figure 9.27: Moignard cell data represented by t-SNE. The plot on the left was obtained by choosing two dimensions for t-SNE at a perplexity of 30. The plot on the right was obtained by choosing three dimensions; we can see the third t-SNE axis represented here as the horizontal axis.

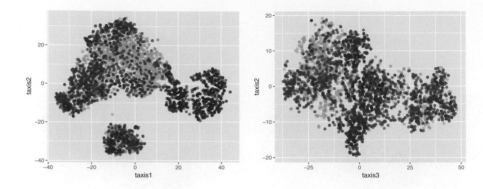

cell type

- 4SG
- 4SGF−
- HF
- NP
- PS

precision of interpoint distances is often better at smaller ranges. Several examples of such methods are covered in Exercise 9.6 at the end of this chapter.

▶ Question **9.17** Why do we take the difference between the 1 and the exponential? What happens when the distance between x and y is very big?   ◀

t-SNE. This widely used method adds flexibility in the kernel defined in (9.2) and allows the σ^2 parameter to vary locally (with a normalization step so that they sum to one). Thus we obtain a distribution that serves as the probability that pairs of points in the high-dimensional space are neighbors. The t-SNE method then uses this probability distribution to construct a representation of the dataset in low dimensions. This method is not robust and has the property of separating clusters of points artificially; it can, however, clarify a complex situation. One can think of it as similar to a network layout algorithm. It stretches the data to clarify relations, but the distances between points cannot be interpreted as being on the same scales in different parts of the plane. Here is an example of the output of t-SNE on the Moignard cell data.

Perplexity is a tunable parameter of t-SNE. It is a measure of precision; it quantifies how well the probability model predicts the data.

```
library("Rtsne")
restsne = Rtsne(blom, dims = 2, perplexity = 30, verbose = FALSE,
                max_iter = 900)
dftsne = as_tibble(restsne$Y[, 1:2]) %>%
                        setNames(paste0("taxis", 1:2))
ggplot(dftsne,aes(x = taxis1, y = taxis2, color = cellt)) +
  geom_point(aes(color = cellt), alpha = 0.6) +
    scale_color_manual(values = colsn) + guides(color = FALSE)
```

In this case, in order to see the subtle differences between MDS and t-SNE, it is really necessary to use 3D plotting. First, we generate the 3D t-SNE representation.

```
restsne3 = Rtsne(blom, dims = 3, perplexity = 30, verbose = FALSE,
                 max_iter = 900)
dftsne3 = as_tibble(restsne3$Y[, 1:3]) %>%
              setNames(paste0("taxis", 1:3))
ggplot(dftsne3,aes(x = taxis3, y = taxis2, group = cellt)) +
        geom_point(aes(color = cellt), alpha = 0.6) +
          scale_colour_manual(values = colsn) + guides(color = FALSE)
```

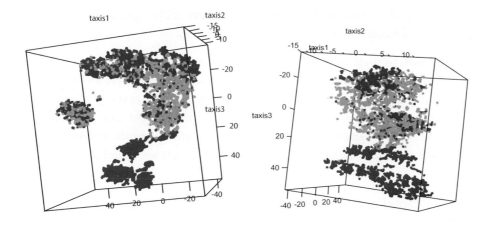

Figure 9.28: Moignard cell data colored according to the cell type (blue: PS, green: NP, yellow: HF, red: 4SG, purple: 4SFG⁻) in the three-dimensional t-SNE layout. We can see that the purple cells (4SFG⁻) segregate at the outer shell on the top of the point cloud. The right panel is (roughly) a 90 degree left-hand rotation of the left panel around the taxis3 axis.

▶ Task   Use the *rgl* package to look at the three t-SNE dimensions and add the correct cell type colors to the display.   ◀

Two of these 3D snapshots are shown in Figure 9.28; we see a much stronger grouping of the purple points than in the MDS plots.

Note.   A site worth visiting in order to appreciate the sensitivity of the t-SNE method to the complexity and σ parameters can be found at `http://distill.pub/2016/misread-tsne`.

There are several other nonlinear methods for estimating nonlinear trajectories followed by points in the relevant state spaces. Here are a few examples:

RDRToolbox   Local linear embedding (**LLE**) and **isomap** are methods that solve this problem.

diffusionMap   This package models connections between points as a Markovian kernel.

kernlab   Kernel methods.

LPCM-package   Local principal curves.

9.6   Multitable techniques

Current studies often attempt to quantify variation in microbial, genomic and metabolic measurements across different experimental conditions. As a result, it is common to perform multiple assays on the same biological samples and ask what features – microbes, genes or metabolites, for example – are associated with different sample conditions. There are many ways to approach these questions; which to apply depends on the study's focus.

9.6.1   Covariation, inertia, co-inertia and the RV coefficient

We define inertia as a sum of distances with "weighted" points, similar to the moment of inertia in physics. This definition enables us to compute the **inertia** of counts in a

Another generalization of variance-inertia is the useful phylogenetic diversity index (computing the sum of distances between a subset of taxa through the tree). Other useful generalizations include using the variability of points on a graph taken from standard spatial statistics.

Some precautions must be taken when using the Mantel coefficient; see a critical review in Guillot and Rousset (2013).

contingency table as the weighted sum of the squares of distances between observed and expected frequencies (as in the chi-squared statistic).

If we want to study two standardized variables measured at the same 10 locations together, we use their **covariance**. If x represents the standardized pH, and y the standardized humidity, we measure their covariation using the mean $\mathrm{cov}(x, y) = \mathrm{mean}(x1 * y1 + x2 * y2 + x3 * y3 + \cdots + x10 * y10)$. If x and y covary in the same direction, this value will be big. We saw how useful the correlation coefficient we defined in Chapter 8 was to our multivariate analyses. Multitable generalizations will be just as useful.

9.6.2   Mantel coefficient and a test of distance correlation

The Mantel coefficient, one of the earliest versions of **matrix association**, developed and used by Henry Daniels, F.N. David and coauthors (Josse and Holmes, 2016), is very popular, especially in ecology. Given two dissimilarity matrices D^X and D^Y, make these matrices into vectors in the way the R `dist` function does, and compute their correlation. This is defined mathematically as

$$r_{\mathrm{m}}(X, Y) = \frac{\sum_{i=1}^{n} \sum_{j=1, j\neq i}^{n} (d_{ij}^X - \bar{d}^X)(d_{ij}^Y - \bar{d}^Y)}{\sqrt{\sum_{i,j,j\neq i}(d_{ij}^X - \bar{d}^X)^2 \sum_{i,j,j\neq i}(d_{ij}^Y - \bar{d}^Y)^2}},$$

where $\bar{d}^X$ (resp. $\bar{d}^Y$) is the mean of the lower diagonal terms of the dissimilarity matrix associated to X (resp. to Y). This formulation shows us that it is a measure of linear correlation between distances. It has been widely used for testing two sets of distances; for instance, one distance, D^X, could be computed using the soil chemistry at 17 different locations. The other distance, D^Y, could record plant abundance dissimilarities using a Jaccard index between the same 17 locations.

The correlation's significance is often assessed via a simple permutation test; see Josse and Holmes (2016) for a review with historical background and modern incarnations. The coefficient and associated tests are implemented in several R packages, such as *ade4* (Chessel et al., 2004), *vegan* and *ecodist* (Goslee and Urban, 2007).

RV coefficient.   A global measure of similarity between two data tables, as opposed to two vectors, can be defined by a generalization of covariance provided by an inner product between tables that gives the RV coefficient, a number between 0 and 1, like a correlation coefficient, but for tables:

$$\mathrm{RV}(A, B) = \frac{\mathrm{Tr}(A^{\mathrm{T}} B A B^{\mathrm{T}})}{\sqrt{\mathrm{Tr}(A^{\mathrm{T}} A)} \sqrt{\mathrm{Tr}(B^{\mathrm{T}} B)}}$$

Several other measures of matrix correlation are available in the package *MatrixCorrelation*.

If we do ascertain a link between two matrices, we then need to find a way to understand that link. One such method is explained next.

9.6.3   Canonical correlation analysis (CCA)

The CCA method is similar to PCA, as it was developed by Hotelling in the 1930s to search for associations between two sets of continuous variables X and Y. Its goal is to find a linear projection of the first set of variables that maximally correlates with a linear projection of the second set of variables.

Finding correlated functions (covariates) of two views of the same phenomenon by discarding the representation-specific details (noise) is expected to reveal the underlying hidden yet influential factors responsible for the correlation.

Canonical correlation algorithm.   Let us consider two matrices X and Y of size $n \times p$ and $n \times q$, respectively. The columns of X and Y correspond to variables and the rows correspond to the same n experimental units. The jth column of the matrix X is denoted by X_j; likewise the kth column of Y is denoted by Y_k. Without loss of generality, it will be assumed that the columns of X and Y are standardized (mean 0 and variance 1).

We denote by S_{XX} and S_{YY} the sample covariance matrices for variable sets X and Y, respectively, and by $S_{XY} = S_{YX}^T$ the sample cross-covariance matrix between X and Y.

Classical CCA assumes first that $p \leqslant n$ and $q \leqslant n$, then that matrices X and Y are of full column rank p and q, respectively. In the following, the principle of CCA is presented as a problem solved through an iterative algorithm. The first stage of CCA consists in finding two vectors $a = (a_1, \ldots, a_p)^T$ and $b = (b_1, \ldots, b_q)^T$ that maximize the correlation between the linear combinations U and V defined as

$$U = Xa = a_1 X_1 + a_2 X_2 + \cdots + a_p X_p,$$
$$V = Yb = b_1 Y_1 + b_2 Y_2 + \cdots + a_q Y_q,$$

where the vectors a and b are normalized so that $\text{var}(U) = \text{var}(V) = 1$. In other words, the problem consists of finding a and b such that $\rho_1 = \text{cor}(U, V) = \max_{a,b} \text{cor}(Xa, Yb)$ subject to $\text{var}(Xa) = \text{var}(Yb) = 1$.

The resulting variables U and V are called the first canonical variates, and ρ_1 is referred to as the first canonical correlation.

Note.   Higher-order canonical variates and canonical correlations can be found via a stepwise procedure. For $s = 1, \ldots, p$, we can successively find positive correlations $\rho_1 \geqslant \rho_2 \geqslant \cdots \geqslant \rho_p$ with corresponding vectors $(a^1, b^1), \ldots, (a^p, b^p)$, by maximizing

$$\rho_s = \text{cor}(U^s, V^s) = \max_{a^s, b^s} \text{cor}(Xa^s, Yb^s) \qquad \text{subject to} \quad \text{var}(Xa^s) = \text{var}(Yb^s) = 1$$

under the additional restrictions $\text{cor}(U^s, U^t) = \text{cor}(V^s, V^t) = 0$, for $1 \leqslant t < s \leqslant p$.

We can think of CCA as a generalization of PCA where the variance we maximize is the "covariance" between the two matrices; see Holmes (2006) for more details.

9.6.4   Sparse canonical correlation analysis (sCCA)

We will see many examples of regularization and the danger of overfitting in Chapter 12.

When the number of variables in each table is very large, finding two very correlated vectors can be too easy and unstable: we have too many degrees of freedom. Then it is beneficial to add a **penalty** to keep the number of non-zero coefficients to a minimum. This approach is called sparse canonical correlation analysis (sparse CCA or sCCA), a method well suited to both exploratory comparisons between samples and the identification of features with interesting **co**variation. We will use an implementation from the *PMA* package.

Here we study a dataset collected by Kashyap et al. (2013) with two tables. One is an abundance table of metabolites and another is a contingency table of bacterial abundances. There are 12 samples, so $n = 12$. The metabolite table has measurements on $p = 637$ features and the bacterial abundances have a total of $q = 20{,}609$ OTUs, which we will filter down to around 200. We start by loading the data and the libraries.

```
mb_path = "../data/metabolites.csv"
library("genefilter")
load("../data/microbe.rda")
metab   = read.csv(mb_path, row.names = 1) %>% as.matrix
```

We first filter down to bacteria and metabolites of interest, removing ("by hand") those that are zero across many samples and giving an upper threshold of 50 to the large values. We transform the data to weaken the heavy tails.

```
metab   = metab[rowSums(metab == 0) <= 3, ]
microbe = prune_taxa(taxa_sums(microbe) > 4, microbe)
microbe = filter_taxa(microbe, filterfun(kOverA(3, 2)), TRUE)
metab = log(1 + metab, base = 10)
X = as.matrix(otu_table(microbe))
X = log(1 + X, base=10)
```

The second step in our preliminary analysis is to look for any association between the two matrices using the RV.test from the *ade4* package.

```
colnames(metab)=colnames(X)
pca1 = dudi.pca(t(metab), scal = TRUE, scann = FALSE)
pca2 = dudi.pca(t(X), scal = TRUE, scann = FALSE)
rv1 = RV.rtest(pca1$tab, pca2$tab, 999)
rv1

## Monte-Carlo test
## Call: RV.rtest(df1 = pca1$tab, df2 = pca2$tab, nrepet = 999)
##
## Observation: 0.8400429
##
## Based on 999 replicates
## Simulated p-value: 0.001
## Alternative hypothesis: greater
##
##      Std.Obs Expectation    Variance
## 6.130593084 0.316031253 0.007305954
```

We can now apply sparse CCA. This method compares sets of features across high-dimensional data tables, where there may be more measured features than samples. In the process, it chooses a subset of available features that capture the most covariance – these are the features that reflect signals present across multiple tables. We then apply PCA to this selected subset of features. In this sense, we use sparse CCA as a screening procedure rather than as an ordination method in its own right.

In the implementation of CCA below, the parameters `penaltyx` and `penaltyz` are **sparsity** penalties. Smaller values of `penaltyx` will result in fewer selected microbes; similarly, `penaltyz` modulates the number of selected metabolites. We tune them manually to facilitate subsequent interpretation – we generally prefer greater sparsity than the default parameters would provide.

```
library("PMA")
ccaRes = CCA(t(X), t(metab), penaltyx = 0.15, penaltyz = 0.15)
## 123456789
ccaRes
## Call: CCA(x = t(X), z = t(metab), penaltyx = 0.15, penaltyz = 0.15)
##
##
## Num non-zeros u's:   5
## Num non-zeros v's:   16
## Type of x:    standard
## Type of z:    standard
## Penalty for x: L1 bound is   0.15
## Penalty for z: L1 bound is   0.15
## Cor(Xu,Zv):   0.9904707
```

This output shows that there is a linear combination of 5 microbial taxa and a linear combination of 16 metabolites that have a strong correlation (0.99).

With these parameters, 5 bacteria and 16 metabolites were selected based on their ability to explain covariation between the tables. Furthermore, these features result in a correlation of 0.99 between the two tables. We interpret this as meaning that the microbial and metabolomic data reflect similar underlying signals, and that these signals can be approximated well by the selected features. Be wary of the correlation value, however, since the scores are far from the usual bivariate normal cloud. Furthermore, note that it is possible that other subsets of features could explain the data just as well – sparse CCA minimizes redundancy among the features it chooses, but makes no guarantee that these are the "true" features in any sense.

Nonetheless, we can still use these 21 features to compress information from the two tables without much loss. In order to relate the observed metabolites and OTUs to characteristics of the samples on which they were measured, we use them as input to an ordinary PCA. We have omitted the code used to generate Figure 9.29 and refer the reader to the online material accompanying the book or the workflow published in Callahan et al. (2016a).

Figure 9.29 displays the PCA *triplot*, where we show different types of samples and the multidomain features (metabolites and OTUs). This plot lets us compare across the measured samples – triangles for knockout and circles for wild-type – and characterizes the influence of the different features – diamonds with text labels. For example, we see

Figure 9.29: A PCA triplot produced from the CCA-selected features from multiple data types (metabolites and OTUs).

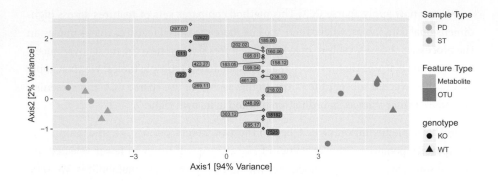

that the main variation in the data is between PD and ST samples, which correspond to the different diets. Furthermore, large values for 15 of the features are associated with ST status, while small values for 5 of them indicate PD status.

The advantage of the sparse CCA screening is now clear: we can display most of the variation across samples using a relatively simple plot, and can avoid plotting the hundreds of additional points that would be needed to display all the features.

9.6.5   Canonical (or constrained) correspondence analysis (CCpnA)

Notational overload for CCA. Originally invented by ter Braak (1985) and called canonical correspondence analysis, this method will here be called constrained correspondence analysis and abbreviated CCpnA to avoid confusion with canonical correlation analysis (CCA). However, several R packages, such as *ade4* and *vegan*, use the name cca for their correspondence analysis function.

The term "constrained correspondence analysis" conveys the idea that this method is similar to a constrained regression. The method attempts to force the latent variables to be correlated with the environmental variables provided as "explanatory".

CCpnA creates biplots where the positions of samples are determined by similarity in both species signatures and environmental characteristics. In contrast, principal components analysis or correspondence analysis looks only at species signatures. More formally, it ensures that the resulting CCpnA directions lie in the span of the environmental variables. For thorough explanations, see ter Braak (1985) and Greenacre (2007).

This method can be run using the function ordinate in *phyloseq*. In order to use the covariates from the sample data, we provide an extra argument specifying which of the features to consider.

Here, we take the data that we denoised using *dada2* in Chapter 5. We will see more details about creating the *phyloseq* object in Chapter 10. For the time being, we use the otu_table component containing a contingency table of counts for different taxa. We will compute the constrained correspondence analyses that explain the taxa abundances by age and family relationship (both variables are contained in the sample_data slot of the ps1 object).

We would like to make two-dimensional plots showing only the four most abundant taxa (making the biplot easier to read).

```
ps1=readRDS("../data/ps1.rds")
ps1p=filter_taxa(ps1, function(x) sum(x) > 0, TRUE)
psCCpnA = ordinate(ps1p, "CCA",
                   formula = ps1p ~ ageBin + family_relationship)
```

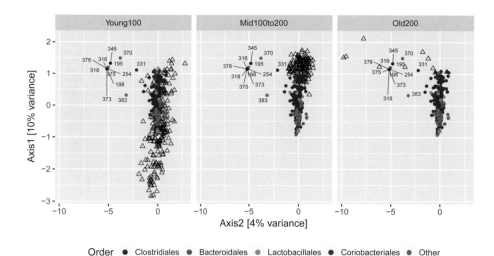

Figure 9.30: The mouse and taxa scores generated by CCpnA. The sites (mice samples) are triangles; species are dots. The separate panels indicate different age groups.

To access the positions for the biplot, we use the `scores` function in *vegan*. Furthermore, to facilitate figure annotation, we also join the site scores with the environmental data in the `sample_data` slot. Of the 23 total taxonomic orders, we explicitly annotate by coloring the four most abundant – this makes the biplot easier to read.

```
evalProp = 100 * psCCpnA$CCA$eig[1:2] / sum(psCCpnA$CA$eig)
ggplot() +
 geom_point(data = sites,aes(x =CCA2, y =CCA1),shape =2,alpha=0.5) +
 geom_point(data = species,aes(x =CCA2,y =CCA1,col = Order),size=0.5)+
 geom_text_repel(data = species %>% filter(CCA2 < -2),
                 aes(x = CCA2, y = CCA1, label = otu_id),
                 size = 1.5, segment.size = 0.1) +
 facet_grid(. ~ ageBin) +
 guides(col = guide_legend(override.aes = list(size = 3))) +
 labs(x = sprintf("Axis2 [%s%% variance]", round(evalProp[2])),
      y = sprintf("Axis1 [%s%% variance]", round(evalProp[1]))) +
 scale_color_brewer(palette = "Set1") + theme(legend.position="bottom")
```

▶ Task Look up the extra code for creating the `tax` and `species` objects in the online resources accompanying the book. Then make the analog of Figure 9.30 but using litter as the faceting variable. ◀

Figures 9.30 and 9.31 show the plots of these annotated scores, splitting sites by their age bin and litter membership, respectively. Note that to keep the appropriate aspect ratio in the presence of faceting, we took the vertical axis as our first canonical component. We labeled individual bacteria that are outliers along the second CCpnA direction.

Evidently, the first CCpnA direction distinguishes between mice in the two main age bins. Dots on the left and right of the biplot represent bacteria that are characteristic of younger and older mice, respectively. The second CCpnA direction splits off the few mice in the oldest age group; it also partially distinguishes between the two litters. Those samples low in the second CCpnA direction have more of the outlier bacteria than the others.

Figure 9.31: The analog to Figure 9.30, faceting by litter membership rather than age bin.

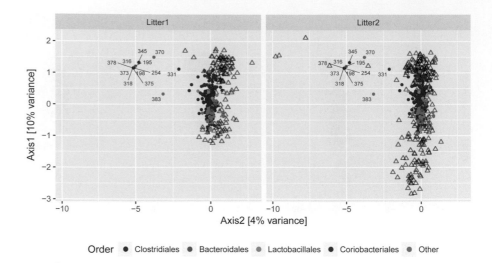

This CCpnA analysis supports the conclusion that the main difference between the microbiome communities of the different mice lies along the age axis. However, in situations where the influence of environmental variables is not so strong, CCA can have more power in detecting such associations. In general, it can be applied whenever it is desirable to incorporate *supplemental data*, but in a way that (1) is less aggressive than supervised methods and (2) can use several environmental variables at once.

9.7   Summary of this chapter

Heterogeneous data A mixture of many continuous and a few categorical variables can be handled by adding the categorical variables as supplementary information to the PCA. This is done by projecting the mean of all points in a group onto the map.

Using distances Relations between data objects can often be summarized as interpoint distances (whether distances between trees, images, graphs or other complex objects).

Ordination A useful representation of these distances is available through a method similar to PCA called multidimensional scaling (MDS), otherwise known as PCoA (principal coordinate analysis). It can be helpful to think of the outcomes of these analyses as uncovering latent variables. In the case of clustering, the latent variables are categorical; in ordination, they are latent variables like time or environmental gradients like distance to the water. This is why these methods are often called ordination.

Robust versions When interpoint distances are wildly different, robust methods give stability. Non-metric multidimensional scaling (NMDS) aims to produce coordinates such that the order of the interpoint distances is respected as closely as possible.

Correspondence analysis This is a method for computing low-dimensional projections that explain dependencies in categorical data. It decomposes chi-squared distance in much the same way that PCA decomposes variance. Correspondence analysis is usually the best way to follow up on a significant chi-squared test. Once we have confirmed significant dependencies between different levels of categories, we can map them and interpret proximities on this map using plots and biplots.

Permutation test for distances Given two sets of distances between the same points, we can measure whether they are related using the Mantel permutation test.

Generalizations of variance and covariance When dealing with more than one matrix of measurements on the same data, we can generalize the notion of covariance and correlations to vectorial measurements of co-inertia.

Canonical correlation This is a method for finding a few linear combinations of variables from each table that are as correlated as possible. When using this method on matrices with large numbers of variables, we use a regularized version with an L_1 penalty that reduces the number of non-zero coefficients.

9.8   Further reading

Interpretation of PCoA maps and nonlinear embeddings can be enhanced in the same way as for PCA using generalizations of the supplementary point method; see Trosset and Priebe (2008) or Bengio et al. (2004). We saw in Chapter 7 how we can project one categorical variable onto a PCA. The correspondence analysis framework actually allows us to mix several categorical variables with any number of continuous variables. This is done through an extension called multiple correspondence analysis (MCA), whereby we can do the same analysis on a large number of binary categorical variables and obtain useful maps. The trick here is to turn the continuous variables into categorical variables first. For extensive examples using R, see for instance the book by Pagès (2016).

A simple extension to PCA that allows for **nonlinear** principal curve estimates instead of principal directions defined by eigenvectors was proposed in Hastie and Stuetzle (1989) and is available in the package *princurve*.

Finding curved subspaces containing a high density of data for dimensions higher than 1 is now called manifold embedding and can be done through Laplacian eigenmaps (Belkin and Niyogi, 2003), local linear embedding as in Roweis and Saul (2000), or using the isomap method (Tenenbaum et al., 2000). For textbooks covering nonlinear unsupervised learning methods, see Hastie et al. (2008, Chapter 14) or Izenman (2008).

A review of many multitable correlation coefficients, and their use in applications, can be found in Josse and Holmes (2016).

9.9   Exercises

▶ Exercise **9.1** Let's take another look at the Phylochip data, replacing the original expression values by presence or absence. We threshold the data to retain only those that have a value of at least 8.633 in at least eight samples.[4]

[4] These values were chosen to retain about 3000 taxa, similar to our choice of threshold in Section 9.3.1.

```
ibd.pres=matrix(0,ncol=28,nrow=8634)
enuf=which(assayIBD[,1:28]>8.633,arr.ind=TRUE)
ibd.pres[enuf]=1
sums28=apply(ibd.pres,1,sum)
useful=which(sums28>7)
length(useful)
## [1] 3006
```

Perform a correspondence analysis on these binary data and compare the plot you obtain to what we saw in Figure 9.12.   ◄

▶ Exercise **9.2** **Correspondence analysis on color association tables.** Table 9.4 gives data collected by looking at the number of `google` query results when two words were typed in. The results are in the thousands of hits. For instance, the `quiet blue` pair returned 2,150,000 hits. Perform a correspondence analysis of these data. What do you notice when you look at the two-dimensional biplot?   ◄

Table 9.4: Contingency table of co-occurring terms from search engine results.

	black	blue	green	gray	orange	purple	white
quiet	2770	2150	2140	875	1220	821	2510
angry	2970	1530	1740	752	1040	710	1730
clever	1650	1270	1320	495	693	416	1420
depressed	1480	957	983	147	330	102	1270
happy	19300	8310	8730	1920	4220	2610	9150
lively	1840	1250	1350	659	621	488	1480
perplexed	110	71	80	19	23	15	109
virtuous	179	80	102	20	25	17	165

▶ Exercise **9.3** The dates Plato wrote various "books" are not known. We take the sentence endings and use those pattern frequencies as the data.

```
platof=read.table("../data/platof.txt",header=T)
platof[1:4,]

##       Rep Laws Crit Phil Pol Soph Tim
## uuuuu  42   91    5   24  13   26  18
## -uuuu  60  144    3   27  19   33  30
## u-uuu  64   72    3   20  24   31  46
## uu-uu  72   98    2   25  20   24  14

resPlato=dudi.coa(platof,scannf=FALSE,nf=2)
fviz_ca_biplot(resPlato,axes=c(2,1)) + ggtitle("")
fviz_eig(resPlato,geom="bar", width=0.6)+ggtitle("")
```

a. From the biplot in Figure 9.32, can you guess the chronological order of Plato's works? Hint: the first (earliest) is known to be *Republica*. The last (latest) is known to be *Laws*.

b. Which sentence ending did Plato use most frequently early in his life?

```
names(resPlato)

## [1] "tab"  "cw"   "lw"   "eig"  "rank" "nf"   "c1"   "li"
## [9] "co"   "l1"   "call" "N"
```

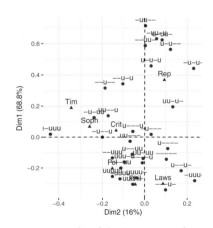

Figure 9.32: Biplot of Plato's sentence endings.

```
sum(resPlato$eig)

## [1] 0.132618

round(100*cumsum(resPlato$eig)/sum(resPlato$eig))

## [1]  69  85  92  96  98 100
```

c. What percentage of the inertia (chi-squared distance) is explained by the map in Figure 9.32?   ◄

▶ Exercise **9.4** Let's look at two datasets, one a perturbed version of the other, with both presenting gradients, as often seen in ecological data.

a. Read in the two species count matrices `lakelike` and `lakelikeh`, which are stored as the object `lakes.RData`.
b. Now compare the output of PCA and CA on the two datasets through plots and the eigenvalues. What do you notice?   ◄

▶ Exercise **9.5** We analyzed the normalized Moignard data in Section 9.5.1. Now redo the analysis with the `Raw` data (in file `nbt.3154-S3-raw.csv`) and compare the output with that obtained using the normalized values.   ◄

▶ Exercise **9.6** We are going to explore the use of kernel methods.

a. Compute kernelized distances taking *kernlab* for the Moignard data taking various values for the σ tuning parameter in the definition of the kernel. Then perform MDS on these kernelized distances. What difference is there in variability explained by the first four components of kernel multidimensional scaling?
b. Make interactive three-dimensional representations of the components. Is there a projection where you see a branch for the purple points?   ◄

▶ Exercise **9.7 Higher resolution study of cell data.** Take the original expression data `blom` that we generated in Section 9.5.1. Map the intensity of expression of each of the top 10 most variable genes onto the 3D plot made with the diffusion mapping. Which dimension, or which one of the principal coordinates (1,2,3,4), can be seen as the one that clusters the **4SG** (red) points the most?   ◄

▶ Exercise **9.8** Here we explore more refined distances and diffusion maps that can show cell development trajectories, as in Figure 9.33.

The diffusion map method restricts the estimation of distances to local points, thus further pursuing the idea that often only local distances should be represented precisely and as points become farther apart, they are not being measured with the same "reference". This method also uses the distances as input but then creates local probabilistic transitions as indicators of similarity. These are combined into an affinity matrix for which the eigenvalues and eigenvectors are also computed, much as in standard MDS.

Compare the output of the `diffuse` function from the *diffusionMap* package on both the 11 and 12 distances computed between the cells available in the `dist2n.euclid` and `dist1n.11` objects from Section 9.5.1.   ◄

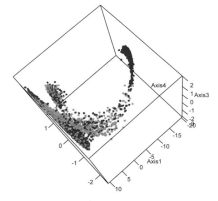

Figure 9.33: Output from a three-dimensional diffusion map projection.

CHAPTER 10

Networks and Trees

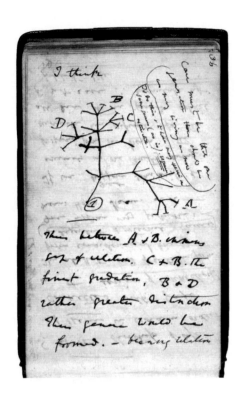

Networks and trees are often used to represent both biological data and knowledge about a system. Phylogenetic trees were used to represent family relationships between species even before Darwin's famous notebook sketch. Networks are often used to schematize complex interactions between proteins involved in diseases, as in Figure 10.1.

We saw in Chapter 2 that we can model state transitions as a Markov chain and these can be usefully represented as directed graphs with weights on the edges. Metabolic pathways can be modeled with nodes representing chemical metabolites and edges representing chemical reactions. Mutation history trees are used in cancer genomics to infer lineages of mutations. Transmission networks are important in studying the epidemiology of infectious diseases.

As real networks can be very large, we will need special methods for representing and visualizing them. This chapter will focus on ways of integrating graphs into a data analysis workflow.

10.1 Goals for this chapter

In this chapter we will:

- Use the formal definition of a graph's components – edges, vertices, layout – to see how we can manipulate them in R using adjacency matrices and lists of edges.
- Transform a graph object from *igraph* into an object that can be visualized according to the layers approach in *ggplot2* using *ggnetwork*. We will experiment with covariates that we attach to graph edges and nodes.
- Learn that graphs are useful ways to encode prior knowledge about a system and see how they enable us to go from simple gene set analyses to meaningful biological recommendations by mapping significance scores onto the network to detect perturbation *hotspots*.
- Build phylogenetic trees starting from DNA sequences and then visualize these trees with the specifically designed R packages *ape* and *ggtree*.

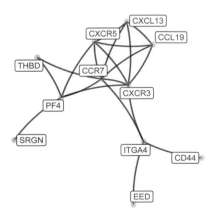

Figure 10.1: This graph represents genetic interactions that appeared to be modified in cancer patients where perturbations appeared in a chemokine signaling network.

- Combine a phylogenetic tree built from microbiome 16S rRNA data with covariates to show how the hierarchical relationship between taxa can increase power in multiple hypothesis testing.
- Learn that a special tree called a minimum spanning tree (MST) is very useful for testing relations between a graph and other covariates. We will show different versions of this approach, known as the Friedman–Rafsky test. We'll study both co-occurrence of bacteria in mice litters and strain similarities in HIV contagion networks.

10.2   Graphs

10.2.1   What is a graph and how can it be encoded?

A **graph** is formed by a set, called V, of nodes or vertices and a set, E, of edges between these vertices. Edges are provided as unordered pairs of nodes in undirected graphs (i.e., graphs in which the edges have no orientation) and as ordered pairs for **directed** or oriented graphs.

An **adjacency matrix** A is the matrix representation of E. It is a square matrix with as many rows as nodes in the graph and contains a non-zero entry in the ith row and jth column if there is an edge between the ith and jth nodes.

▶ Question **10.1** For graphs with undirected edges, what is special about the adjacency matrix A?   ◀

▶ Solution **10.1**   The adjacency matrix is symmetric, i.e., $A = A^{\mathrm{T}}$. This can be seen visually in Figure 10.2.   ☐

```
library("igraph")
edges1 = matrix(c(1,3,2,3,3,4,4,5,4,6),byrow=TRUE,ncol=2)
g1 = graph_from_edgelist(edges1,directed=FALSE)
plot(g1, vertex.size=25,edge.width=5, vertex.color="coral")
```

▶ Question **10.2** Can you give an alternative way of reading the graph from an edge set dataframe?   ◀

▶ Solution **10.2**

```
edges = "1,3\n2,3\n3,4\n4,6\n4,5"
sg   = graph_from_data_frame(read.csv(textConnection(edges),
                        header = FALSE), directed = FALSE)
sg
## IGRAPH d03d854 UN-- 6 5 --
## + attr: name (v/c)
## + edges from d03d854 (vertex names):
## [1] 1--3 2--3 3--4 4--6 4--5
```
☐

Elements of a simple graph

- Nodes or vertices: these are the circles with numbers in them in Figure 10.3.
- Edges or connections: these segments join the nodes and can be directed or not.

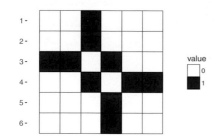

Figure 10.2: The adjacency matrix of the small undirected graph represented in Figure 10.3. We see that A is a symmetric $n{\times}n$ matrix of 0s and 1s.

- Edge lengths or weights: when not specified, we suppose these are all 1 and compute the distance between two nodes on the graph as the number of edges traversed to get from one to the other. In many situations, however, we have meaningful edge lengths or strengths of connection between nodes that we can use in both the plots and analyses.

We call a weighted directed graph a **network**. Networks have adjacency matrices A that are $n{\times}n$ matrices of positive numbers corresponding to the edge lengths.

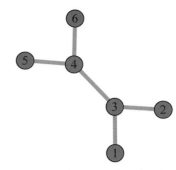

Figure 10.3: A small undirected graph with numbered nodes.

Graph statistics

For large graphs, some authors like to summarize overall graph structure such as vertex degrees (the number of edges connected to the vertex), centrality or betweenness. We focus here on combining graphs with many other sources of data and will not delve deeply into these summary statistics, though they are available in the various packages (*network*, *igraph*) that we do use.

If the number of edges is similar to the number of nodes (written $\#E \sim O(\#V)$), we say that the graph is **sparse**. Some graphs have many nodes, for instance the package *ppiData* contains a predicted protein interaction (`ppipred`) graph on about 2500 proteins with 20,000 edges. A complete adjacency matrix for this graph requires 6,250,000 elements. In fact, a list of edges and weights is sufficient: this only uses 60,000 elements. So storing a large graph as an adjacency matrix can be wasteful. If a graph is **sparse**, we can use sparse encodings similar to those implemented in the package *Matrix*.

On the other hand, if the number of edges is approximately a quadratic function of the nodes (written $\#E \sim O(\#V^2)$), our graph is **dense**. Memory space then becomes an issue for the storage of large graphs.

An **enriched** graph can contain:

Arrows and directed edges In directed graphs, we differentiate between in-degrees and out-degrees and can identify graphs that have cycles, i.e., a path through the edges that returns to its starting node.

Annotation variables on nodes and edges The strength of a link in a graph can be visualized by the width of the edge. Covariates can be added to nodes. A continuous covariate can be associated to the size of the node in the graphical representation. A categorical value can be associated to the color.

Graph layout

We will see several examples where the same graph is plotted in different ways, either for aesthetic or for practical reasons. Different representations are made through the choice of the **graph layout**.

When the edges have lengths representing distances, the problem of finding a 2D representation of the graph is the same as the multidimensional scaling problem we saw in Chapter 9. It is often solved in a similar way, by spreading out the vertex points as much as possible. In the simple case of edges without lengths, the algorithms can choose different criteria; we'll see that Fruchterman-Reingold is often the default choice. It is based on a model in which similar points attract and repel each other as if under the effect of physical forces.

▶ **Task** Use the *igraph* package to do the following:

(a)   Create a dense random graph with 12 nodes and more than 50 edges.

(b)   Experiment plotting the graph with different layouts.

Place the nodes on a circle, or represent the graph as symmetrically as possible, avoiding any overlapping nodes or edges.   ◀

Graphs from data

Usually data do not arrive in the form of graphs. Graphical or network representations are often the result of transforming other data types.

From distances Graphs can simplify distance matrices by rounding the smaller distances down to zero. This requires defining a threshold t and then making edges between points whose distances are smaller than the threshold t; these are often called geometric graphs.

From binary data Some data arrive naturally as 0–1 matrices; for instance, presence or absence of the different finches in the Galapagos Islands gives a 0–1 table. We could build a special graph between the finch-vertices and the island-vertices that is equivalent to the table. That graph is called a **bipartite graph**; there are no edges between taxa or any between sites. An example is shown in Figure 10.4.

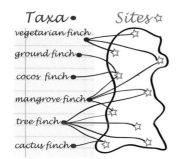

Figure 10.4: This **bipartite** graph connects each taxon to the sites where it was observed.

▶ **Question 10.3** Load the `finch` data from the *networksis* package and experiment with plotting the data to highlight that this is a bipartite network by modifying the following lines of code.

```
library("networksis")
data(finch)
plot(finch, vertex.col = c(rep(2, 13), rep(3, 17)),
    vertex.cex = 2.5, displaylabels=TRUE)
```
◀

▶ **Question 10.4** Make a dataframe from the g1 graph using the *ggnetwork* package, then plot g1 using `ggplot` and the special added elements `geom_edges`, `geom_nodes` and `geom_nodetext`.   ◀

▶ **Solution 10.4** An example of using *ggnetwork* with its various elements:

```
library(ggnetwork)
g1df=ggnetwork(g1)
ggf=ggplot(g1df,aes(x=x, y=y, xend=xend, yend=yend))+
 geom_edges()+geom_nodes(aes(x=x, y=y),size=6,color="#8856a7")+
 geom_nodetext(aes(label = vertex.names),size=4,color="white")+
 theme_blank() + theme(legend.position="none")
```
□

Example: a four-state Markov chain

In Chapter 2 we saw how a Markov chain can summarize transitions between nucleotides (considered the states of the system). This is often schematized by a graph. The *igraph* package enables many choices for graph "decoration".

```
library("markovchain")
statesNames = c("A", "C", "G","T")
T1MC = new("markovchain", states = statesNames, transitionMatrix =
   matrix(c(0.2,0.1,0.4,0.3,0,1,0,0,0.1,0.2,0.2,0.5,0.1,0.1,0.8,0.0),
      nrow = 4,byrow = TRUE, dimnames=list(statesNames,statesNames)))
plot(T1MC, edge.arrow.size = 0.2, vertex.color="purple",
      edge.arrow.width = 2.2, edge.width = 5, edge.color = "blue",
      edge.curved = TRUE, edge.label.cex = 2.5, vertex.size= 32,
      vertex.label.cex = 3.5, edge.loop.angle = 3,
      vertex.label.family="sans", vertex.label.color = "white")
```

Markov chains are idealized models of dynamical systems, and the states are represented by the nodes in the graph. The transition matrix gives us the weights on the directed edges (arrows) between the states.

▶ Question **10.5** In which state do you think this Markov chain will end? ◀

▶ Task (a) Try changing your `set.seed` function. Does the plot change?
(b) Access the help for this particular `plot`.
(c) Redo the graph and label the edges with transition probabilities in green and vertices in brown. ◀

We will see how to build a complete example of an annotated state space Markov chain graph in Exercise 10.3.

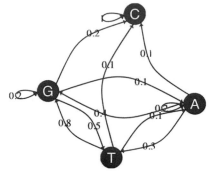

Figure 10.5: A four-state *Markov chain* with arrows representing possible transitions between states.

10.2.2 Graphs with many layers: labels on edges and nodes

Here is an example of plotting a graph downloaded from the STRING database `https://string-db.org` with *annotations* at the vertices.

```
library("ggnetwork")
datf=read.table("../data/string_graph.txt",header=TRUE)
grf=graph_from_data_frame(datf[,c("node1", "node2")],directed=FALSE)
E(gr)$weight = 1
V(gr)$size = centralization.degree(gr)$res
ggdf=ggnetwork(grf,layout= "fruchtermanreingold",cell.jitter = 0)
ggf=ggplot(ggdf,aes(x=x, y=y, xend=xend, yend=yend))+
geom_edges(color="black", curvature=0.1, size=0.95, alpha=0.8)+
geom_nodes(aes(x=x, y=y),size=3,alpha=1/2, color="orange") +
geom_nodetext(aes(label = vertex.names), size=4, color="#8856a7") +
theme_blank() +theme(legend.position="none")
print(ggf)
```

Figure 10.6 shows the full perturbed chemokine subnetwork discovered in the study of breast cancer metastasis using GXNA (Nacu et al., 2007) and reported by Yu et al. (2012).

Figure 10.6: This chemokine subnetwork was uncovered in Yu et al. (2012) using differential gene expression patterns in sorted T cells mapped onto a STRING-generated graph. The structure among the genes CXCR3, CXCL13, CCL19, CSCR5 and CCR7 in the right-hand corner is called a *clique*.

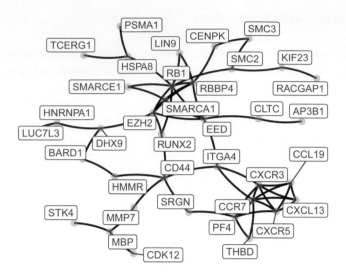

A long unstructured laundry list of possibly differentially expressed genes can be daunting.

10.3   From gene set enrichment to networks

In Chapter 8, we studied methods for finding a list of **differentially expressed** genes. Small sample sizes, coupled with efforts to maintain low FDRs, often result in low power to detect differential expression. Therefore, obtaining a long list of genes that can be confidently declared as differentially expressed is, initially, a triumph. However, understanding the underlying biology requires more than just a laundry list of significant players in a biological system. We need structure.

10.3.1   Methods using predefined gene sets (GSEA)

One of the earliest approaches to finding structure was to look for gene attributes that are **overrepresented** or **enriched** in the laundry list of significant genes. These gene classes are often based on gene ontology categories (e.g., genes that are involved in organ growth, or genes that are involved in feeding behavior). The **Gene Ontology** (GO) is a collection of three ontologies that describe genes and gene products. These ontologies are restricted vocabularies that have the structure of directed acyclic graphs (DAGs). The most specific terms are the leaves of the graph. The GO graph consists of nodes (here, gene ontology terms) and edges from more specific terms (children) to less specific (parents): these edges are directed. Nodes and edges can have multiple attributes that can be visualized. The main purpose of using GO annotations for a particular set of genes designated as significant in an experiment is to look for the **enrichment** of a GO term in this list. We will give this term a statistical meaning below. Many other useful lists of important gene sets exist.

▶ Task   Find a useful database of gene sets.   ◀

For instance, the `MsigDB Molecular Signature Database` (Liberzon et al., 2011) contains many gene sets that can be accessed from within R using the Bioconductor package *GSEABase* command `getBroadSets`.

```
library("GSEABase")
##Not run, this requires a login to the website.
fl  =  system.file("extdata","Broad.xml",package="GSEABase")
gss  =  getBroadSets(fl) # read entire msigdb
organism(gss[[1]])
[1] "Human"
table(sapply(gss, organism))
```

10.3.2 Gene set analysis with two-way table tests

Here, we start by explaining a basic approach often called **Fisher's "exact" test** or **hypergeometric testing**.

Define a universe of candidate genes that are potentially significant; say this universe is of size N. We also have a record of the genes that actually *did* come out significant, of which we suppose there were m.

We make a toy model involving balls in boxes, with a total of N balls corresponding to the genes identified in the gene universe. These genes are split into different functional categories: suppose that of $N = 1000$ genes, 500 are yellow, 100 are blue and 400 are red. A subset of $m = 75$ genes are labeled as *significant*. Suppose among these significantly interesting genes, there are 25 yellow, 25 blue and 25 red. Is the blue category enriched or overrepresented?

We use hypergeometric two-way table testing to account for the fact that some categories are extremely numerous and others are rarer.

▶ Question **10.6** Run a Monte Carlo experiment with 20,000 simulations and compute the p-value of having 25 blues under the null hypothesis that no category is overrepresented in the significant set. ◀

▶ Solution **10.6** Under the null, the 75 significant genes are sampled randomly from our unequal boxes as follows.

```
universe = c(rep("Yellow",500),rep("Blue",100),rep("Red",400))
countblue=rep(0,20000)
for (i in (1:20000))
{
pick75=sample(universe,75,replace=FALSE)
countblue[i]=length(which(pick75=="Blue"))
}
summary(countblue)
##    Min. 1st Qu.  Median    Mean 3rd Qu.    Max.
##   0.000   6.000   7.000   7.482   9.000  19.000
```

The histogram in Figure 10.7 – for the blue gene – shows that having a value as large as 25 under the null model would be extremely rare. □

In the general case, the gene universe is an urn with N balls, and there is a proportion of k/N blue balls. If we pick the m significant balls at random, we expect to see $m{\times}k/N$ blue balls in the significant set.

Table 10.1: Although the same number of each category of gene is found in the *significant* set, both the simulation in Question 10.6 and the theory of testing in two-way tables show us that the blue category is enriched.

	Yellow	Blue	Red
Significant	25	25	25
Universe	500	100	400

exact

These tests are called "exact" because they're nonparametric and based on exhaustive enumerations, *not* because we're sure of the answer – this is statistics after all.

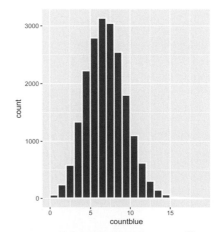

Figure 10.7: Even in 20,000 simulations, no blue count comes close to being 25. We can reject a blue count of 25 as having happened by chance and conclude that the blue category is *enriched*.

Figure 10.8: This graph shows the correspondence between GO terms and significantly changed genes in a study on differential expression in endothelial cells from two steady-state tissues (brain and heart; see Nolan et al., 2013). After normalization, a differential expression analysis was performed, giving a list of genes. A gene-annotation enrichment analysis of the set of differentially expressed genes (adjusted p-value < 0.05) was then performed with the *GOplot* package.

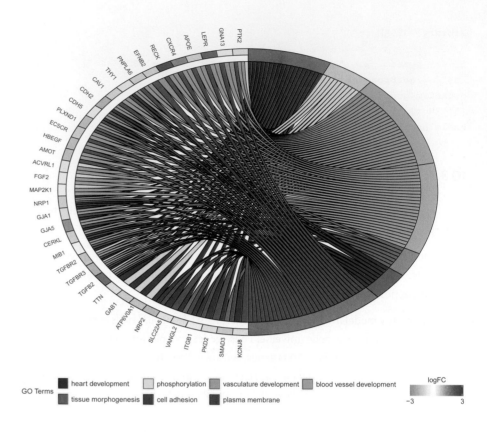

Plotting gene enrichment networks with *GOplot*

In Figure 10.8 we show an attractive way to summarize the connections between the gene functional categories and the significant gene set.

```r
library("GOplot")
data("EC")
circ = circle_dat(EC$david, EC$genelist)
chord = chord_dat(circ, EC$genes, EC$process)
GOChord(chord, limit = c(0, 5))
```

In fact, the Gene Ontology graph does not necessarily capture meaningful *gene interactions*, as genes from different processes often interact productively. A large amount of information remains unused: for example, all significant genes are usually given equal weight, despite the potentially large variations in their p-values.

10.3.3 Significant subgraphs and high-scoring modules

We have at our disposal more than just the Gene Ontology. There are many different databases of gene networks from which we can choose a *known skeleton* graph onto which we project significance scores such as p-values from our differential expression experiment. We will follow an idea first suggested by Ideker et al. (2002) and further developed by Nacu et al. (2007). A careful implementation with many improvements is available as the Bioconductor package *BioNet* (Beisser et al., 2010). These methods all search for the subgraphs or modules of a scored-skeleton network that seem to be particularly **perturbed**.

Each gene node in the network is assigned a score that can be calculated either from a *t*-statistic or from a p-value. Often pathways contain both upregulated and downregulated genes; as pointed out in Ideker et al. (2002), this can be captured by taking absolute values of the test statistic or just incorporating scores computed from the p-values.[1] Beisser et al. (2010) modeled the p-values of the genes as we did in Chapter 6, as a mixture of p-values from "non-perturbed" genes, which will be uniformly distributed, and non-uniformly distributed p-values from the perturbed genes. The signal in the data is modeled using a beta distribution for the p-values following Pounds and Morris (2003).

> [1] We'll want something like $-\log p$, so that small p-values give large scores.

Given our node-scoring function, we search for connected **hotspots** in the graph, i.e., a subgraph of genes with high combined scores.

Using a subgraph search algorithm

Finding the maximal scoring subgraph of a generic graph is known to be intractable in general (we say it is an NP-hard problem), so various approximate algorithms have been proposed. Ideker et al. (2002) suggested using simulated annealing; however, this is slow and tends to produce large subgraphs that are difficult to interpret. Nacu et al. (2007) started with a seed vertex and gradually expanded around it. Beisser et al. (2010) started the search with a so-called minimum spanning tree (MST), a graph we will study later in this chapter.

10.3.4   An example with the BioNet implementation

To illustrate the method, we show data from the *BioNet* package.

The `dataLym` object contains the relevant p-values and *t*-statistics for 3583 genes. We access them and start the analysis.

> The `interactome` data contain a connected component of the network comprising 2034 different gene products and 8399 interactions. This constitutes the skeleton graph with which we will work; see Beisser et al. (2010).

```
library("BioNet")
library("DLBCL")
data(dataLym)
data(interactome)
interactome

## A graphNEL graph with undirected edges
## Number of Nodes = 9386
## Number of Edges = 36504

pval=dataLym$t.pval
names(pval)  =  dataLym$label
subnet  =  subNetwork(dataLym$label, interactome)
subnet  =  rmSelfLoops(subnet)
subnet

## A graphNEL graph with undirected edges
## Number of Nodes = 2559
## Number of Edges = 7788
```

The package actually gives a different name to π_0: it uses λ and calls it the *mixture parameter*.

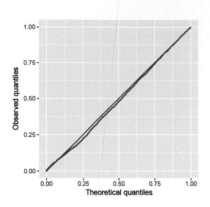

Figure 10.9: The QQ-plot shows the quality of the fit of the beta–uniform mixture model to the data. The red points have theoretical quantiles from the beta distribution as x-coordinates and observed quantiles as y-coordinates. Proximity of the red points to the blue diagonal shows how well the model fits – this model fits nicely.

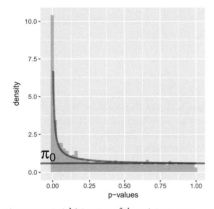

Figure 10.10: A histogram of the mixture components for the p-values, the beta in red and the uniform in blue; π_0 is the mixing proportion assigned to the null component, whose distribution should be uniform.

[2] Because they are contemporary, the trees are often represented so that the leaves are all the same distance from the root.

Fit a beta–uniform model. We will fit the set of p-values with the type of mixture we studied in Chapter 4, having a uniform component from the null with probability π_0 and a beta distribution (proportional to ax^{a-1}) for the p-values corresponding to the alternatives (Pounds and Morris, 2003):

$$f(x|a, \pi_0) = \pi_0 + (1 - \pi_0)ax^{a-1} \qquad \text{for } 0 < x \leqslant 1;\ 0 < a < 1.$$

Let's run the model with an fdr of 0.001. Fit diagnostics are shown in Figures 10.9 and 10.10.

```
fb=fitBumModel(pval, plot = FALSE)
fb

## Beta-Uniform-Mixture (BUM) model
##
## 3583 pvalues fitted
##
## Mixture parameter (lambda): 0.482
## shape parameter (a):  0.180
## log-likelihood: 4471.8

scores=scoreNodes(subnet, fb, fdr = 0.001)
```

Then we run a heuristic search for a high-scoring subgraph.

```
hotSub  =  runFastHeinz(subnet, scores)
hotSub

## A graphNEL graph with undirected edges
## Number of Nodes = 153
## Number of Edges = 243

logFC=dataLym$diff
names(logFC)=dataLym$label
```

▶ Question **10.7** We made Figure 10.11 with the following code.

```
plotModule(hotSub,layout=layout.davidson.harel, scores = scores,
                  diff.expr = logFC)
```

Using the function `igraph.from.graphNEL`, transform the module object and plot it using the *ggnetwork* method shown in Section 10.2.2.   ◀

10.4   Phylogenetic trees

One really important use of graphs in biology is the construction of phylogenetic trees. Trees are graphs with no **cycles** (the official word for loops, whether self-loops or loops that go through several vertices). Phylogenetic trees are usually rooted binary trees that have labels only on the leaves corresponding to contemporary[2] taxa at the tips. The inner nodes correspond to **ancestral** taxa that have to be inferred from the **contemporaneous** data on the tips. Many methods use aligned DNA sequences from the different (almost contemporary) species or populations to infer or estimate the tree. The tips of the tree are usually called **OTUs** (operational taxonomic units) because these methods work with many types of data at the tips.

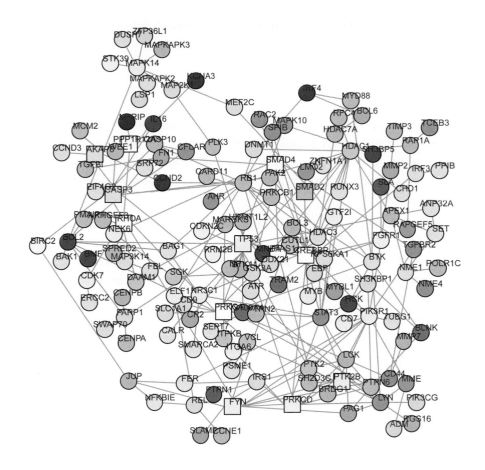

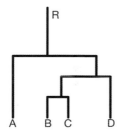

Figure 10.11: The functional subgraph found as maximally enriched differential expression between ABC and GCB B-cell lymphoma. The nodes are colored in red and green: green shows an upregulation in ACB and red an upregulation in GBC. The shape of the nodes depicts the score: rectangles indicate a negative score, circles a positive score.

Figure 10.12: As mathematical objects, hierarchical clustering trees (studied in Chapter 5) are the same as phylogenetic trees. They are **rooted binary** trees with labels at the tips.

The statistical **parameter** of interest in these analyses is the rooted binary tree with OTU labels on its leaves (see Holmes (1999, 2003b) for details).

The example of HIV

HIV is a virus that protects itself by evolving very rapidly (several mutations can appear within months). Its evolution can thus be followed in real time; compare this with the evolution of large organisms that has happened over millions of years. HIV trees are built for medical purposes, such as the detection and understanding of drug resistance. They are estimated for individual genes. Different genes can show differences in their evolutionary histories and thus produce different **gene trees**. The phylogenetic tree in Figure 10.13 shows times when the virus switched from monkeys to humans (Wertheim and Worobey, 2009).

Special elements in phylogenies

Most phylogenetic trees are shown rooted: the "root" is usually found by including an outgroup in the tree tips, as we will see later.

- Characters that are derived from this common ancestry are called homologous (geneticists doing population studies replace the term *homology* with *identity by descent*, IBD).

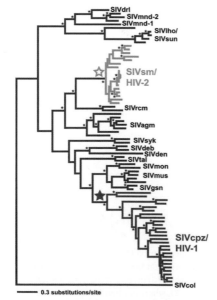

Figure 10.13: This phylogenetic tree describes the history of different HIV/SIV strains in Africa. Figure from Wertheim and Worobey (2009).

- Sisters on the tree defined by a common ancestor are called clades or monophyletic groups: they have more than just *similarities* in common.

10.4.1 Markovian models for evolution

To infer what happened in the ancestral species from contemporary data collected on the tips of the tree, we have to make assumptions about how substitutions and deletions occur through time. The models we use are all Markovian and are said to be time-homogeneous, because we assume the mutation rate is constant across history.

Assuming a constant mutation rate is called the **molecular clock** hypothesis. This assumption allows us to avoid what is known as **non-identifiability** (i.e., we can't tell the difference between the many possible mutational histories given the observed data).

Continuous Markov chain and generator matrix

We're going to use the Markov chain we saw in Figure 10.5 on the states A, C, G, T; however, now we consider that the changes of state, i.e., mutations, occur at random times. The gaps between these mutational events will follow an exponential distribution. These continuous-time **Markov chains** have the following properties:

No memory $P(Y(u + t) = j | Y(t) = i)$ does not depend on times before t.

Time homogeneity The mutation process is time-homogeneous, which translates the fact that the probability $P(Y(h + t) = j | Y(t) = i)$ does not depend on t but only on h, the time between the events, and on i and j.

Linearity The instantaneous transition rate is approximately linear in form:

$$P_{ij}(h) = q_{ij}h + o(h), \quad \text{for } j \neq i,$$
$$P_{ii}(h) = 1 - q_i(h) + o(h), \qquad q_i = \sum_{j \neq i} q_{ij}.$$

The error term is written here as $o(h)$: we read this as little o of h, which means that this term grows much more slowly than h.

We call q_{ij} the instantaneous transition rate. These rates define matrices as in Table 10.2.

Exponential distribution Times between changes are exponentially distributed.

Li (1997) gives a clear description of the exact mathematical model and explains why the transitions can be described by the instantaneous change probability matrix called the **generator**. In the simplest possible model, called the Jukes–Cantor model, all the mutations are equally likely; see Table 10.2, *left*. A slightly more flexible model, called the Kimura model, is shown in Table 10.2, *right*.

▶ **Question 10.8** Why do we say the Kimura model is more flexible? ◀

▶ **Solution 10.8** The Jukes–Cantor model has only one parameter, and it supposes all transitions and transversions are equally likely. The Kimura model has one parameter for transitions and another for transversions (mutations occurring from purine to pyrimidine, or vice versa). □

Vocabulary overload here! Transitions in this context mean mutational changes within the purines (A<->G) or within the pyrimidines (C <-> T); whereas when we talked about Markov chains earlier, our **transition** matrix contained all probabilities of any state changes.

The most flexible model is called the Generalized Time Reversible (GTR) model; it has six free parameters.

We next show an example of data simulated according to these generative models from a known tree.

$$Q = \begin{array}{c} \\ A \\ T \\ C \\ G \end{array} \begin{array}{cccc} A & T & C & G \\ -3\alpha & \alpha & \alpha & \alpha \\ \alpha & -3\alpha & \alpha & \alpha \\ \alpha & \alpha & -3\alpha & \alpha \\ \alpha & \alpha & \alpha & -3\alpha \end{array} \qquad Q = \begin{array}{c} \\ A \\ T \\ C \\ G \end{array} \begin{array}{cccc} A & T & C & G \\ -\alpha-2\beta & \beta & \beta & \alpha \\ \beta & -\alpha-2\beta & \alpha & \beta \\ \beta & \alpha & -\alpha-2\beta & \beta \\ \alpha & \beta & \beta & -\alpha-2\beta \end{array}$$

Table 10.2: Two examples of rate matrices. On the left, the Jukes–Cantor (JC69) model; on the right, the Kimura (K80) two-parameter model.

10.4.2   Simulating data and plotting a tree

Suppose we already know our phylogenetic tree and want to simulate the evolution of the nucleotides down this tree. First, we visualize the tree tree1 using ggtree, loading the tree and the relevant packages.

```
library("phangorn")
library("ggtree")
load("../data/tree1.RData")
```

▶ Task   Use the ggtree function to plot tree1. Make the tips of the tree green triangles and the ancestral nodes red circles.   ◀

```
ggtree(tree1,lwd=2,color="coral",alpha=0.8,right=TRUE) +
            geom_tiplab(size=7,angle=90,offset=0.05) +
geom_point(aes(shape=isTip, color=isTip), size=5, alpha=0.6)
```

Now we generate sequences from our tree, in Figure 10.14. Each sequence starts with a new nucleotide letter generated randomly at the root; mutations may occur as we go down the tree. You can see in Figure 10.15 that the colors are not equally represented. This is because the frequency at the root was chosen to be different from the uniform; see the following code.

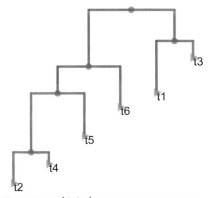

Figure 10.14: This is the tree we use as our *true* parameter. We generate nucleotides one at a time from the root and "drop" them down the tree. With some probability proportional to the edge lengths, mutations occur down the branches.

```
seqs6=simSeq(tree1,l=60,type="DNA",bf=c(1/8,1/8,3/8,3/8),rate=.1)
seqs6

## 6 sequences with 60 character and 27 different site patterns.
## The states are a c g t

mat6=as.character(seqs6)
mat6df=data.frame(mat6)
p=ggtree(tree1,lwd=1.2)+geom_tiplab(aes(x=branch),size=5,vjust=2)
gheatmap(p,mat6df[,1:60],offset=0.01,colnames=FALSE)
```

▶ Question 10.9   Experiment with the code above. Change the bf and rate arguments in the simSeq function to make mutations more likely. Do you think sequences generated with a very high mutation rate would make it easier to infer the tree that generated them?   ◀

▶ Solution 10.9   Very high mutation rates result in mutations overwriting themselves and make inference more difficult. After a certain time and a certain number of mutations, it may be very difficult to see what was happening at the root; see Mossel (2003) for details. Of course, there is a sweet spot, because enough mutations must occur in order for us to resolve the tree branches.   □

Figure 10.15: The tree on the left was used to generate the sequences on the right according to a Jukes–Cantor model. The nucleotide frequencies generated at the root were quite unequal, with A and C generated more rarely. As the sequences percolate down the tree, mutations occur; they are more likely to occur on the longer branches.

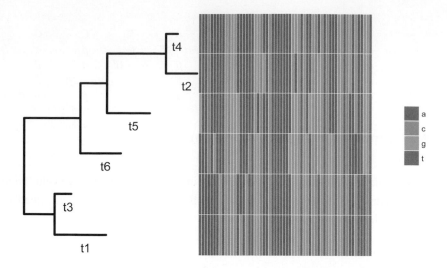

▶ **Question 10.10** **Estimation bias: distance underestimation.**

(a) If we only count the number of changes between two sequences using a simple Hamming distance, but there has been much evolutionary change between the two, why do we underestimate the distance between the sequences?

(b) Will the bias be larger for smaller evolutionary distances?   ◀

The standard Markovian models of evolution we saw above allow us to improve these estimates.

10.4.3   Estimating a phylogenetic tree

When the true tree parameter is known, probabilistic generative models of evolution tell us which patterns to expect in the sequences. As we have seen in earlier chapters, statistics means going back from the data to reasonable estimates of the parameters. Here the tree itself and the branch lengths, and even the evolutionary rates, can be considered to be the parameters.

There are several approaches to estimation: tree "building" is no exception. Here are the main ones:

Nonparametric estimate: the parsimony tree   Parsimony is a nonparametric method that minimizes the number of changes necessary to explain the data. Its solution is the same as that of the Steiner tree problem (see Figure 10.16).

Parametric estimate: the maximum likelihood tree   In order to estimate the tree using a maximum likelihood or Bayesian approach, one needs a model for molecular evolution that integrates mutation rates and branch edge lengths. ML estimation (e.g., `Phyml`, `FastML`, `RaxML`) uses efficient optimization algorithms to maximize the likelihood of a tree under the model assumptions.

Bayesian posterior distributions for trees   Bayesian estimation software such as MrBayes (Ronquist et al., 2012) and BEAST (Bouckaert et al., 2014) uses MCMC to find

"In solving a problem of this sort, the grand thing is to be able to reason backward. That is a very useful accomplishment, and a very easy one, but people do not practice it much. In the everyday affairs of life it is more useful to reason forward, and so the other comes to be neglected. There are fifty who can reason synthetically for one who can reason analytically." From **A Study In Scarlet***, by Sir Arthur Conan Doyle.*

posterior distributions of the phylogenies. Bayesian methods are not directly integrated into R and require the user to import the collections of trees generated by Monte Carlo methods in order to summarize them and make confidence statements; see Chakerian and Holmes (2012) for simple examples.

Semiparametric approach: distance-based methods These methods, called neighbor joining and UPGMA, are similar to the hierarchical clustering algorithms we encountered in Chapter 5. However, the distance estimation steps use the parametric evolutionary models of Table 10.2; this "parametric" part is why we call the method semiparametric.

The neighbor-joining algorithm itself uses Steiner points as the summary of two combined points and proceeds iteratively as in hierarchical clustering. It can be quite fast and is often a good starting point for more time-consuming methods.

Let's start by estimating the tree from the data `seqs6` using the `nj` (neighbor-joining) algorithm on DNA distances based on the one-parameter Jukes–Cantor model. We make Figure 10.17 using the `ggtree` function.

```
tree.nj = nj(dist.ml(seqs6,"JC69"))
ggtree(tree.nj)+geom_tiplab(size=7)+ggplot2::xlim(0, 0.8)
```

▶ **Question 10.11** Generate the maximum likelihood scores of tree1 given the `seqs6` data and compare them to those of the neighbor-joining tree. ◀

▶ **Solution 10.11**

```
fit = pml(tree1, seqs6, k=4)
```
□

▶ **Question 10.12** When we align amino acids from which we want to infer a tree, we use (20×20) transition matrices. Methods for estimating the phylogenetic tree are very similar. Try this in *phangorn* with an HIV amino acid sequence downloaded from `https://www.hiv.lanl.gov/content/sequence/NEWALIGN/align.html`.

◀

The quality of the tree estimates depends on the number of sequences per taxa and the distance to the root. We can evaluate the quality of the estimates either by using parametric and nonparametric bootstraps, or by performing Bayesian tree estimation using MCMC. For examples of how to visualize and compare the sampling distributions of trees, see Chakerian and Holmes (2012).

10.4.4 Application to 16S rRNA data

In Chapter 5 we saw how to use a probabilistic clustering method to denoise 16S rRNA sequences. We can now reload these denoised sequences and *preprocess* them before building their phylogeny.

```
library("dada2")
seqtab = readRDS("../data/seqtab.rds")
seqs = getSequences(seqtab)
names(seqs) = seqs
```

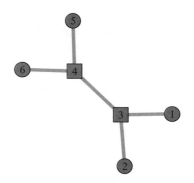

Figure 10.16: A Steiner tree; the inner points are represented as squares. The method for creating the shortest tree that passes through all outer points 1, 2, 5, 6 is to create two inside ("ancestor") points 3 and 4.

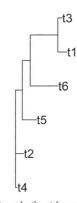

Figure 10.17: Trees built with a neighbor-joining algorithm are very fast to compute and are often used as initial values for more expensive estimation procedures such as maximum likelihood or parsimony.

[3] In order to keep all the information and be able to compare sequences from different experiments, we use the sequences themselves as their labels (Callahan et al., 2017).

[4] See the download link on the dada2 website: https://benjjneb.github.io/dada2/training.html.

One of the benefits of using well-studied marker loci such as the 16S rRNA gene is the ability to taxonomically classify the sequenced variants.[3] The *dada2* package includes a naive Bayesian classifier method for this purpose (Wang et al., 2007). This classifier compares sequence variants to training sets of classified sequences. Here we use the RDP v16 training set (Cole et al., 2009).[4] Let's run the following code.

```
fastaRef = "../tmp/rdp_train_set_16.fa.gz"
taxtab = assignTaxonomy(seqtab, refFasta = fastaRef)
```

We then obtain a table of taxonomic information.

```
taxtab = readRDS(file= "../data/taxtab16.rds")
dim(taxtab)
## [1] 268    6
```

▶ Question **10.13** Write one line of code using the `%>%` operator that shows just the first six rows of the taxonomic information without the row names. ◀

▶ Solution **10.13**

```
taxtab %>% `rownames<-`(NULL) %>% head
##      Kingdom    Phylum          Class          Order
## [1,] "Bacteria" "Bacteroidetes" "Bacteroidia" "Bacteroidales"
## [2,] "Bacteria" "Bacteroidetes" "Bacteroidia" "Bacteroidales"
## [3,] "Bacteria" "Bacteroidetes" "Bacteroidia" "Bacteroidales"
## [4,] "Bacteria" "Bacteroidetes" "Bacteroidia" "Bacteroidales"
## [5,] "Bacteria" "Bacteroidetes" "Bacteroidia" "Bacteroidales"
## [6,] "Bacteria" "Bacteroidetes" "Bacteroidia" "Bacteroidales"
##      Family               Genus
## [1,] "Porphyromonadaceae" NA
## [2,] "Porphyromonadaceae" NA
## [3,] "Porphyromonadaceae" NA
## [4,] "Porphyromonadaceae" "Barnesiella"
## [5,] "Bacteroidaceae"     "Bacteroides"
## [6,] "Porphyromonadaceae" NA
```

▶ Question **10.14** What is the difference between taxonomic and phylogenetic information? ◀

Note that as the `seqs` data are randomly generated, they are "cleaner" than the real data we will have to handle. In particular, naturally occurring raw sequences have to be **aligned**. This is necessary, as there are often extra nucleotides in some sequences, a consequence of what we call *indel* events.[5] Also, mutations occur and appear as substitutions of one nucleotide by another.

[5] A nucleotide is **in**serted or **del**eted, and it is often hard to distinguish which took place.

Here is an example of what the first few characters of aligned sequences look like.

```
readLines("../data/mal2.dna.txt") %>% head(12) %>% cat(sep="\n")
##     11   1620
## Pre1      GTACTTGTTA GGCCTTATAA GAAAAAAGT- TATTAACTTA AGGAATTATA
## Pme2      GTATCTGTTA AGCCTTATAA AAAGATAGT- T-TAAATTAA AGGAATTATA
## Pma3      GTATTTGTTA AGCCTTATAA GAGAAAGTA TATTAACTTA AGGA-TTATA
## Pfa4      GTATTTGTTA GGCCTTATAA GAAAAAAGT- TATTAACTTA AGGAATTATA
## Pbe5      GTATTTGTTA AGCCTTATAA GAAAAA--T- TTTTAAATTAA AGGAATTATA
```

```
## Plo6          GTATTTGTTA AGCCTTATAA GAAAAAAGT- TACTAACTAA AGGAATTATA
## Pfr7          GTACTTGTTA AGCCTTATAA GAAAGAAGT- TATTAACTTA AGGAATTATA
## Pkn8          GTACTTGTTA AGCCTTATAA GAAAAGAGT- TATTAACTTA AGGAATTATA
## Pcy9          GTACTCGTTA AGCCTTTTAA GAAAAAAGT- TATTAACTTA AGGAATTATA
## Pvi10         GTACTTGTTA AGCCTTTTAA GAAAAAAGT- TATTAACTTA AGGAATTATA
## Pga11         GTATTTGTTA AGCCTTATAA GAAAAAAGT- TATTAATTTA AGGAATTATA
```

We will perform this multiple alignment on our `seqs` data using the *DECIPHER* package (Wright, 2015).

```
library("DECIPHER")
alignment=AlignSeqs(DNAStringSet(seqs), anchor = NA, verbose = FALSE)
```

We use the *phangorn* package to build the MLE tree (under the GTR model), but will use the neighbor-joining tree as our starting point.

```
phangAlign = phangorn::phyDat(as(alignment, "matrix"), type = "DNA")
dm = phangorn::dist.ml(phangAlign)
treeNJ = phangorn::NJ(dm) # Note, tip order != sequence order
fit = phangorn::pml(treeNJ, data = phangAlign)
fitGTR = update(fit, k = 4, inv = 0.2)
fitGTR = phangorn::optim.pml(fitGTR, model = "GTR", optInv = TRUE,
        optGamma = TRUE,  rearrangement = "stochastic",
        control = phangorn::pml.control(trace = 0))
```

10.5   Combining a phylogenetic tree into a data analysis

We now need to combine the phylogenetic tree, the denoised read abundances and the supplementary information that was provided about the samples from which the reads were gathered. This **sample** information is often provided as a spreadsheet (or `.csv`) and (mis)named *meta*data. This data integration step is facilitated by the specialized containers and accessors that *phyloseq* provides.

We read in the sample data from the `.csv` file.

```
mimarksPathClean = "../data/MIMARKS_Data_clean.csv"
samdf = read.csv(mimarksPathClean, header=TRUE)
```

Then the full suite of data for this study – the sample-by-sequence feature table, the sample (meta)data, the sequence taxonomies, and the phylogenetic tree – are combined into a single object.

```
library("phyloseq")
physeq = phyloseq(tax_table(taxtab), sample_data(samdf),
   otu_table(seqtab, taxa_are_rows = FALSE), phy_tree(fitGTR$tree))
```

This block of code will usually be executed only once. When the object is created, we save it and do all the manipulations starting from that container.

We have already encountered several cases of combining heterogeneous data into special data classes (in particular in Chapter 8, where we studied the `pasilla` data).

▶ **Task**   Look at the detailed *phyloseq* documentation. Try a few **filtering operations**. For instance, make a subset of the data that contains the tree, taxa abundance table, and sample and taxa information for only those samples that have more than 5000 reads.
◀

This can be done in one line.

```
ps1 = prune_samples(rowSums(otu_table(ps0)) > 5000, ps0)
```

We can also make data transformations while maintaining the integrity of the links between all the data components.

▶ **Question 10.15**   What do the following lines of code do?

```
prev0 = apply(X = otu_table(ps0),
              MARGIN = ifelse(taxa_are_rows(ps0), yes = 1, no = 2),
              FUN = function(x){sum(x > 0)})
prevdf = data.frame(Prevalence = prev0,
                    TotalAbundance = taxa_sums(ps0),
                    tax_table(ps1))
keepPhyla = table(prevdf$Phylum)[table(prevdf$Phylum) >  5]
prevdf1   = subset(prevdf, Phylum %in% names(keepPhyla))
ps2v      = subset_taxa(ps1v, Phylum %in% names(keepPhyla))
```
◀

Plotting abundances for certain bacteria is easy using barcharts: *ggplot2* commands have been hardwired into one-line calls in the *phyloseq* package, which makes performing these types of exploratory plots painless. There is even an interactive *Shiny-phyloseq* browser-based tool (McMurdie and Holmes, 2015). We do not give full details here but refer the reader to the online vignettes.

10.5.1   Hierarchical multiple testing

Hypothesis testing can identify individual bacteria whose abundance relates to sample variables of interest. A standard approach is similar to the one we used in Chapter 6. Compute a test statistic for each taxon individually, then jointly adjust p-values to ensure a false discovery rate below a given upper bound. However, this procedure does not exploit any structure among the tested hypotheses – for example, it is likely that if one *ruminococcus* species is strongly associated with age, then others are as well. To integrate this information, Benjamini and Yekutieli (2003) and Benjamini and Bogomolov (2014) propose a hierarchical testing procedure in which taxonomic groups are tested only if higher levels are found to be be associated. In the case where many related species have a slight signal, this pooling of information can increase power.

We apply this method to test the association between microbial abundance and age. Before computing the test statistic, it is appropriate to start by using the normalization protocols we discussed in Chapter 8 following Love et al. (2014) for RNA-Seq data and McMurdie and Holmes (2014) for 16S rRNA generated count data and available in the *DESeq2* package.

```
library("DESeq2")
library("phyloseq")
ps1 = readRDS("../data/ps1.rds")
ps_dds = phyloseq_to_deseq2(ps1,
    design = ~ ageBin + family_relationship)
geo_mean_protected = function(x) {
            if (all(x == 0)) {return (0) }
    exp(mean(log(x[x != 0])))
  }
geoMeans = apply(counts(ps_dds), 1, geo_mean_protected)
ps_dds = estimateSizeFactors(ps_dds, geoMeans = geoMeans)
ps_dds = estimateDispersions(ps_dds)
abund = getVarianceStabilizedData(ps_dds)
```

We use the *structSSI* package to perform the hierarchical testing (Sankaran and Holmes, 2014). For more convenient printing, we first shorten the name of each taxon.

```
rownames(abund) = substr(rownames(abund), 1, 5)
    %>% make.names(unique = TRUE)
```

Unlike standard multiple hypothesis testing, the hierarchical testing procedure needs univariate tests for each higher level taxonomic group, not just every taxon. A helper function, `treePValues`, is available for this; it expects an edge list that encodes parent–child relationships, with the first row specifying the root node.

```
library("structSSI")
el = phy_tree(ps1)$edge
el0 = el
el0 = el0[rev(seq_len(nrow(el))), ]
el_names = c(rownames(abund), seq_len(phy_tree(ps1)$Nnode))
el[, 1] = el_names[el0[, 1]]
el[, 2] = el_names[el0[, 2]]
unadj_p = treePValues(el, abund, sample_data(ps1)$ageBin)
```

We can now make our FDR calculations using the hierarchical testing procedure. The test results are guaranteed to control several variants of FDR, but at different levels (for details, see Benjamini and Yekutieli, 2003; Benjamini and Bogomolov, 2014; Sankaran and Holmes, 2014).

▶ Task   Try the following code, including the **interactive** plotting command that will open a browser window.

```
hfdr_res = hFDR.adjust(unadj_p, el, 0.75)
summary(hfdr_res)
#plot(hfdr_res, height = 5000) # not run: opens in a browser   ◀
```

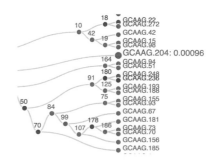

Figure 10.18: A screenshot of a subtree with many differentially abundant microbes, as determined by the hierarchical testing procedure. Currently the user is hovering over the node associated with microbe GCGAG.204; this causes the adjusted p-value to appear.

The plot opens in a new browser – a static screenshot of a subtree is displayed in Figure 10.18. Nodes are shaded according to p-values, from blue to orange, representing the strongest to weakest associations. Gray nodes were never tested in order to focus power on more promising subtrees. Scanning the full tree, it becomes clear that the association between age group and taxonomic abundances is present in only a few isolated taxonomic groups, in which it is quite strong. To give context to these results, we can retrieve the taxonomic identity of the rejected hypotheses.

```
library("dplyr")
options(digits=3)
tax = tax_table(ps1)[, c("Family", "Genus")] %>% data.frame()
tax$seq = rownames(abund)
hfdr_res@p.vals$seq = rownames(hfdr_res@p.vals)
tax %>% left_join(hfdr_res@p.vals[,-3]) %>%
  arrange(adjp) %>% head(9) %>% dplyr::select(1,2,4,5)
##              Family          Genus   unadjp      adjp
## 1 Lachnospiraceae           <NA> 2.15e-82  4.30e-82
## 2 Lachnospiraceae       Roseburia 1.31e-75  2.62e-75
## 3 Lachnospiraceae Clostridium_XlVa 4.00e-59  8.01e-59
## 4 Lachnospiraceae           <NA> 3.84e-50  7.68e-50
## 5 Lachnospiraceae Clostridium_XlVa 1.21e-49  2.42e-49
## 6 Lachnospiraceae           <NA> 8.54e-49  1.71e-48
## 7 Ruminococcaceae   Ruminococcus 9.37e-47  1.87e-46
## 8 Lachnospiraceae Clostridium_XlVa 5.91e-43  1.18e-42
## 9 Lachnospiraceae       Roseburia 2.33e-36  4.67e-36
```

It seems that the most strongly associated bacteria all belong to family *Lachnospiraceae*.

10.6 Minimum spanning trees

A very simple and useful graph is the so-called **minimum spanning tree (MST)**. Given distances between vertices, the MST is the tree that spans all the points and has minimum total length (it's the blue graph in Figure 10.19).

Greedy algorithms work well for computing the MST and R offers many implementations: `mstree` in *ade4*, `mst` in *ape*, `spantree` in *vegan* and `mst` in *igraph*.

Here we take the DNA sequence distances between strains of HIV from patients all over the world and construct their minimum spanning tree. The result is shown in Figure 10.20.

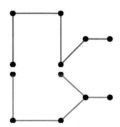

Figure 10.19: A **spanning tree** is a tree that goes through all nodes at least once. The graph with red edges is such a tree. The graph with blue edges is a minimum spanning tree.

```
load("../data/dist2009c.RData")
country09=attr(dist2009c,"Label")
mstree2009=ape::mst(dist2009c)
gr09=graph.adjacency(mstree2009, mode="undirected")
gg=ggnetwork(gr09, arrow.gap=0, layout = "fruchtermanreingold")
ggplot(gg, aes(x = x, y = y, xend = xend, yend = yend)) +
  geom_edges(color = "black",alpha=0.5,curvature = 0.1) +
  geom_nodes(aes(color = vertex.names), size = 2) + theme_blank() +
  geom_nodetext(aes(label = vertex.names), color="black",size=2.5) +
  theme(plot.margin = unit(c(0, 1, 1, 6), "cm"))+
  guides(color=guide_legend(keyheight=0.09,keywidth=0.09,
      title="Countries")) + theme(legend.position = c(0, 0.14),
      legend.background = element_blank(),
      legend.text=element_text(size=7))
```

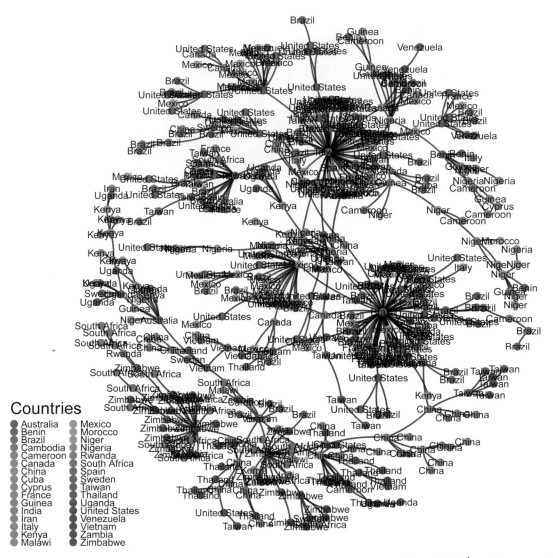

Figure 10.20: The minimum spanning tree computed from DNA distances between HIV sequences from samples taken in 2009 and whose country of origin was known, data as published in the `HIVdb` database (Rhee et al., 2003).

▶ **Question 10.16** Make the network plot again, but replace `geom_nodetext` with labels that repel each other to minimize the overlapping node labels. ◀

▶ **Solution 10.16**

```
ggplot(gg, aes(x = x, y = y, xend = xend, yend = yend)) +
  geom_edges(color = "black",alpha=0.5,curvature = 0.1) +
  geom_nodes(aes(color = vertex.names), size = 2) +
  geom_nodetext_repel(aes(label = vertex.names),
        color="black", size=2) +
  theme_blank() +
  guides(color=guide_legend(keyheight=0.3, keywidth=0.3,
        override.aes = list(size=6), title="Countries"))
```

It might be preferable to use a **graph layout** that incorporates the known geographic coordinates. We may thus see how the virus jumped large distances across the world through traveler mobility. We introduce approximate country coordinates, which we then **jitter** slightly to avoid too much overlapping. The result is shown in Figure 10.21.

Figure 10.21: A minimum spanning tree between HIV cases using a **jitter** of the geographic location of each case to reduce overlapping of points; the DNA distances between patient strains were used as the input to an undirected minimum spanning tree algorithm.

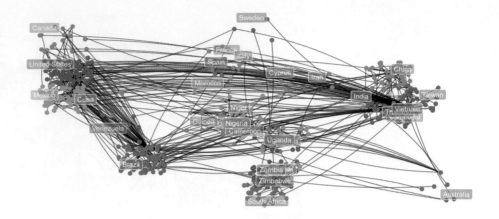

```
library("rworldmap")
mat = match(country09,countriesLow$NAME)
lat2009 =countriesLow$LAT[mat]
lon2009 =countriesLow$LON[mat]
coords2009 = data.frame(lat=lat2009, lon=lon2009,country=country09)
x=jitter(coords2009$lon,amount=15)
y=jitter(coords2009$lat,amount=8)
layoutCoordinates =cbind(x,y)
labc=names(table(country09)[which(table(country09)>1)])
matc=match(labc,countriesLow$NAME)
latc=countriesLow$LAT[matc]
lonc=countriesLow$LON[matc]
dfc=data.frame(latc,lonc,labc)
dfctrans=dfc
dfctrans[,1]=(dfc[,1]+31)/(93)
dfctrans[,2]=(dfc[,2]+105)/(238)
ggeo09=ggnetwork(gr09, arrow.gap=0, layout = layoutCoordinates)
ggplot(ggeo09, aes(x = x, y = y, xend = xend, yend = yend)) +
  geom_edges(color ="black", alpha=0.5,curvature = 0.1) +
  geom_nodes(aes(color = vertex.names), size = 2) +
  theme_blank() +
  geom_label(data=dfctrans,aes(x=lonc, xend=lonc, y=latc, yend=latc,
          label=labc,fill=labc),colour = "white",alpha=0.5,size=3) +
  theme(legend.position="none")
```

The input to the minimum spanning tree algorithm is a distance matrix or a graph with a length edge attribute. Figure 10.21 is the minimum spanning tree between cases of HIV for which strain information was made available through the HIVdb database of Rhee et al. (2003). The DNA distances were computed using the Jukes–Cantor mutation model.

▶ Question **10.17** The analysis above provides an **undirected** network of connections. In fact, several implementations of the minimum spanning tree (for instance, `mstree` in *ade4*) provide a directed path through the points that can give meaningful information on the spread of diseases. Make a directed network version of the above maps.   ◀

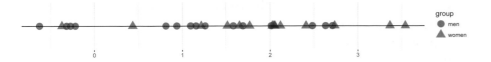

Figure 10.22: Seeing the number of "runs" in a
one-dimensional, two-sample, nonparametric
Wald–Wolfowitz test can indicate whether the
two groups have the same distribution.

Minimum spanning trees can be a very useful component of a simple nonparametric test for detecting differences between factors that are mapped onto its vertices.

10.6.1   MST-based testing: the Friedman–Rafsky test

Graph-based two-sample tests[6] were introduced in Friedman and Rafsky (1979) as a generalization of the Wald–Wolfowitz runs test (see Figure 10.22). Our previous examples show graph vertices associated with covariates such as country of origin. Here we test whether the covariate is significantly **associated** to the graph structure.

[6] These are tests that assess whether two samples are drawn from the same distribution.

The **Friedman–Rafsky** tests for two or multiple sample segregations on a minimum spanning tree. It was conceived as a generalization of the univariate Wald–Wolfowitz runs test. Suppose we are comparing two samples, say men and women, whose coordinates represent a measurement of interest. We color the two groups blue and red, as in Figure 10.22. The Wald–Wolfowitz test looks for long runs of the same color that would indicate that the two groups have different distributions.

Instead of looking for consecutive values of one type ("runs"), we count the number of connected nodes of the same type.

Once the minimum spanning tree has been constructed, the vertices are assigned "colors" according to the different levels of a categorical variable. We call **pure** those edges whose two nodes have the same level of the factor variable. We use S_O, the number of pure edges, as our test statistic. To evaluate whether our observed value could have occurred by chance when the groups have the same distribution, we permute the vertex labels (colors) randomly and recount how many pure edges there are. This label swapping is repeated many times, creating our null distribution for S.

10.6.2   Example: bacteria sharing between mice

Here we illustrate the idea on a collection of samples from mice whose stools were analyzed for their microbial content. We read in a dataset with many mice and many taxa. We compute the *Jaccard distance* and then use the `mst` function from the *igraph* package. We annotate the graph with the relevant covariates, as shown in the code below.

```
ps1  = readRDS("../data/ps1.rds")
sampledata = data.frame( sample_data(ps1))
d1 = as.matrix(phyloseq::distance(ps1, method="jaccard"))
gr = graph.adjacency(d1,  mode = "undirected", weighted = TRUE)
net = igraph::mst(gr)
V(net)$id = sampledata[names(V(net)), "host_subject_id"]
V(net)$litter = sampledata[names(V(net)), "family_relationship"]
```

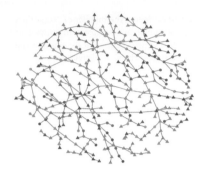

F003 ●	F006 ●	M001 ●	M004 ●	litter ●	Litter1 ▲
F004 ●	F007 ●	M002 ●	M005 ●		
F005 ●	F008 ●	M003 ●	M006 ●		

Figure 10.23: The minimum spanning tree based on Jaccard dissimilarity and annotated with the mouse ID and litter factors.

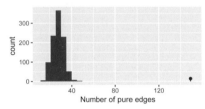

Figure 10.24: The permutation histogram of the number of pure edges in the network obtained from the minimum spanning tree with Jaccard similarity.

We make a `ggnetwork` object from the resulting `igraph`-generated minimum spanning tree and then plot it, as shown in Figure 10.23.

```
gnet=ggnetwork(net)
ggplot(gnet, aes(x = x, y = y, xend = xend, yend = yend))+
  geom_edges(color = "darkgray") +
  geom_nodes(aes(color = id, shape = litter)) + theme_blank()+
  theme(legend.position="bottom")
```

Now we compute the null distribution and p-value for the test; this is implemented in the *phyloseqGraphTest* package.

```
library("phyloseqGraphTest")
gt = graph_perm_test(ps1, "host_subject_id", distance="jaccard",
                     type="mst",  nperm=1000)
gt$pval
## [1] 0.000999
```

We can take a look at the complete histogram of the null distribution generated by permutations.

```
plot_permutations(gt)
```

Different choices for the skeleton graph

It is not necessary to use an MST for the skeleton graph that defines the edges. Graphs made by linking nearest neighbors (Schilling, 1986) or distance thresholding work as well.

The Bioconductor package *phyloseq* has functionality for creating graphs based on thresholding a distance matrix through the function `make_network`. We create a network by creating an edge between samples whose Jaccard dissimilarity is less than a given threshold, which we set in the code below via the parameter `max.dist`. We use the *ggnetwork* package to add attributes to the vertices indicating which particular mouse the sample came from and which litter the mouse was in. We see that in the resulting network, shown in Figure 10.25, there is grouping of the samples by both mouse and litter.

```
net = make_network(ps1, max.dist = 0.35)
sampledata = data.frame(sample_data(ps1))
V(net)$id = sampledata[names(V(net)), "host_subject_id"]
V(net)$litter = sampledata[names(V(net)), "family_relationship"]
netg = ggnetwork(net)
```

```
ggplot(netg, aes(x = x, y = y, xend = xend, yend = yend)) +
  geom_edges(color = "darkgray") +
  geom_nodes(aes(color = id, shape = litter)) + theme_blank()+
    theme(plot.margin = unit(c(0, 5, 2, 0), "cm"))+
    theme(legend.position = c(1.4, 0.3),legend.background =
        element_blank(),legend.margin = margin(0, 3, 0, 0, "cm"))+
      guides(color = guide_legend(ncol=2))
```

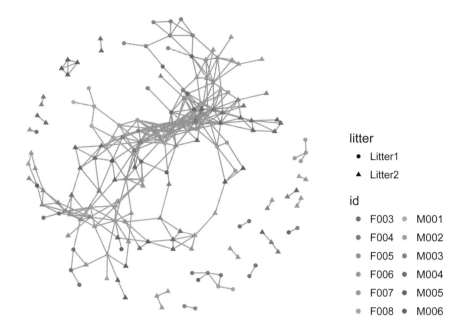

litter
- ● Litter1
- ▲ Litter2

id
●	F003	●	M001
●	F004	●	M002
●	F005	●	M003
●	F006	●	M004
●	F007	●	M005
●	F008	●	M006

Figure 10.25: A *co-occurrence* network created by using a threshold on the Jaccard dissimilarity matrix. The colors represent which mouse the sample came from; the shape represents which litter the mouse was in.

Note that no matter which graph we build between the samples, we can approximate a null distribution by permuting the labels of the nodes of the graph. However, sometimes it will be preferable to adjust the permutation distribution to account for known structure between the covariates.

10.6.3 Friedman–Rafsky test with nested covariates

In the test in the previous section, we took a rather naive approach and showed that there were significant differences between individual mice (the `host_subject_id` variable). Here we perform a slightly different permutation test to find out: if we control for the difference between mice, is there a litter (the `family_relationship` variable) effect? The setup of the test is similar; it is how the permutations are generated that differs. We maintain the nested structure of the two factors using the `grouping` argument. We permute the `family_relationship` labels but keep the `host_subject_id` structure intact.

```
gt = graph_perm_test(ps1, "family_relationship",
        grouping = "host_subject_id",
        distance = "jaccard", type = "mst", nperm= 1000)
gt$pval
## [1] 0.002
```

This test has a small p-value, and we reject the null hypothesis that the two samples come from the same distribution. From the plot of the minimum spanning tree in Figure 10.27, we see by eye that the samples group by litter more than we would expect by chance.

```
plot_permutations(gt)
```

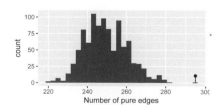

Figure 10.26: The permutation histogram obtained from the minimum spanning tree with Jaccard similarity.

▶ Question **10.18** The *k*-nearest neighbor graph is obtained by putting an edge between two samples whenever one of them is in the set of *k*-nearest neighbors of the other. Redo the test with the graph using nearest neighbors defined by the Jaccard distance. What would you conclude?   ◀

▶ **Solution 10.18**

```
gtnn1 = graph_perm_test(ps1, "family_relationship",
                        grouping = "host_subject_id",
                        distance = "jaccard", type = "knn", knn = 1)
gtnn1$pval
## [1] 0.01
```

Figure 10.27 shows that pairs of samples having edges between them in this nearest neighbor graph are much more likely to be from the same litter.

```
plot_test_network(gtnn1)
```
                                                                                          □

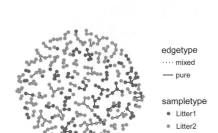

edgetype
···· mixed
— pure

sampletype
● Litter1
● Litter2

Figure 10.27: The graph obtained from a nearest neighbor graph with Jaccard similarity.

Note: The dual graph.   In the examples above, we sought to show the relationships between samples through their shared taxa. It can also be of interest to ask the question about taxa: do some of the taxa co-occur more often than one would expect? This approach can help in studying microbial "communities" as they assemble in the **microbiome**. The methods we developed above all apply to this use case: all one really does is transpose the data. It is always preferable with sparse data, such as the microbiome, to use Jaccard and not build correlation networks that might be appropriate in other settings.

10.7   Summary of this chapter

Annotated graphs.   We learned how to store and plot data that have more structure than simple arrays: graphs have edges and nodes that can also be associated to extra annotations that can be displayed usefully.

Important examples of graphs and useful R packages.   We started with specific examples such as Markov chain graphs, phylogenetic trees and minimum spanning trees. We saw how to use the *ggnetwork* and *igraph* packages to visualize graphs and show as much information as possible by using specific graph layout algorithms.

Combining graphs with statistical data.   We incorporated a known "skeleton" graph into differential expression analyses. This can be used to pinpoint perturbation hotspots in a network. We saw how evolutionary models defined along rooted binary trees serve as the basis for phylogenetic tree estimation and how we can incorporate these trees as supplementary information in a differential abundance analysis using the R packages *structSSI* and *phyloseq*.

Linking co-occurrence to other variables. Graph and network tools also enable the creation of networks from co-occurrence data and can be used to visualize and test the effect of factor covariates. We encountered the Friedman–Rafsky test which provides an easy way of testing dependencies of a variable with the edge structure of a skeleton graph.

Context and intepretation aides. We saw ways of incorporating interactions of players in a network and demonstrated how useful it is to combine this information with statistical scores. This often provides biological insight in the analysis of complex biological systems.

Previous knowledge or outcome? We saw that graphs can be useful for encoding our previous knowledge: metabolic network information, gene ontologies and phylogenetic trees of known bacteria are all available in standard databases. It is beneficial in a study to incorporate all known information, and doing this by combining skeleton networks with observed data enhances our understanding of experimental results in the context of what is already known. On the other hand, the graph can be the outcome that we want to predict and we build graphs from data (phylogenetic trees, co-occurrence networks and minimum spanning trees).

10.8 Further reading

For complete developments and many important consequences of the evolutionary models used for phylogenetic trees, see the books by Li (1997) and Li and Graur (1991). Felsenstein (2004) is the classic text on estimating phylogenetic trees.

Paradis (2011), written by the author of the *ape* package, contains many use cases and details about manipulation of trees in R. A review of bootstrapping for phylogenetic trees can be found in Holmes (2003a).

We can use a tree as well as abundances in contingency table data through an extension of PCoA-MDS called DPCoA (double principal coordinate analysis). For **microbiome data**, the phylogenetic tree provides distances between taxa; these distances serve as the basis for the first PCoA. A second PCoA enables projection of the weighted sample points. This procedure has proved very effective in microbial ecology applications; see Purdom (2011) or Fukuyama et al. (2012) for details.

Graphs can be used to predict vertex covariates. There is a large field of applied statistics and machine learning that considers the edges in a graph as a response variable for which one can make predictions based on covariates or partial knowledge of the graph; these include **ERGMs** (exponential random graph models; Robins et al. 2007) and kernel methods for graphs (Schölkopf et al., 2004).

For theoretical properties of the Friedman–Rafsky test and more examples, see Bhattacharya (2015).

A full list of Bioconductor packages that deal with graphs and networks is available at `http://www.bioconductor.org/packages/release/BiocViews.html#___GraphAndNetwork`.

10.9   Exercises

▶ Exercise **10.1** Create a function that plots a graph starting from an adjacency matrix. Show how it works on an example. ◀

▶ Exercise **10.2** The relationships between gene functions are organized hierarchically into a graph called the Gene Ontology graph. The biological processes are organized at finer and finer scales. Take one of the databases providing Gene Ontology information for the organisms you are interested in. Choose a gene list and build the gene ontology graph for that list.

Hint: some examples can be found in the packages *GOstats*, *FGNet* and *eisa*. ◀

▶ Exercise **10.3 Markov chain graph of transitions between states of the vaginal microbiota.** In DiGiulio et al. (2015) the authors use an *igraph* plot to represent the transitions rates between community state types (CSTs) using the *markovchain* package. Load the data and the transition rates and state names into an object of the special class `markovchain` and tailor the layout carefully to include the percentage of preterm births as a covariate for the vertices (make the vertex size proportional to this variable); include the size of transitions between states as the width of the arrows. ◀

▶ Exercise **10.4 Protein interaction networks.** Read the Wikipedia article on the STRING database (https://www.string-db.org). The protein Cyclin B1 is encoded by the CCNB1 gene. You can read about in the Wikipedia article on *Cyclin B1*.

Use the STRING site to generate a text file (call it `ccnb1datsmall.txt`) of edges around the CCNB1 gene. Choose nodes that are connected by evidence of co-expression with a confidence higher than 0.9. Collect no more than 50 interactions and additional nodes that are two steps away from CCNB1 in the graph. ◀

▶ Exercise **10.5** Read `ccnb1datsmall.txt` into R and make a plot of the graph using one of the graph visualization methods covered in this chapter. ◀

▶ Exercise **10.6** Make a heatmap showing the adjacency matrix of the graph created in Exercise 10.5. ◀

▶ Exercise **10.7** These visualizations show the strongest interactions in the two-step neighborhood of `CCNB1`. Both the plotted graph and the heatmap image show the same data: there seems to be a cluster of proteins that are all similar to `CCNB1`, and there is also another cluster in the other proteins. Many of the proteins in the CCNB1 cluster are co-expressed at the same time as each other. Why might this be the case?

Conversely, proteins that are co-expressed with a protein that is co-expressed with CCNB1 (two steps away) do not tend to be co-expressed with each other.

Is it easier for you to see this in one of the figures (the plot or the heatmap) than the other? ◀

▶ **Exercise 10.8** Compare the use of *ape* and *phangorn* in the analysis of HIV GAG data. Compute the Jukes–Cantor distances between the sequences using both packages and compare them to the Hamming distances.

```
library("ape")
library("phangorn")
GAG=read.dna("../data/DNA_GAG_20.txt")
```
◀

▶ **Exercise 10.9** Look up the *Bray-Curtis dissimilarity*, a statistic used in ecology, on Wikipedia. Use it to perform a Friedman–Rafsky type test with a "two-nearest neighbor" graph.
◀

CHAPTER 11

Image Data

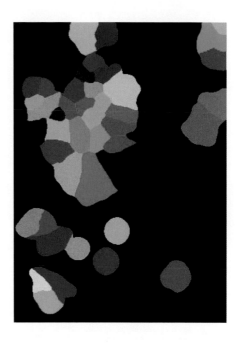

Images are a rich source of data. In this chapter, we will see how quantitative information can be extracted from images, and how we can use statistical methods to summarize and understand the data. The goal of the chapter is to show that getting started working with image data is easy – if you are able to handle the basic R environment, you are ready to start working with images. That said, this chapter is not a general introduction to image analysis. The field is extensive; it touches many areas of signal processing, information theory, mathematics, engineering and computer science, and there are excellent books that present a systematic overview.

We will mainly study series of two-dimensional images, in particular, images of cells. We will learn how to identify the cells' positions and shapes and how to quantitatively measure characteristics of the identified shapes and patterns, such as sizes, intensities, color distributions and relative positions. Such information can then be used in downstream analyses: for instance, we can compare cells between different conditions, say under the effect of different drugs, or in different stages of differentiation and growth; or we can measure how the objects in the image relate to each other, e.g., whether they like to cluster together or repel each other, or whether certain characteristics tend to be shared between neighboring objects, indicative of cell-to-cell communication. In the language of genetics, what this means is that we can use images as complex phenotypes or as multivariate quantitative traits.

We will not here touch upon image analysis in more than two dimensions: we won't consider 3D segmentation and registration, or temporal tracking. These are sophisticated tasks for which specialized software would likely perform better than what we could assemble in the scope of this chapter.

There are similarities between data from high-throughput imaging and other high-throughput data in genomics. Batch effects tend to play a role, for instance, because of changes in staining efficiency, illumination or many other factors. We'll need to take appropriate precautions in our experimental design and analysis choices. In principle, the intensity values in an image can be calibrated in physical units corresponding, say, to radiant energy or fluorophore concentration; however, this is not always done in practice in biological imaging, and perhaps also is not needed. Somewhat easier to achieve, and clearly valuable, is a calibration of the spatial dimensions of the image, i.e., the conversion factor between pixel units and metric distances.

11.1   Goals for this chapter

In this chapter we will:

- Learn how to read, write and manipulate images in R.
- Understand how to apply filters and transformations to images.
- Combine these skills to do segmentation and feature extraction; we will use cell segmentation as an example.
- Learn how to use statistical methods to analyze spatial distributions and dependencies.
- Get to know the most basic distribution for a spatial point process: the homogeneous Poisson process.
- Recognize whether data fit the basic homogeneous Poisson assumption or show evidence of clumping or exclusion.

11.2   Loading images

A useful toolkit for handling images in R is the Bioconductor package *EBImage* (Pau et al., 2010). We start out by reading in a simple picture to demonstrate the basic functions.

```
library("EBImage")
imagefile = "../data/mosquito.png"
mosq = readImage(imagefile)
```

EBImage currently supports three image file formats: `jpeg`, `png` and `tiff`. Above, we loaded a sample image from the *MSBdata* package. When you are working with your own data, you do not need that package, just provide the name(s) of your file(s) to the `readImage` function. As you will see later in this chapter, `readImage` can read multiple images in one go, which are then all assembled into a single image data object. For this to work, the images need to have the same dimensions and color mode.

▶ Question **11.1** The *RBioFormats* package[1] provides functionality for reading and writing many more image file formats. How many different file formats are supported?   ◄

▶ Solution **11.1** See the manual page of the `read.image` function in the *RBioFormats* package (note that this is distinct from `EBImage::readImage`) and the online documentation of the Bio-Formats project on the website of the Open Microscopy Environment, `http://www.openmicroscopy.org/site/support/bio-formats5.5/supported-formats.html`.   □

11.3   Displaying images

Let's visualize the image that we just read in. The basic function is `display`.

```
display(mosq)
```

[1] As of September 2018, it is only available on github, although the author plans to provide it through Bioconductor.

The `display` command opens the image in a window of your web browser (as set by `getOption("browser")`). Using the mouse or keyboard shortcuts, you can zoom in and out of the image, pan and cycle through multiple image frames.

Alternatively, we can also display the image using R's built-in plotting by calling `display` with the argument `method = "raster"`. The image then goes to the current device. In this way, we can combine image data with other plotting functionality, for instance, to add text labels.

```
display(mosq, method = "raster")
text(x = 85, y = 800, label = "A mosquito",
     adj = 0, col = "orange", cex = 1.5)
```

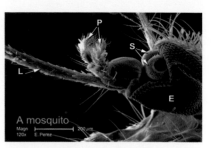

Figure 11.1: Mosquito discovered dead in the suburbs of Decatur, Georgia. Credit: CDC/Janice Haney Carr.

The resulting plot is shown in Figure 11.1. As usual, the graphics displayed in an R device can be saved using the *base* R function `dev.print` or `dev.copy`.

Note that we can also read and view color images; see Figure 11.2.

```
imagefile = "../data/hiv.png"
hivc = readImage(imagefile)
display(hivc)
```

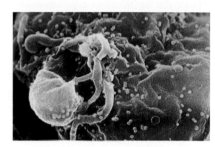

Figure 11.2: Scanning electron micrograph of HIV-1 virions budding from a cultured lymphocyte. Credit: CDC/C. Goldsmith, P. Feorino, E.L. Palmer, W.R. McManus.

Furthermore, if an image has multiple frames, they can be displayed all at once in a grid arrangement by specifying the function argument `all = TRUE` (see Figure 11.3).

```
nuc = readImage("../data/nuclei.tif")
display(1 - nuc, method = "raster", all = TRUE)
```

Or we can just view a single frame, for instance, the second one.

```
display(1 - nuc, method = "raster", frame = 2)
```

▶ Question **11.2** Why did we pass the argument `1 - nuc` to the `display` function in the code for Figure 11.3? How does it look if we display `nuc` directly? ◀

11.4 How are images stored in R?

Let's dig into what's going on by first identifying the class of the image object.

```
class(mosq)
## [1] "Image"
## attr(,"package")
## [1] "EBImage"
```

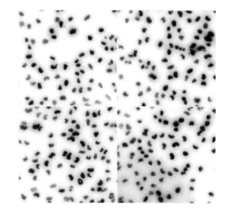

Figure 11.3: Tiled display of four images of cell nuclei from the *EBImage* package.

So we see that this object has the class *Image*. This is not one of the base R classes; rather, it is defined by the package *EBImage*. We can find out more about this class through the help browser or by typing `class ? Image`. The class is derived from the base R class *array*, so you can do with *Image* objects everything that you can do with R arrays; in addition, they have some extra features and behaviors.[2]

[2] In R parlance, the extra features are called **slots** and the behaviors are called methods; methods are a special kind of function.

▶ Question **11.3** How can you find out what the slots of an *Image* object are and which methods can be applied to it? ◀

▶ **Solution 11.3** The class definition is easy; it is accessed with `showClass("Image")`. Finding all the methods applicable to the *Image* class by an analogous call to an R function is painful; your best bet is to consult the manual page of the class to see which methods the author chose to mention.   □

The dimensions of the image can be extracted using the `dim` method, just as for regular arrays.

```
dim(mosq)
## [1] 1400  952
```

In object-oriented terminology, redefining a method in this way, to change its parameters, is called *overloading*.

The `hist` method has been redefined compared to the ordinary `hist` function for arrays; it uses different and possibly more useful defaults (Figure 11.4).

```
hist(mosq)
```

If we want to directly access the data matrix as an R *array*, we can use the accessor function `imageData`.

```
imageData(mosq)[1:3, 1:5]
##             [,1]      [,2]      [,3]      [,4]      [,5]
## [1,] 0.1960784 0.1960784 0.1960784 0.1960784 0.1960784
## [2,] 0.1960784 0.1960784 0.1960784 0.1960784 0.1960784
## [3,] 0.1960784 0.1960784 0.2000000 0.2039216 0.2000000
```

Image histogram: 1332800 pixels

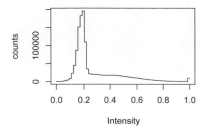

Figure 11.4: Histogram of the pixel intensities in `mosq`. Note that the range is between 0 and 1.

A useful summary of an *Image* object is printed if we simply type the object's name.

```
mosq
## Image
##   colorMode    : Grayscale
##   storage.mode : double
##   dim          : 1400 952
##   frames.total : 1
##   frames.render: 1
##
## imageData(object)[1:5,1:5]
##             [,1]      [,2]      [,3]      [,4]      [,5]
## [1,] 0.1960784 0.1960784 0.1960784 0.1960784 0.1960784
## [2,] 0.1960784 0.1960784 0.1960784 0.1960784 0.1960784
## [3,] 0.1960784 0.1960784 0.2000000 0.2039216 0.2000000
## [4,] 0.1960784 0.1960784 0.2039216 0.2078431 0.2000000
## [5,] 0.1960784 0.2000000 0.2117647 0.2156863 0.2000000
```

Now let us look at the color image.

```
hivc
## Image
##   colorMode    : Color
##   storage.mode : double
##   dim          : 1400 930 3
##   frames.total : 3
##   frames.render: 1
##
```

```
## imageData(object)[1:5,1:6,1]
##      [,1] [,2] [,3] [,4] [,5]
## [1,]    0    0    0    0    0
## [2,]    0    0    0    0    0
## [3,]    0    0    0    0    0
## [4,]    0    0    0    0    0
## [5,]    0    0    0    0    0
```

The two images differ by their property `colorMode`, which is `Grayscale` for `mosq` and `Color` for `hivc`. What is the point of this property? It turns out to be convenient when we are dealing with stacks of images. If `colorMode` is `Grayscale`, then the third and higher dimensions of the array are considered as separate image frames corresponding, for instance, to different z-positions, time points, replicates, etc. On the other hand, if `colorMode` is `Color`, then the third dimension is assumed to hold different color channels, and only the fourth and higher dimensions – if present – are used for multiple image frames. In `hivc`, there are three color channels, which correspond to the red, green and blue intensities of our photograph. However, this is not necessarily the case: there can be any number of color channels.

▶ Question **11.4** Describe how R stores the data `nuc`. ◀

▶ **Solution 11.4**
```
nuc
dim(imageData(nuc))
```

We see that we have four frames in total, which correspond to the four separate images (`frames.render`). □

11.5 Writing images to file

Saving images directly to disk in the array representation that we saw in the previous section produces large file sizes – in most cases, needlessly large. It is common to use compression algorithms to reduce storage consumption. There are two main types of image[3] compression:

- Lossless compression: it is possible to exactly reconstruct the original image data from the compressed file. Simple principles of lossless compression are: (i) do not spend more bits on representing a pixel than needed (e.g., the pixels in the `mosq` image have a range of 256 grayscale values, and this could be represented by eight bits, although `mosq` stores them in a 64-bit numeric format[4]); and (ii) identify patterns (such as those that you saw above in the printed pixel values for `mosq` and `hivc`) and represent them much more compactly by writing down rules instead.
- Lossy compression: additional savings are made compared with lossless compression by dropping details that a human viewer would be unlikely to notice anyway.

An example of a storage format with lossless compression is PNG;[5] an example of lossy compression is the JPEG[6] format. While JPEG is fine for your holiday pictures, it is good practice to store scientific images in a lossless format.

[3] This is also true for movies and music.

[4] While this is somewhat wasteful of memory, it is more compatible with the way the rest of R works and is rarely a limiting factor on modern computer hardware.

[5] See *Portable Network Graphics* on Wikipedia.

[6] See *JPEG* on Wikipedia.

Figure 11.5: The original mosquito image (top left) and three different image transformations (subtraction, multiplication, power transformation).

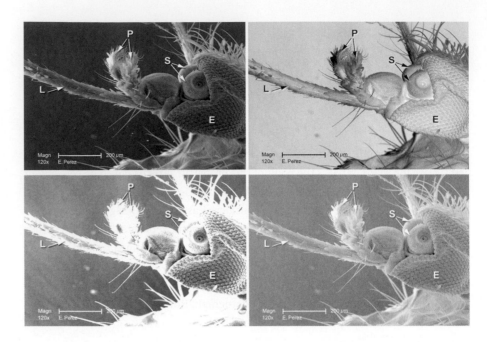

We read the image `hivc` from a file in PNG format, so let's now write it out as a JPEG file. The lossiness is specified by the *quality* parameter, which can lie between 1 (worst) and 100 (best).

```
writeImage(hivc, "hivc.jpeg", quality = 85)
```

Similarly, we could have written the image as a TIFF file and chosen among several compression algorithms (see the manual page of the `writeImage` and `writeTiff` functions). The package *RBioFormats* lets you write to many additional image file formats.

▶ Question **11.5** How big is the `hivc` object in R's memory? How big is the JPEG file? How much RAM would you expect a three-color, 16-megapixel image to occupy?   ◀

▶ Solution **11.5**

```
object.size(hivc) %>% format(units = "Mb")
## [1] "29.8 Mb"
(object.size(hivc)/prod(dim(hivc))) %>% format %>% paste("per pixel")
## [1] "8 bytes per pixel"
file.info("hivc.jpeg")$size
## [1] 296241
16 * 3 * 8
## [1] 384
```

11.6   Manipulating images

Now that we know that images are stored as arrays of numbers in R, our method of manipulating images becomes clear – simple algebra! For example, we can take our original image, shown again in the top left of Figure 11.5, and flip the bright areas to dark, and vice versa, by multiplying the image by −1 (see Figure 11.5, top right).

```
mosqinv = normalize(-mosq)
```

▶ Question **11.6** What does the function `normalize` do? ◀

We could also adjust the contrast through multiplication (see Figure 11.5, bottom left) and the gamma-factor through exponentiation (see Figure 11.5, bottom right).

```
mosqcont = mosq * 3
mosqexp = mosq ^ (1/3)
```

Furthermore, we can crop, threshold and transpose images with matrix operations (Figures 11.6–11.8).

```
mosqcrop   = mosq[100:438, 112:550]
mosqthresh = mosq > 0.5
mosqtransp = transpose(mosq)
```

▶ Question **11.7** What data type is `mosqthresh`, the result of the thresholding? ◀

▶ Solution **11.7** It is an *Image* object whose pixels are binary values represented by an R array of type *logical*. You can inspect the object by typing its name into the console. □

▶ Question **11.8** Instead of the `transpose` function as above, could we also have used R's *base* function `t`? ◀

▶ Solution **11.8** The values of `t(mosq)` and `transpose(mosq)` happen to be the same, but `transpose` is preferable because it also works with color and multiframe images. □

11.7 Spatial transformations

We just saw one type of spatial transformation, transposition, but there are many others, including:

```
mosqrot    = EBImage::rotate(mosq, angle = 30)
mosqshift  = translate(mosq, v = c(40, 70))
mosqflip   = flip(mosq)
mosqflop   = flop(mosq)
```

In the code above, the function `rotate`[7] rotates the image clockwise by the specified angle, and `translate` moves the image by the specified two-dimensional vector (pixels that end up outside the image region are cropped, and pixels that enter into the image region are set to zero). The functions `flip` and `flop` reflect the image around the central horizontal and vertical axes, respectively. The results of these operations are shown in Figure 11.9.

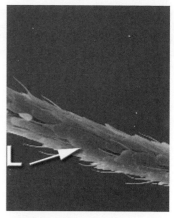

Figure 11.6: Cropping: `mosqcrop`.

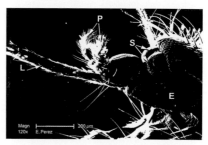

Figure 11.7: Threshold: `mosqthresh`.

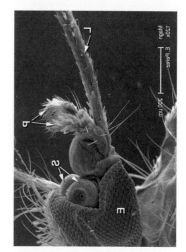

Figure 11.8: Transposition: `mosqtransp`.

[7] Here we call the function with its namespace qualifier `EBImage::` to avoid confusion with a function of the same name in the namespace of the *spatstat* package, which we will attach later.

Figure 11.9: Spatial transformations: rotation (top left), translation (top right), reflection about the central horizontal axis (`flip`, bottom left), reflection about the central vertical axis (`flop`, bottom right).

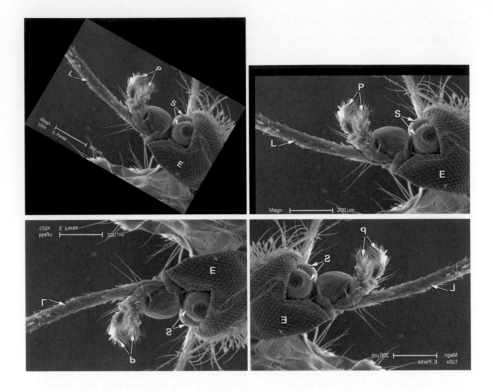

11.8 Linear filters

Let's now switch to an application in cell biology. We load images of human cancer cells that were studied in Laufer et al. (2013). They are shown in Figure 11.10.

```
imagefiles = file.path("..", "data", c("image-DAPI.tif",
  "image-FITC.tif", "image-Cy3.tif"))
cells = readImage(imagefiles)
```

The *Image* object `cells` is a three-dimensional array of size 340×490×3, where the last dimension indicates that there are three individual grayscale frames. Our goal now is to computationally identify and quantitatively characterize the cells in these images. That by itself would be a modest goal, but note that the dataset of Laufer et al. contains over 690,000 images, each of which has 2048×2048 pixels. Here, we are looking at three of these, out of which a small region was cropped. Once we know how to achieve our stated goal, we can apply our abilities to such large image collections, and that is no longer a modest aim!

11.8.1 Interlude: the intensity scale of images

However, before we can start with real work, we need to deal with a slightly mundane data conversion issue. This is, of course, not unusual. Let us inspect the **dynamic range** (the minimum and maximum values) of the images.

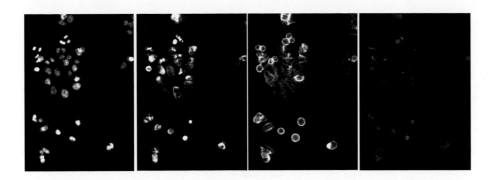

Figure 11.10: Human colon cancer cells (HCT116). The four images show the same cells: the leftmost image corresponds to DAPI staining of the cells' DNA, the second to immunostaining against α-tubulin, the third to actin. They are displayed as grayscale images. The rightmost image is obtained by overlaying the three images as color channels of an RGB image (red: actin, green: α-tubulin, blue: DNA).

```
apply(cells, 3, range)
##         image-DAPI   image-FITC    image-Cy3
## [1,] 0.001586938  0.002899214  0.001663233
## [2,] 0.031204700  0.062485695  0.055710689
```

We see that the maximum values are small numbers well below 1. The reason for this is that the `readImage` function recognizes that the `TIFF` images use 16-bit integers to represent each pixel, and it returns the data – as is common for numeric variables in R – in an array of double precision floating-point numbers, with the integer values (whose theoretical range is from 0 to $2^{16} - 1 = 65{,}535$) stored in the mantissa of the floating-point representation and the exponents chosen so that the theoretical range is mapped to the interval $[0, 1]$. However, the scanner that was used to create these images used only the lower 11 or 12 bits, and this explains the small maximum values in the images. We can rescale these data to approximately cover the range $[0, 1]$ as follows.[8]

```
cells[,,1]   = 32 * cells[,,1]
cells[,,2:3] = 16 * cells[,,2:3]
apply(cells, 3, range)
##         image-DAPI  image-FITC   image-Cy3
## [1,] 0.05078202  0.04638743  0.02661173
## [2,] 0.99855039  0.99977111  0.89137102
```

Keep in mind that these multiplications, with a multiple of two, have no impact on the underlying precision of the stored data.

[8] The function `normalize` provides a more flexible interface to the scaling of images.

11.8.2   Noise reduction by smoothing

Now we are ready to start analyzing the images. As our first goal is **segmentation** of the images in order to identify the individual cells, we can start by removing local artifacts or noise from the images through smoothing. An intuitive approach is to define a window of a selected size around each pixel and average the values within that window. After applying this procedure to all pixels, the new, smoothed image is obtained. Mathematically, we can express this as

$$f^*(x, y) = \frac{1}{N} \sum_{s=-a}^{a} \sum_{t=-a}^{a} f(x + s, y + t), \tag{11.1}$$

where $f(x, y)$ is the value of the pixel at position x, y, and a determines the window size, which is $2a + 1$ in each direction. The number of pixels over which we averaged is $N = (2a + 1)^2$, and f^* is the new, smoothed image.

More generally, we can replace the moving average by a weighted average, using a weight function w, which typically has highest weight at the window midpoint ($s = t = 0$) and then decreases toward the edges:

$$(w * f)(x, y) = \sum_{s=-\infty}^{+\infty} \sum_{t=-\infty}^{+\infty} w(s, t) f(x + s, y + s). \tag{11.2}$$

For notational convenience, we let the summations range from $-\infty$ to ∞, even if in practice the sums are finite as w has only a finite number of non-zero values. In fact, we can think of the weight function w as another image, and this operation is also called *convolution* of the images f and w, indicated by the the symbol $*$. In *EBImage*, the two-dimensional convolution is implemented by the function `filter2`, and the auxiliary function `makeBrush` can be used to generate weight functions w.

```
w = makeBrush(size = 51, shape = "gaussian", sigma = 7)
nucSmooth = filter2(getFrame(cells, 1), w)
```

▶ Question **11.9** What does the weight matrix `w` look like? ◀

▶ Solution **11.9** See Figure 11.11.

```
library("tibble")
library("ggplot2")
tibble(w = w[(nrow(w)+1)/2, ]) %>%
  ggplot(aes(y = w, x = seq(along = w))) + geom_point()
```

In fact, the `filter2` function does not directly perform the summation expressed in Equation (11.2). Instead, it uses the fast Fourier transformation in a way that is mathematically equivalent and computationally more efficient.

The convolution in Equation (11.2) is a *linear* operation, in the sense that we have $w * (c_1 f_1 + c_2 f_2) = c_1 w * f_1 + c_2 w * f_2$ for any two images f_1, f_2 and numbers c_1, c_2. There is beautiful and powerful theory underlying linear filters (Vetterli et al., 2014).

To proceed we now use smaller smoothing bandwidths than were displayed in Figure 11.12 for demonstration. Let's use a `sigma` of one pixel for the DNA channel and three for actin and tubulin.

```
cellsSmooth = Image(dim = dim(cells))
sigma = c(1, 3, 3)
for(i in seq_along(sigma))
  cellsSmooth[,,i] = filter2( cells[,,i],
        filter = makeBrush(size = 51, shape = "gaussian",
                sigma = sigma[i]) )
```

The smoothed images have reduced pixel noise, yet still have the needed resolution.

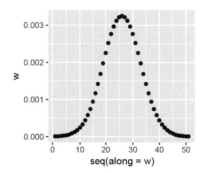

Figure 11.11: The middle row of the weight matrix, `w[26, ]`.

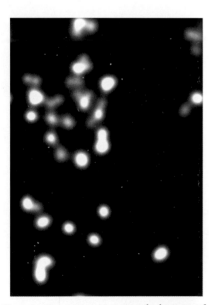

Figure 11.12: `nucSmooth`, a smoothed version of the DNA channel in the image object `cells` (the original version is shown in the leftmost panel of Figure 11.10).

11.9   Adaptive thresholding

The idea of adaptive thresholding is that, unlike the straightforward thresholding we performed for Figure 11.7, the threshold is allowed to vary between different regions of the image. In this way, one can anticipate **spatial dependencies** in the underlying background signal caused, for instance, by uneven illumination or by stray signals from nearby bright objects. In fact, we have already seen an example of uneven background in the bottom right image of Figure 11.3.

Our colon cancer images (see Figure 11.10) do not have such artifacts, but for demonstration, let's simulate uneven illumination by multiplying the image with a two-dimensional bell function `illuminationGradient`, which has highest value in the middle and falls off to the sides (see Figure 11.13).

```
py = seq(-1, +1, length.out = dim(cellsSmooth)[1])
px = seq(-1, +1, length.out = dim(cellsSmooth)[2])
illuminationGradient = Image(
    outer(py, px, function(x, y) exp(-(x^2+y^2))))
nucBadlyIlluminated = cellsSmooth[,,1] * illuminationGradient
```

We now define a smoothing window, `disc`, whose size is 21 pixels, and therefore bigger than the nuclei we want to detect, but small compared to the length scales of the illumination artifact. We use it to compute the image `localBackground` and the thresholded image `nucBadThresh` (both shown in Figure 11.13).

```
disc = makeBrush(21, "disc")
disc = disc / sum(disc)
localBackground = filter2(nucBadlyIlluminated, disc)
offset = 0.02
nucBadThresh = (nucBadlyIlluminated - localBackground > offset)
```

Having seen that this procedure might work, let's do the same for the actual (not artificially degraded) image, as we need this for the next steps.

```
nucThresh =
    (cellsSmooth[,,1] - filter2(cellsSmooth[,,1], disc) > offset)
```

By comparing each pixel's intensity to a background determined from the values in a local neighborhood, we assume that the objects are relatively sparsely distributed in the

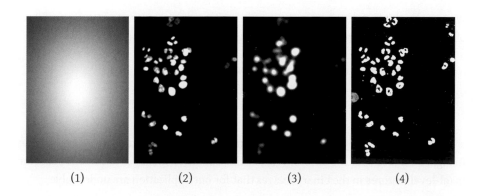

(1)   (2)   (3)   (4)

Figure 11.13: From left to right: (1) `illuminationGradient`, a function that has its maximum at the center and falls off toward the sides, and that simulates uneven illumination sometimes seen in images. (2) `nucBadlyIlluminated`, the image that results from multiplying the DNA channel in `cellsSmooth` with `illuminationGradient`. (3) `localBackground`, the result of applying a linear filter with a bandwidth that is larger than the objects to be detected. (4) `nucBadThresh`, the result of adaptive thresholding. The nuclei at the periphery of the image are reasonably well identified, despite the drop-off in signal strength.

Figure 11.14: Different steps in segmentation of the nuclei.

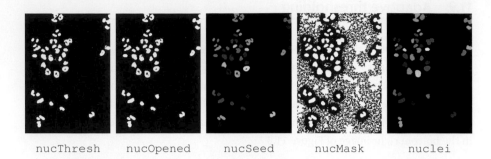

nucThresh   nucOpened   nucSeed   nucMask   nuclei

image, so that the signal distribution in the neighborhood is dominated by background. For the nuclei in our images, this assumption makes sense; for other situations, you may need to make different assumptions. The adaptive thresholding that we have done here uses a linear filter, `filter2`, and therefore amounts to (weighted) local averaging. Other distribution summaries, e.g., the median or a low quantile, tend to be preferable, even if they are computationally more expensive. For local median filtering, *EBimage* provides the function `medianFilter`.

11.10   Morphological operations on binary images

The thresholded image `nucThresh` (shown in the left panel of Figure 11.14) is not yet satisfactory. The boundaries of the nuclei are slightly rugged, and there is noise at the single-pixel level. An effective and simple way to remove these nuisances is given by a set of morphological operations, together called *opening* (Serra, 1983).

Provided a binary image (with values, say 0 and 1, representing background and foreground pixels) and a binary mask (which is sometimes also called the structuring element), these operations work as follows:[9]

- `erode`: For every foreground pixel, put the mask around it, and if any pixel under the mask is from the background, then set all these pixels to background.
- `dilate`: For every background pixel, put the mask around it, and if any pixel under the mask is from the foreground, then set all these pixels to foreground.
- `open`: Perform `erode` followed by `dilate`.

[9] An example of a mask is a disk with a given radius, or more precisely the set of pixels within a certain distance of a center pixel.

We can also think of these operations as filters; however, in contrast to the linear filters of Section 11.8, they operate on binary images only, and there is no linearity.

Let us apply morphological opening to our image.

```
nucOpened = EBImage::opening(nucThresh,
                kern = makeBrush(5, shape = "disc"))
```

The result of this operation is subtle, and you will have to zoom in on the images in Figure 11.14 to spot the differences, but this operation manages to smooth out some pixel-level features in the binary images that for our application are undesirable.

11.11   Segmentation of a binary image into objects

The binary image `nucOpened` represents a segmentation of the image into foreground and background pixels, but not into individual nuclei. We can take one step further and extract individual objects defined as connected sets of pixels. In *EBImage*, there is a handy function for this purpose, `bwlabel`.

```
nucSeed = bwlabel(nucOpened)
table(nucSeed)
```

```
## nucSeed
##        0        1        2        3        4        5        6        7        8
## 155408      511      330      120      468      222      121      125      159
##        9       10       11       12       13       14       15       16       17
##      116      520      115      184      179      116      183      187      303
##       18       19       20       21       22       23       24       25       26
##      226      164      309      194      148      345      287      203      379
##       27       28       29       30       31       32       33       34       35
##      371      208      222      320      443      409      493      256      169
##       36       37       38       39       40       41       42       43
##      225      376      214      228      341      269      119      315
```

The function returns an image, `nucSeed`, of integer values, where 0 represents the background and the numbers from 1 to 43 index the different identified objects.

▶ Question **11.10** What are the numbers in the above table?   ◀

▶ Solution **11.10** The numbers correspond to the area (in pixels) of each of the objects. We could use this information to remove objects that are too large or too small compared with what we expect.   □

To visualize such images, the function `colorLabels` is convenient; it converts the (grayscale) integer image into a color image, using a distinct, arbitrarily chosen color for each object.

```
display(colorLabels(nucSeed))
```

This is shown in the middle panel of Figure 11.14. The result is already encouraging, although we can spot two types of errors:

- some neighboring objects were not properly separated, and
- some objects contain holes.

Indeed, we could change the occurrences of these by playing with the disc size and the parameter `offset` in Section 11.9. Making the offset higher reduces the probability that two neighboring objects touch and are seen as one object by `bwlabel`; on the other hand, a higher offset leads to even more and bigger holes. Lowering the offset has the opposite effects.

Segmentation is a rich and diverse field of research and engineering, with a large body of literature, software tools (Schindelin et al., 2012; de Chaumont et al., 2012; Carpenter et al., 2006; Held et al., 2010) and practical experience in the image analysis and machine learning communities. What the adequate approach is to a given task depends hugely on the data and the underlying question, and there is no universally best method. It is typically difficult even to obtain a "ground truth" or "gold standard" by which to evaluate an analysis: relying on manual annotation of a modest number of selected images is not uncommon. Despite the bewildering array of choices, it is easy to get going, and we need not be afraid of starting out with a simple solution, which we can successively refine. Improvements can usually be gained from methods that allow inclusion of more prior knowledge of the expected shapes, sizes and relationships between the objects to be identified.

For statistical analyses of high-throughput images, we may choose to be satisfied with a simple method that does not rely on too many parameters or assumptions yet results in perhaps a suboptimal but rapid and good enough result (Rajaram et al., 2012). In this spirit, let us proceed with what we have. First, we generate a lenient foreground mask, which surely covers all nuclear stained regions, even though it also covers some regions between nuclei. To do so, we simply apply a second, less stringent, adaptive thresholding.

```
nucMask = cellsSmooth[,,1] - filter2(cellsSmooth[,,1], disc) > 0
```

Next, we apply another morphological operation, `fillHull`, which fills holes that are surrounded by foreground pixels.

```
nucMask = fillHull(nucMask)
```

To improve `nucSeed`, we can now *propagate* its segmented objects until they fill the mask defined by `nucMask`. Boundaries between nuclei, in those places where the mask is connected, can be drawn by Voronoi tessellation, which is implemented in the function `propagate` and will be explained in the next section.

```
nuclei = propagate(cellsSmooth[,,1], nucSeed, mask = nucMask)
```

The result is displayed in the rightmost panel of Figure 11.14.

11.12   Voronoi tessellation

Voronoi tessellation is useful if we have a set of seed points (or regions) and want to partition the space that lies between these seeds in such a way that each point in the space is assigned to its closest seed. As this is an intuitive and powerful idea, we'll use this section for a short digression on it.

Let us consider a basic example. We use the image `nuclei` as seeds. To call the function `propagate`, we also need to specify another image; for now we just provide a trivial image consisting of all zeros, and we set the parameter `lambda` to a large positive value (we will come back to these choices).

```
zeros       = Image(dim = dim(nuclei))
voronoiExamp = propagate(seeds = nuclei, x = zeros, lambda = 100)
voronoiPaint = paintObjects(voronoiExamp, 1 - nucOpened)
```

▶ Question **11.11** How do you select partition elements from the tessellation?   ◀

▶ **Solution 11.11** The result, `voronoiExamp`, of the above call to `propagate` is simply an image of integers whose values indicate the different partitions.

```
head(table(voronoiExamp))

## voronoiExamp
##    1    2    3    4    5    6
## 5644 4736  371 5963 3336 1378

ind = which(voronoiExamp == 13, arr.ind = TRUE)
head(ind, 3)

##        row col
## [1,] 112 100
## [2,] 113 100
## [3,] 114 100
```
□

The result is shown in Figure 11.15. This looks interesting, but perhaps not yet as useful as the image `nuclei` in Figure 11.14. We note that the basic definition of Voronoi tessellation, which we gave above, allows for two generalizations:

- By default, the space that we partition is the full rectangular image area – but we could restrict ourselves to any arbitrary subspace. This is akin to finding the shortest distance from each point to the next seed, not in a simple landscape, but in one that is interspersed by lakes and rivers (that you cannot cross), so that all paths need to remain on the land. The function `propagate` allows for this generalization through its `mask` parameter.
- By default, we think of the space as flat – but in fact it could have hills and canyons, so that the distance between two points in the landscape depends not only on their x- and y-positions but also on the ascents and descents, up and down in the z-direction, that lie in between. We can think of z as an "elevation". You can specify such a landscape to `propagate` through its x argument.

Mathematically, we say that instead of the simple default case (a flat rectangle, or image, with a Euclidean metric on it), we perform the Voronoi segmentation on a Riemannian manifold that has a special shape and a special metric. Let's use the notation x and y for the column and row coordinates of the image, and z for the elevation. For two neighboring points, defined by coordinates (x, y, z) and $(x + dx, y + dy, z + dz)$, the distance ds between them is thus not obtained by the usual Euclidean metric on the 2D image, i.e.,

$$ds^2 = dx^2 + dy^2, \tag{11.3}$$

but instead by

$$ds^2 = \frac{2}{\lambda + 1}\left[\lambda\left(dx^2 + dy^2\right) + dz^2\right], \tag{11.4}$$

where the parameter $\lambda \geqslant 0$ is a real number. To understand this, let's look at some important cases:

$$\begin{aligned}
\lambda = 1: \quad & ds^2 = dx^2 + dy^2 + dz^2, \\
\lambda = 0: \quad & ds^2 = 2\,dz^2, \\
\lambda \to \infty: \quad & ds^2 = 2\left(dx^2 + dy^2\right).
\end{aligned} \tag{11.5}$$

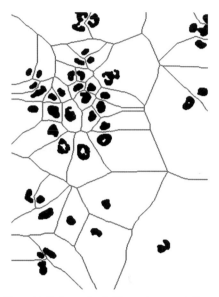

Figure 11.15: Example of a Voronoi segmentation, indicated by the gray lines, using the nuclei (indicated by black regions) as seeds.

For $\lambda = 1$, the metric becomes the isotropic Euclidean metric, i.e., a movement in the z-direction is equally "expensive" or "far" as in the x- or y-direction. In the extreme case of $\lambda = 0$, only the z-movements matter, while lateral movements (in the x- or y-direction) do not contribute to the distance. In the other extreme case, $\lambda \to \infty$, only lateral movements matter, and movement in the z-direction is "free". Distances between points farther apart are obtained by summing ds along the shortest path between them. The parameter λ serves as a convenient control of the relative weighting between sideways movement (along the x- and y-axes) and vertical movement. Intuitively, if you imagine yourself as a hiker in such a landscape, by choosing λ you can specify how much you are prepared to climb up and down to overcome a mountain, as opposed to walking around it. When we used `lambda = 100` in our call to `propagate` at the begin of this section, this value was effectively infinite, so we were in the third boundary case of Equation (11.5).

For the purpose of cell segmentation, these ideas were put forward by Jones et al. (2005) and Carpenter et al. (2006), who also wrote the efficient algorithm that is used by `propagate`.

▶ Task   Explore the effect of using different values of λ.   ◀

11.13   Segmenting the cell bodies

To determine a mask of cytoplasmic area in the images, let us explore a different way of thresholding, this time using a global threshold, which we find by fitting a mixture model to the data. The histograms show the distributions of the pixel intensities in the actin image. We look at the data on the logarithmic scale in Figure 11.16, and in Figure 11.17 zoom in on the region where most of the data lie.

```
hist(log(cellsSmooth[,,3]) )
hist(log(cellsSmooth[,,3]), xlim = -c(3.6, 3.1), breaks = 300)
```

Looking at the histograms for many images, we can set up the following model for the purpose of segmentation: the signal in the cytoplasmic channels of the *Image* `cells` is a mixture of two distributions, a log-normal background and a foreground with another, unspecified, rather flat, but mostly non-overlapping distribution.[10] Moreover, the majority of pixels are from the background. We can then find robust estimates for the location and width parameters of the log-normal component from the half-range mode (implemented in the package *genefilter*) and from the root mean square of the values that lie left of the mode.

```
library("genefilter")
bgPars = function(x) {
  x    = log(x)
  loc  = half.range.mode( x )
  left = (x - loc)[ x < loc ]
  wid  = sqrt( mean(left^2) )
  c(loc = loc, wid = wid, thr = loc + 6*wid)
}
```

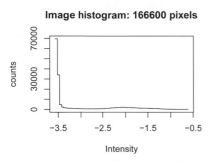

Figure 11.16: Histogram of the actin channel in `cellsSmooth` after taking the logarithm.

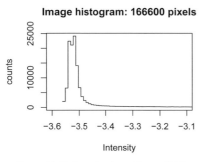

Figure 11.17: Zooming in on Figure 11.16.

[10] This is an application of the ideas we saw in Chapter 4 on mixture models.

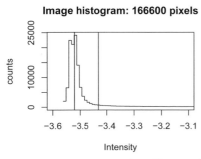

Figure 11.18: As in Figure 11.17, but with `loc` and `thr` shown by vertical lines.

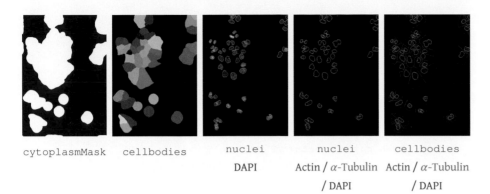

cytoplasmMask	cellbodies	nuclei	nuclei	cellbodies
		DAPI	Actin / α-Tubulin / DAPI	Actin / α-Tubulin / DAPI

Figure 11.19: Steps in the segmentation of the cell bodies.

```
cellBg = apply(cellsSmooth, MARGIN = 3, FUN = bgPars)
cellBg
##           [,1]        [,2]        [,3]
## loc -2.90176965 -2.94427499 -3.52191681
## wid  0.00635322  0.01121337  0.01528207
## thr -2.86365033 -2.87699477 -3.43022437
```

The function defines as a threshold `thr` the location `loc` plus six widths `wid`.[11]

```
hist(log(cellsSmooth[,,3]), xlim = -c(3.6, 3.1), breaks = 300)
abline(v = cellBg[c("loc", "thr"), 3], col = c("brown", "red"))
```

We can now define `cytoplasmMask` by the union of all those pixels that are above the threshold in the actin or tubulin image, or that we have already classified as nuclear in the image `nuclei`:

```
cytoplasmMask = (cellsSmooth[,,2] > exp(cellBg["thr", 2])) |
    nuclei | (cellsSmooth[,,3] > exp(cellBg["thr", 3]))
```

The result is shown in the leftmost panel of Figure 11.19. To define the cellular bodies, we can now simply extend the nucleus segmentation within this mask by the Voronoi tessellation-based propagation algorithm of Section 11.12. This method makes sure that there is exactly one cell body for each nucleus, and the cell bodies are delineated in such a way that a compromise is reached between compactness of cell shape and following the actin and α-tubulin intensity signal in the images. In the terminology of the `propagate` algorithm, cell shape is kept compact by the x- and y-components of the distance metric (11.4), and the actin signal is used for the z-component. The parameter λ controls the trade-off.

```
cellbodies = propagate(x = cellsSmooth[,,3], seeds = nuclei,
                    lambda = 1.0e-2, mask = cytoplasmMask)
```

As an alternative representation to the `colorLabel` plots, we can also display the segmentations of nuclei and cell bodies on top of the original images using the `paintObjects` function; the images `nucSegOnNuc`, `nucSegOnAll` and `cellSegOnAll` that are computed below are shown, respectively, in the three rightmost panels of Figure 11.19.

[11] The choice of the number six here is ad hoc; we could make the choice of threshold more objective by estimating the weights of the two mixture components and assigning each pixel to either foreground or background based on its posterior probability according to the mixture model. More advanced segmentation methods use the fact that this is really a **classification** problem and include additional features and more complex classifiers to separate foreground and background regions.

```
cellsColor = rgbImage(red   = cells[,,3],
                      green = cells[,,2],
                      blue  = cells[,,1])

nucSegOnNuc = paintObjects(nuclei, tgt = toRGB(cells[,,1]),
                           col = "#ffff00")
nucSegOnAll = paintObjects(nuclei, tgt = cellsColor,
                           col = "#ffff00")
cellSegOnAll = paintObjects(cellbodies, tgt = nucSegOnAll,
                            col = "#ff0080")
```

11.14   Feature extraction

Now that we have the segmentations `nuclei` and `cellbodies` together with the original image data `cells`, we can compute various descriptors, or features, for each cell. We saw at the start of Section 11.11 how to use the base R function `table` to determine the total number and sizes of the objects. Let us now take this further and compute the mean intensity of the DAPI signal (`cells[, , 1]`) in the segmented nuclei, the mean actin intensity (`cells[, , 3]`) in the segmented nuclei and the mean actin intensity in the cell bodies.

```
meanNucInt      = tapply(cells[,,1], nuclei, mean)
meanActIntInNuc = tapply(cells[,,3], nuclei, mean)
meanActIntInCell = tapply(cells[,,3], cellbodies, mean)
```

We can visualize the features in pairwise scatterplots (Figure 11.20). We see that they are correlated with each other, although each feature also carries independent information.

```
library("GGally")
ggpairs(tibble(meanNucInt, meanActIntInNuc, meanActIntInCell))
```

With a little more work, we could also compute more sophisticated summary statistics – e.g., the ratio of nucleus area to cell body area; or entropies, mutual information and correlation of the different fluorescent signals in each cell body – as more or less abstract measures of cellular morphology. Such measures can be used, for instance, to detect subtle drug-induced changes of cellular architecture.

While it is easy and intuitive to perform these computations using basic R idioms, as in the `tapply` expressions above, the package *EBImage* also provides the function `computeFeatures`, which efficiently computes a large collection of features that have been commonly used in the literature (a pioneering reference is Boland and Murphy, 2001). Details about this function are described on its manual page, and an example application is worked through in the *HD2013SGI* vignette. Below, we compute features for intensity, shape and texture of each cell from the DAPI channel using the nucleus segmentation (`nuclei`) and from the actin and tubulin channels using the cell body segmentation (`cytoplasmRegions`).

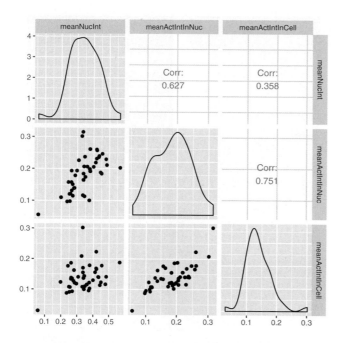

Figure 11.20: Pairwise scatterplots of per-cell intensity descriptors.

```
F1 = computeFeatures(nuclei,      cells[,,1], xname = "nuc",
                                              refnames = "nuc")
F2 = computeFeatures(cellbodies, cells[,,2], xname = "cell",
                                              refnames = "tub")
F3 = computeFeatures(cellbodies, cells[,,3], xname = "cell",
                                              refnames = "act")
dim(F1)
## [1] 43 89
```

F1 is a *matrix* with 43 rows (one for each cell) and 89 columns (one for each of the computed features).

```
F1[1:3, 1:4]

##    nuc.0.m.cx nuc.0.m.cy nuc.0.m.majoraxis nuc.0.m.eccentricity
## 1   119.5523   17.46895          44.86819            0.8372059
## 2   143.4511   15.83709          26.15009            0.6627672
## 3   336.5401   11.48175          18.97424            0.8564444
```

The column names encode the type of feature, as well the color channel(s) and segmentation mask on which it was computed. We can now use multivariate analysis methods – like those we saw in Chapters 5, 7 and 9 – for many different tasks, such as:

- detecting cell subpopulations (clustering);
- classifying cells into predefined cell types or phenotypes (classification); and
- seeing whether the absolute or relative frequencies of the subpopulations or cell types differ between images that correspond to different biological conditions.

In addition to these "generic" machine learning tasks, we also know the spatial positions of the cells, and in the following we will explore some ways to make use of these in our analyses.

Figure 11.21: A biopsy of an enlarged lymph node revealed an intact capsule and obliterated sinuses (upper-left panel, stained with hematoxylin and eosin, original magnification ×100). The infiltrate was composed of an admixture of small lymphocytes, macrophages and plasma cells (upper-right panel, hematoxylin and eosin, original magnification ×400). The infiltrate was composed of a mixture of CD3-positive T cells (including both CD4- and CD8-positive cells) and CD20-positive B cells. Numerous macrophages were also CD4 positive. From Hurley et al., *Diagnostic Pathology* (2008) 3:13.

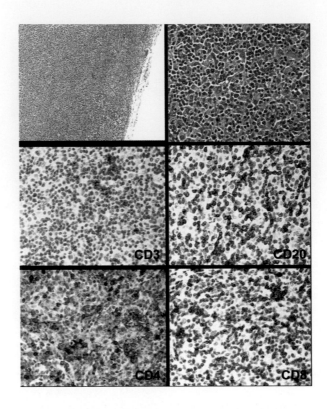

▶ **Task** Use explorative multivariate methods to visualize the matrices $F1, F2, F3$: PCA, heatmap. What's special about the "outlier" cells?   ◀

11.15   Spatial statistics: point processes

In the previous sections, we saw ways of using images of cells to extract their positions and various shape and morphological features. We'll now explore spatial distributions of the position. In order to have interesting data to work on, we'll change datasets and look at breast cancer lymph node biopsies.

11.15.1   Case study: interaction between immune cells and cancer cells

The lymph nodes function as an immunologic filter for the bodily fluid known as lymph. They filter antigens out of the lymph before returning it to the circulation. Lymph nodes are found throughout the body and are composed mostly of T cells, B cells, dendritic cells and macrophages. The nodes drain fluid from most of our tissues. The lymph ducts of the breast usually drain to one lymph node first, before draining through the rest of the lymph nodes underneath the arm. That first lymph node is called the *sentinel* lymph node. In a similar fashion to the spleen, the macrophages and dendritic cells that capture antigens present these foreign materials to T and B cells, consequently initiating an immune response.

T lymphocytes are usually divided into two major subsets that are functionally and phenotypically different:

- CD4+ T cells, or T helper cells, are pertinent coordinators of immune regulation. The main function of T helper cells is to augment or potentiate immune responses by the secretion of specialized factors that activate other white blood cells to fight off infection.

• CD8+ T cells, or T killer/suppressor cells, are important in directly killing certain tumor cells, viral-infected cells and sometimes parasites. CD8+ T cells are also important for the downregulation of immune responses.

Both types of T cells can be found throughout the body. They often depend on the secondary lymphoid organs (the lymph nodes and spleen) as sites where activation occurs.

Dendritic cells, or CD1a cells, are antigen-presenting cells that process antigen and present peptides to T cells.

Typing the cells can be done by staining them with protein antibodies that provide specific signatures. For instance, different types of immune cells have different proteins expressed, mostly in their cell membranes.

We'll look at data by Setiadi et al. (2010). After segmenting the image shown in Figure 11.22 using the segmentation method *GemIdent* (Holmes et al., 2009), the authors obtained the coordinates and the type of all the cells in the image. We call this type of data a *marked point process*, and it can be seen as a simple table with three columns.

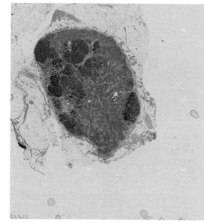

Figure 11.22: A stained lymph node. This image is the basis for the spatial data in `brcalymphnode`. From Setiadi et al. (2010).

```
library("readr")
library("dplyr")
cellclasses = c("T_cells", "Tumor", "DCs", "other_cells")
brcalymphnode = lapply(cellclasses, function(k) {
    read_csv(file.path("..", "data",
             sprintf("99_4525D-%s.txt", k))) %>%
    transmute(x = globalX,
              y = globalY,
              class = k)
}) %>% bind_rows %>% mutate(class = factor(class))

brcalymphnode

## # A tibble: 209,462 x 3
##         x     y class
##     <int> <int> <fct>
##  1   6355 10382 T_cells
##  2   6356 10850 T_cells
##  3   6357 11070 T_cells
##  4   6357 11082 T_cells
##  5   6358 10600 T_cells
##  6   6361 10301 T_cells
##  7   6369 10309 T_cells
##  8   6374 10395 T_cells
##  9   6377 10448 T_cells
## 10   6379 10279 T_cells
## # ... with 209,452 more rows

table(brcalymphnode$class)

##
##         DCs other_cells     T_cells       Tumor
##         878       77081      103681       27822
```

Figure 11.23: Scatterplot of the x- and y-positions of the T and tumor cells in `brcalymphnode`. The locations were obtained by a segmentation algorithm from a high-resolution version of Figure 11.22. Some rectangular areas in the T-cells plot are suspiciously empty; this could be because the corresponding image tiles within the overall composite image went missing or were not analyzed.

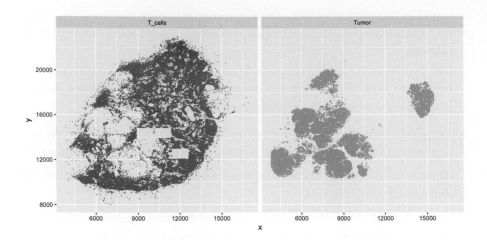

We see that there are over 100,000 T cells, around 28,000 tumor cells and only several hundred dendritic cells. Let's plot the x- and y-positions of the cells (Figure 11.23).

```
ggplot(filter(brcalymphnode, class %in% c("T_cells", "Tumor")),
    aes(x = x, y = y, col = class)) + geom_point(shape = ".") +
    facet_grid( . ~ class) + guides(col = FALSE)
```

▶ Question **11.12** Compare Figures 11.22 and 11.23. Why are the y-axes inverted relative to each other?   ◀

▶ Solution **11.12**   Figure 11.22 follows the convention for image data, where the origin is in the top-left corner of the image, while Figure 11.23 follows the convention for Cartesian plots, with the origin at the bottom left.   □

To use the functionality of the *spatstat* package, it is convenient to convert our data in `brcalymphnode` into an object of class *ppp*; we do this by calling the eponymous function.

```
library("spatstat")
```

```
ln = with(brcalymphnode,
  ppp(x = x, y = y, marks = class, xrange=range(x), yrange=range(y)))
ln
## Marked planar point pattern: 209462 points
## Multitype, with levels = DCs, other_cells, T_cells, Tumor
## window: rectangle = [3839, 17276] x [6713, 23006] units
```

Class *ppp* objects are designed to capture realizations of a **spatial point process**, that is, a set of isolated points located in a mathematical space. In our case, as you can see above, the space is a two-dimensional rectangle that contains the range of the x- and y-coordinates. In addition, the points can be *marked* with certain properties. In `ln`, the mark is simply the *factor* variable `class`. More generally, it could be several attributes, times or quantitative data as well. There are similarities between a marked point process and an image, although for the former, the points can lie anywhere within the space, whereas in an image, the pixels cover the space in a regular, rectangular way.

11.15.2   Convex hull

We have considered a space in which the point process lies as a rectangle. In fact, the space is more confined, and we can compute a tighter region from the convex hull of the points.

```
library("geometry")
coords = cbind(ln$x, ln$y)
chull = convhulln( coords )
```

The heavy lifting is done by the function `convhulln` in the *geometry* package. However, as so often, a bit of data wrangling remains to be done. Namely, the `ppp` function expects the hull to be described by a closed polygonal line, while `convhulln` presents its result as a set of line segments in no particular order. This is because `convhulln` works not only with two-dimensional data but just as well with *d*-dimensional data. The hull is then represented by $(d - 1)$-dimensional simplices. The function's output format reflects this more general setup. Thus, the entries of `chull` are integer indices into the array `coords` that refer to the points defining each simplex. In our case, $d = 2$, and one-dimensional simplices are simply line segments. So we write a little `for`-loop that assembles them into a closed polygonal line, that is, a polygon.

```
pidx = integer(nrow(chull) + 1)
pidx[1:2] = chull[1, ]
chull[1, ] = NA
for(j in 3:length(pidx)) {
  wh = which(chull == pidx[j-1], arr.ind = TRUE)
  stopifnot(nrow(wh )== 1)
  wh[, "col"] = 3 - wh[, "col"] ## 2->1, 1->2
  pidx[j] = chull[wh]
  chull[wh[, "row"], ] = NA
}
pidx = rev(pidx)
```

```
ggplot(tibble(x = ln$x, y = ln$y)[pidx, ], aes(x = x, y = y)) +
  geom_point() + geom_path() + coord_fixed()
```

We can see the polygon in Figure 11.24 and now call `ppp` again, this time with the polygon.

```
ln = with(brcalymphnode,
    ppp(x = x, y = y, marks = class, poly = coords[ pidx, ],
        check = FALSE))
ln
## Marked planar point pattern: 209462 points
## Multitype, with levels = DCs, other_cells, T_cells, Tumor
## window: polygonal boundary
## enclosing rectangle: [3839, 17276] x [6713, 23006] units
```

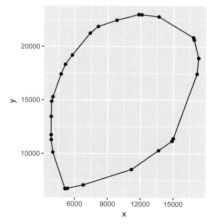

Figure 11.24: Polygon describing the convex hull of the points in `ln`.

11.15.3   Other ways of defining the space for the point process

We do not have to use the convex hull to define the space on which the point process is considered. Alternatively, we could provide an image mask to `ppp` that defines the space based on prior knowledge, or we could use density estimation on the sampled points to identify only a region in which there is high enough point density, ignoring sporadic outliers. These choices are part of the analyst's job when considering spatial point processes.

11.16   First-order effects: the intensity

One of the most basic questions of spatial statistics is whether neighboring points are "clustering", i.e., whether, and to what extent, they are closer to each other than expected "by chance"; or perhaps the opposite – whether they seem to repel each other. There are many examples where this kind of question can be asked, for instance:

- crime patterns within a city,
- disease patterns within a country, or
- soil measurements in a region.

It is usually not hard to find reasons why such patterns exist: good and bad neighborhoods, local variations in lifestyle or environmental exposure, the common geological history of the soil. Sometimes there may also be mechanisms by which the observed events attract or repel each other – the proverbial "broken windows" in a neighborhood, or the tendency of many cell types to stick close to other cells.

The cell example highlights that spatial clustering (or anticlustering) can depend on the objects' attributes (or marks, in the parlance of spatial point processes). It also highlights that the answer can depend on the length scale considered. Even if cells attract each other, they have a finite size and cannot occupy the same space. So there will be some minimal distance between them, on the scale at which they essentially repel each other, while at farther distances, they attract.

To attack these questions more quantitatively, we need to define a probabilistic model of what we expect *by chance*. Let's count the number of points lying in a subregion, say, a circle of area a around a point $p = (x, y)$; call this $N(p, a)$.[12] The mean and covariance of N provide first- and second-order properties. The former is the intensity of the process:

$$\lambda(p) = \lim_{a \to 0} \frac{E[N(p, a)]}{a}.$$
(11.6)

Here we use infinitesimal calculus to define the local intensity $\lambda(p)$. As for time series, a stationary process is one where we have homogeneity throughout the region, i.e., $\lambda(p) =$ const.; then the intensity in an area A is proportional to the area: $E[N(\cdot, A)] = \lambda A$. Later we'll also look at higher-order statistics, such as the spatial covariance

$$\gamma(p_1, p_2) = \lim_{a \to 0} \frac{E\left[(N(p_1, a) - E[N(p_1, a)])\left(N(p_2, a) - E[N(p_2, a)]\right)\right]}{a^2}.$$
(11.7)

If the process is stationary, this will depend only on the relative position of the two points (the vector between them). If it depends only on the distance, i.e., only on the length but not on the direction of the vector, it is called second-order isotropic.

[12] As usual, we use the uppercase notation $N(p, a)$ for the random variable, and the lowercase $n(p, a)$ for its realizations, or samples.

11.16.1 Poisson process

The simplest spatial process is the **Poisson process**. We will use it as a null model against which to compare our data. It is stationary with intensity λ, and there are no further dependencies between occurrences of points in non-overlapping regions of the space. Moreover, the number of points in a region of area A follows a Poisson distribution with rate λA.

11.16.2 Estimating the intensity

To estimate the intensity, divide the area into subregions small enough to see potential local variations of $\lambda(p)$, but big enough to contain a sufficient sample of points. This is analogous to 2D density estimation, and instead of hard region boundaries, we can use a smooth kernel function K:

$$\hat{\lambda}(p) = \sum_i e(p_i)K(p - p_i). \qquad (11.8)$$

The kernel function depends on a smoothing parameter, σ: the larger this is, the larger the regions over which we compute the local estimate for each p. The quantity $e(p)$ is an edge correction factor, and takes into account the estimation bias caused when the support of the kernel (the "smoothing window") falls outside the space on which the point process is defined. The function `density`, which is defined for *ppp* objects in the *spatstat* package, implements Equation (11.8).

```
d = density(subset(ln, marks == "Tumor"), edge=TRUE, diggle=TRUE)
plot(d)
```

The plot is shown in Figure 11.26.

▶ Question **11.13** What does the estimate look like without edge correction?   ◀

▶ Solution **11.13**

```
d0 = density(subset(ln, marks == "Tumor"), edge = FALSE)
plot(d0)
```

Now estimated intensity is smaller toward the edge of the space, reflecting edge bias (see Figure 11.27).   □

The `density` function gives us an estimate of the *intensity* of the point process. A related, but different, task is the estimation of the (conditional) *probability* of being a particular cell class. The function `relrisk` computes a nonparametric estimate of the spatially varying risk of a particular event type. We're interested in the probability that a cell that is present at particular spatial location will be a tumor cell (Figure 11.28).

```
rr = relrisk(ln, sigma = 250)
```

```
plot(rr)
```

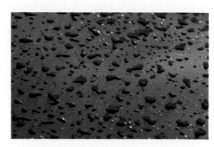

Figure 11.25: Raindrops falling on the floor are modeled by a Poisson process. The number of drops falling on a particular spot only depends on the rate λ (and on the size of the spot), but not on what happens at other spots. Image credit: underworld111/iStock/Getty Images.

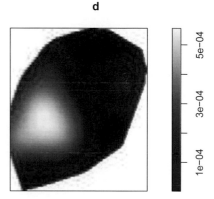

Figure 11.26: Intensity estimate for the cells marked `Tumor` in ppp. The support of the estimate is the polygon that we specified earlier (Figure 11.24).

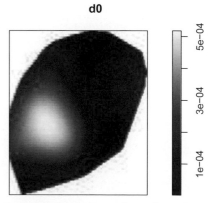

Figure 11.27: As Figure 11.26, but without edge correction.

Figure 11.28: Estimates of the spatially varying probability of each of the cell classes, conditional on there being cells.

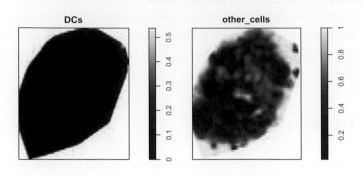

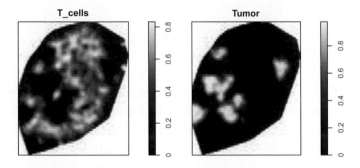

11.17   Second-order effects: spatial dependence

If we pick a point at random in our spatial process, what is the distance W to its nearest neighbor? For a homogeneous Poisson process, the cumulative distribution function of this distance is

$$G(w) = P(W \leqslant w) = 1 - e^{-\lambda \pi w^2}. \tag{11.9}$$

Plotting G gives a way of noticing departure from the homogeneous Poisson process. An estimator of G, which also takes into account edge effects (Baddeley, 1998; Ripley, 1988), is provided by the function `Gest` of the *spatstat* package.

```
gln = Gest(ln)
gln

## Function value object (class 'fv')
## for the function r -> G(r)
## .................................................................
##           Math.label
## r         r
## theo      G[pois](r)
## han       hat(G)[han](r)
## rs        hat(G)[bord](r)
## km        hat(G)[km](r)
## hazard    hat(h)[km](r)
```

```
## theohaz h[pois](r)
##          Description
## r        distance argument r
## theo     theoretical Poisson G(r)
## han      Hanisch estimate of G(r)
## rs       border corrected estimate of G(r)
## km       Kaplan-Meier estimate of G(r)
## hazard   Kaplan-Meier estimate of hazard function h(r)
## theohaz  theoretical Poisson hazard function h(r)
## ..............................................................
## Default plot formula:  .~r
## where "." stands for 'km', 'rs', 'han', 'theo'
## Recommended range of argument r: [0, 20.998]
## Available range of argument r: [0, 52.443]

library("RColorBrewer")
plot(gln, xlim = c(0, 10), lty = 1, col = brewer.pal(4, "Set1"))
```

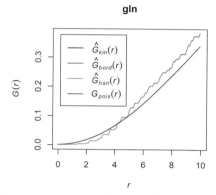

Figure 11.29: Estimates of G, using three different edge-effect corrections – which here happen to lie essentially on top of each other – and the theoretical distribution for a homogenous Poisson process.

The printed summary of the object gln gives an overview of the computed estimates; further explanations are on the manual page of Gest. In Figure 11.29 we see that the empirical distribution function and that of our null model, a homogeneous Poisson process with a suitably chosen intensity, cross at around 4.5 units. Cell-to-cell distances that are shorter than this value are less likely than for the null model. In particular, there are essentially no distances below around 2; this, of course, reflects the fact that our cells have finite size and cannot overlap the same space. There seems to be a trend to avoid very large distances (compared to the Poisson process), perhaps indicative of a tendency of the cells to cluster.

11.17.1 Ripley's K function

The average number of points found near a randomly picked point of the process will indicate fluctuations from the complete spatial randomness model, for which this number grows with the distance r as the area of the circle, πr^2, increases.

The K function (variously called **Ripley's K function** or the *reduced second-moment function*) of a stationary point process is defined so that $\lambda K(r)$ is the expected number of (additional) points within a distance r of a given, randomly picked point. Remember that λ is the intensity of the process, i.e., the expected number of points per unit area. The K function is a second-order moment property of the process.

The definition of K can be generalized to inhomogeneous point processes and written as in Baddeley et al. (2000):

$$K_{\text{inhom}}(r) = \sum_{i,j} \mathbb{1}(d(p_i, p_j) \leq r) \times \frac{e(p_i, p_j, r)}{\lambda(x_i)\lambda(x_j)}, \tag{11.10}$$

where $d(p_i, p_j)$ is the distance between points p_i and p_j, and $e(p_i, p_j, r)$ is an edge-correction factor.[13] For estimation and visualization, it is useful to consider a

[13] See the manual page of Kinhom for more.

transformation of K (and, analogously, of K_{inhom}), the so-called L function:

$$L(r) = \sqrt{\frac{K(r)}{\pi}}. \tag{11.11}$$

For a complete spatial random pattern, the theoretical value is $L(r) = r$. By comparing that to the estimate of L for a dataset, we can learn about interpoint dependence and spatial clustering. The square root in Equation (11.11) has the effect of stabilizing the variance of the estimator, so that L, compared with K, is more appropriate for data analysis and simulations. The computations in the function `Linhom` of the *spatstat* package take a few minutes for our data (Figure 11.30).

```
Lln = Linhom(subset(ln, marks == "T_cells"))
Lln

## Function value object (class 'fv')
## for the function r -> L[inhom](r)
## .................................................................
##              Math.label
## r            r
## theo         L[pois](r)
## border       {hat(L)[inhom]^{bord}}(r)
## bord.modif   {hat(L)[inhom]^{bordm}}(r)
##              Description
## r            distance argument r
## theo         theoretical Poisson L[inhom](r)
## border       border-corrected estimate of L[inhom](r)
## bord.modif   modified border-corrected estimate of L[inhom](r)
## .................................................................
## Default plot formula:  .~.x
## where "." stands for 'bord.modif', 'border', 'theo'
## Recommended range of argument r: [0, 694.7]
## Available range of argument r: [0, 694.7]
```

```
plot(Lln, lty = 1, col = brewer.pal(3, "Set1"))
```

We could now proceed with looking at the L function for other cell types, and for different tumors as well as for healthy lymph nodes. This is what Setiadi and colleagues did in their report (Setiadi et al., 2010): by comparing the spatial grouping patterns of T and B cells between healthy and breast cancer lymph nodes, they saw that B cells appeared to lose their normal localization in the extrafollicular region of the lymph nodes in some tumors.

The pair correlation function. This describes how point density varies as a function of distance from a reference point. It provides a perspective, inspired by physics, for looking at spatial clustering. For a stationary point process, it is defined as

$$g(r) = \frac{1}{2\pi r}\frac{dK}{dr}(r). \tag{11.12}$$

For a stationary Poisson process, the pair correlation function is identically equal to 1. Values of $g(r) < 1$ suggest inhibition between points; values greater than 1 suggest clustering.

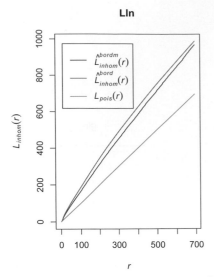

Figure 11.30: Estimate of L_{inhom}, Equations (11.10) and (11.11), of the T-cell pattern.

The *spatstat* package allows us to compute estimates of g even for inhomogeneous processes; if we call `pcf` as below, the definition (11.12) is applied to the estimate of K_{inhom}.

```
pcfln = pcf(Kinhom(subset(ln, marks=="T_cells")))

plot(pcfln, lty = 1)
plot(pcfln, lty = 1, xlim = c(0,10))
```

As we see in Figure 11.31, the T cells cluster, although at very short distances, there is also evidence for avoidance.

▶ Question **11.14** The sampling resolution in the plot of the pair correlation function in the bottom panel of Figure 11.31 is low. How can it be increased?   ◀

11.18   Summary of this chapter

We learned to work with image data in R. Images are basically just arrays, and we can use familiar idioms to manipulate them. We can extract quantitative features from images, and then many of the analytical questions are not unlike those from other high-throughput data: we summarize the features into statistics such as means and variances, do hypothesis testing for differences between conditions, perform analysis of variance, apply dimension reduction, clustering and classification.

Often we want to compute such quantitative features not for the whole image, but for individual objects shown in the image, and then we need to first segment the image to demarcate the boundaries of the objects of interest. We saw how to do this for images of nuclei and cells.

When our interest is in the positions of objects and how these positions relate to each other, we enter the realm of spatial statistics. We explored some of the functionality of the *spatstat* package, encountered the point process class and learned some of the specific diagnostic statistics used for point patterns, such as Ripley's K function.

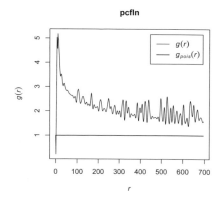

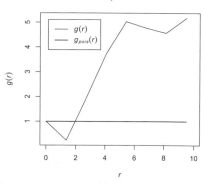

Figure 11.31: Estimate of the pair correlation function, Equation (11.12), of the T-cell pattern.

11.19   Further reading

- There is a vast literature on image analysis. When navigating it, it is helpful to realize that the field is driven by two forces: specific application domains (we saw the analysis of high-throughput cell-based assays) and available computer hardware. Some algorithms and concepts that were developed in the 1970s are still relevant; others have been superseded by more systematic and perhaps more computationally intensive methods. Many algorithms imply certain assumptions about the nature of the data and and scientific questions asked, which may be fine for one application but need a fresh look in another. A classic introduction is *The Image Processing Handbook* (Russ and Neal, 2015), which is now in its seventh edition.
- For spatial point pattern analysis, see Diggle (2013), Ripley (1988), Cressie (1991) or Chiu et al. (2013).

11.20   Exercises

▶ Exercise **11.1** Load some images from your personal photo library into R and try out the manipulations from Section 11.6 on them.   ◀

▶ Exercise **11.2** Explore the effect of the parameter `lambda` in the `propagate` function (Sections 11.12 and 11.13) using a *shiny* app that displays the `cellbodies` image, as in Figure 11.19.   ◀

▶ Exercise **11.3** Use the `fft` function (package *stats*) to compute the periodograms of some of your images from Exercise 11.1.

- How do the periodograms of different images compare?
- How do they change when you apply a filter as in Section 11.8.2?
- Save an image in `jpeg` format with a high compression (low quality) parameter, and load the image again. How did the periodogram change?   ◀

▶ Exercise **11.4** Compute and display the Voronoi tesselation for the European cities from Chapter 9. You can use either their PCA or MDS coordinates in a plane with Euclidean distances, or the latitudes and longitudes with the great circle distance (Haversine formula). Optionally, you can add data for additional places from your favorite parts of the world and overlay political boundaries.   ◀

[14] For instance,
`http://www.digital-embryo.org.`

▶ Exercise **11.5** Download 3D image data from light sheet microscopy,[14] load it into an *EBImage Image* object and explore the data.   ◀

CHAPTER 12

Supervised Learning

A frequent question in biological and biomedical applications is whether a property of interest (say, disease type, cell type, the prognosis of a patient) can be "predicted", given one or more other properties, called the **predictors**. Often we are motivated by a situation in which the property to be predicted is unknown (it lies in the future or is hard to measure), while the predictors are known. The crucial point is that we *learn* the prediction rule – the relationship between predictors and outcome – from a set of *training data* in which the property of interest is known. Once we have the rule, we can either apply it to new data and make actual predictions of unknown outcomes, or we can dissect the rule with the aim of better understanding the underlying biology.

Compared to unsupervised learning and what we have seen in Chapters 5, 7 and 9, where we do not know what we are looking for or how to decide whether our result is "right", we are on much more solid ground with supervised learning: the objective is clearly stated, and we have straightforward criteria to measure how well we are doing.

The central issues in supervised learning[1] are **overfitting** and **generalizability**. Did we just learn the training data "by heart" by constructing a rule that has 100% accuracy on the training data but would perform poorly on any new data? Or did our rule indeed pick up some of the pertinent patterns in the *system* being studied, which will also apply to yet unseen new data? (See Figure 12.1.)

12.1 Goals for this chapter

In this chapter we will:

- See exemplary applications that motivate the use of supervised learning methods.
- Learn what discriminant analysis does.
- Define measures of performance.
- Encounter the curse of dimensionality and see what overfitting is.
- Find out about regularization – in particular, penalization – and understand the concepts of generalizability and model complexity.
- See how to use cross-validation to tune parameters of algorithms.
- Discuss method hacking.

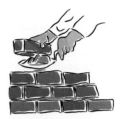

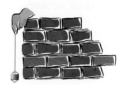

In a supervised learning setting, we have a yardstick or plumbline to help us judge how well we are doing: the response itself.

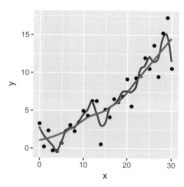

Figure 12.1: An example of *overfitting*: two regression lines are fit to data in the (x, y)-plane (black points). We can think of such a line as a rule that predicts the y-value given an x-value. Both lines are smooth, but the fits differ in what is called their *bandwidth*, which intuitively can be interpreted as their stiffness. The blue line seems overly keen to follow minor wiggles in the data, while the orange line captures the general trend but is less detailed. The effective number of parameters needed to describe the blue line is much higher than for the orange. Also, if we were to obtain additional data, it is likely that the blue line would do a *worse* job than the orange in modeling the new data. We'll formalize these concepts – training error and test set error – later in this chapter. Although exemplified here with line fitting, the concept applies more generally to prediction models.

[1]The terms supervised learning and **statistical learning** can be used more or less interchangeably.

12.2   What are the data?

The basic data structure for both supervised and unsupervised learning is (at least conceptually) a dataframe, where each row corresponds to an object and the columns are different features (usually numerical values) of the objects.[2] While in unsupervised learning we aim to find (dis)similarity relationships between the objects based on their feature values (e.g., by clustering or ordination), in supervised learning we aim to find a mathematical function (or a computational algorithm) that predicts the value of one of the features from the others. Many implementations require that there are no missing values, whereas other methods can be made to work with some amount of missing data.

The feature that we select over all the others with the aim of predicting it is called the **objective** or the **response**. Sometimes the choice is natural, but sometimes it is also instructive to reverse the roles, especially if we are interested in dissecting the prediction function for the purpose of biological understanding, or in disentangling correlations from causation.

The framework for supervised learning covers both continuous and categorical response variables. In the continuous case we also call it **regression**, in the categorical case, **classification**. It turns out that this distinction is not a detail, as it has quite far-reaching consequences for the choice of loss function (Section 12.5) and thus the choice of algorithm (Friedman, 1997).

The first question to consider in any supervised learning task is how the number of objects compares to the number of predictors. The more objects, the better, and much of the hard work in supervised learning has to do with overcoming the limitations of having a finite (and, typically, too small) training set.

▶ Task   Give examples where we have encountered instances of supervised learning with a categorical response in this book.   ◀

12.2.1   Motivating examples

Predicting diabetes type

The `diabetes` dataset (Reaven and Miller, 1979) presents three different groups of diabetes patients and five clinical variables measured on them.

```
library("readr")
library("magrittr")
diabetes = read_csv("../data/diabetes.csv", col_names = TRUE)
diabetes

## # A tibble: 144 x 7
##       id relwt glufast glutest steady insulin group
##    <int> <dbl>   <int>   <int>  <int>   <int> <int>
## 1     1 0.810      80     356    124      55     3
## 2     3 0.940     105     319    143     105     3
```

[2] This description is simplified. Machine learning is a huge field, and lots of generalizations of this simple conceptual picture have been made. Already the construction of relevant features is an art by itself – we have seen examples with images of cells in Chapter 11 – and more generally there are lots of possibilities to extract features from images, sounds, movies, free text, etc. Moreover, a variant of machine learning called **kernel methods** do not need features at all; instead, kernel methods use *distances* or measures of similarity between objects. It may be easier, for instance, to define a measure of similarity between two natural language text objects than to find relevant numerical features to represent them. Kernel methods are beyond the scope of this book.

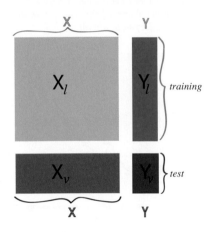

Figure 12.2: In supervised learning, we assign two different roles to our variables. We have labeled the explanatory variables X and the response variable(s) Y. There are also two different sets of observations: the training sets X_ℓ and Y_ℓ and the test sets X_v and Y_v. (The subscripts refer to alternative names for the two sets: "learning" and "validation".)

```
## 3      5 1.00        90    323    240    143    3
## 4      7 0.910      100    350    221    119    3
## 5      9 0.990       97    379    142     98    3
## 6     11 0.900       91    353    221     53    3
## 7     13 0.960       78    290    136    142    3
## 8     15 0.740       86    312    208     68    3
## 9     17 1.10        90    364    152     76    3
## 10    19 0.830       85    296    116     60    3
## # ... with 134 more rows
diabetes$group %<>% factor
```

We used the forward–backward pipe operator `%<>%` to convert the `group` column into a factor. The plot is shown in Figure 12.3.

```
library("ggplot2")
library("reshape2")
ggplot(melt(diabetes, id.vars = c("id", "group")),
       aes(x = value, col = group)) +
  geom_density() + facet_wrap( ~variable, ncol = 1, scales = "free") +
  theme(legend.position="bottom")
```

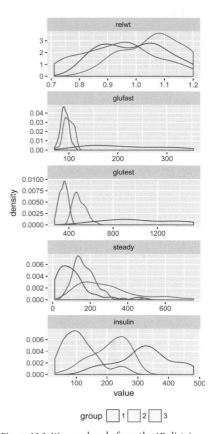

Figure 12.3: We see already from the 1D distributions that some of the individual variables could potentially predict which group a patient is more likely to belong to. Our goal is to combine variables to improve over such 1D prediction models.

Predicting cellular phenotypes

Neumann et al. (2010) observed human cancer cells using live-cell imaging. The cells were genetically engineered so that their histones were tagged with a green fluorescent protein (GFP). A genome-wide RNAi library was applied to the cells, and for each siRNA perturbation, movies of a few hundred cells were recorded for about two days, to see what effect the depletion of each gene had on cell cycle, nuclear morphology and cell proliferation. Their paper reports the use of an automated image classification algorithm that quantified the visual appearance of each cell's nucleus and enabled the prediction of normal mitosis states or aberrant nuclei. The algorithm was trained on data from around 3000 cells that were annotated by a human expert. It was then applied to almost 2 billion images of nuclei (Figure 12.4). Using automated image classification provided scalability (annotating 2 billion images manually would take a long time!) and objectivity.

Predicting embryonic cell states

We will revisit the mouse embryo data (Ohnishi et al., 2014), which we already met in Chapters 3, 5 and 7. We'll try to predict cell state and genotype from the gene expression measurements in Sections 12.3.2 and 12.6.3.

12.3   Linear discrimination

We start with one of the simplest possible discrimination problems:[3] we have objects described by two continuous features (so the objects can be thought of as points in the

[3] Arguably the simplest problem is a single continuous feature, two classes and the task of finding a single threshold to discriminate between the two groups – as in Figure 6.5.

Figure 12.4: The data were images of 2×10^9 nuclei from movies. The images were segmented to identify the nuclei, and numeric features were computed for each nucleus, corresponding to size, shape, brightness and lots of other more or less abstract quantitative summaries of the joint distribution of pixel intensities. From the features, the cells were classified into 16 nucleus morphology classes, represented by the rows of the barplot. Representative images for each class are shown in black and white in the center column. The class frequencies, which are very unbalanced, are shown by the lengths of the bars. From Neumann et al. (2010).

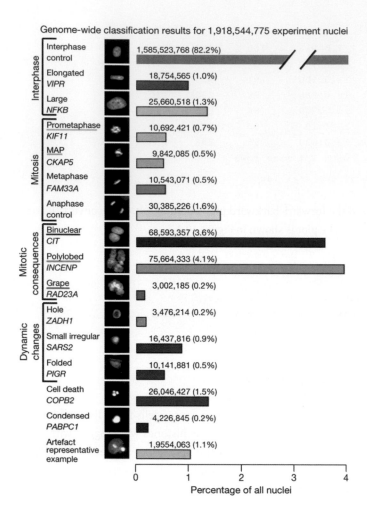

2D plane) and falling into three groups. Our aim is to define class boundaries, which are lines in the 2D space.

12.3.1 Diabetes data

Let's see whether we can predict `group` from the `insulin` and `glutest` variables in the `diabetes` data. It's always a good idea to first visualize the data (Figure 12.5).

```
ggdb = ggplot(mapping = aes(x = insulin, y = glutest)) +
  geom_point(aes(colour = group), data = diabetes)
ggdb
```

We'll start with a method called **linear discriminant analysis (LDA)**. This method is a foundation stone of classification: many of the more complicated (and sometimes more powerful) algorithms are really just generalizations of LDA.

```
library("MASS")
diabetes_lda = lda(group ~ insulin + glutest, data = diabetes)
diabetes_lda
```

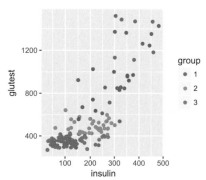

Figure 12.5: Scatterplot of two of the variables in the `diabetes` data. Each point is a sample, and the color indicates the diabetes type as encoded in the `group` variable.

```
## Call:
## lda(group ~ insulin + glutest, data = diabetes)
##
## Prior probabilities of groups:
##         1         2         3
## 0.2222222 0.2500000 0.5277778
##
## Group means:
##     insulin   glutest
## 1 320.9375 1027.3750
## 2 208.9722  493.9444
## 3 114.0000  349.9737
##
## Coefficients of linear discriminants:
##                   LD1         LD2
## insulin -0.004463900 -0.01591192
## glutest -0.005784238  0.00480830
##
## Proportion of trace:
##    LD1    LD2
## 0.9677 0.0323
ghat = predict(diabetes_lda)$class
table(ghat, diabetes$group)

##
## ghat  1  2  3
##    1 25  0  0
##    2  6 24  6
##    3  1 12 70
mean(ghat != diabetes$group)
## [1] 0.1736111
```

▶ Question **12.1** What do the different parts of the above output mean?   ◀

Now let's visualize the LDA result. We are going to plot the prediction regions for each of the three groups. We do this by creating a grid of points and using our prediction rule on each of them. We'll then also dig a bit deeper into the mechanics of LDA and plot the class centers (`diabetes_lda$means`) and ellipses that correspond to the fitted covariance matrix (`diabetes_lda$scaling`). Assembling this visualization requires us to write a bit of code.

```
make1Dgrid = function(x) {
  rg = grDevices::extendrange(x)
  seq(from = rg[1], to = rg[2], length.out = 100)
}
```

Set up the points for prediction, a 100×100 grid that covers the data range.

```
diabetes_grid = with(diabetes,
  expand.grid(insulin = make1Dgrid(insulin),
              glutest = make1Dgrid(glutest)))
```

Do the predictions.

```
diabetes_grid$ghat =
  predict(diabetes_lda, newdata = diabetes_grid)$class
```

Identify the group centers.

```
centers = diabetes_lda$means
```

Compute the ellipse. We start from a unit circle and apply the corresponding affine transformation from the LDA output.

```
unitcircle = exp(1i * seq(0, 2*pi, length.out = 90)) %>%
             {cbind(Re(.), Im(.))}
ellipse = unitcircle %*% solve(diabetes_lda$scaling)
```

Make all three ellipses, one for each group center.

```
ellipses = lapply(seq_len(nrow(centers)), function(i) {
  (ellipse +
   matrix(centers[i, ], byrow = TRUE,
          ncol = ncol(centers), nrow = nrow(ellipse))) %>%
     cbind(group = i)
}) %>% do.call(rbind, .) %>% data.frame
ellipses$group %<>% factor
```

Now we are ready to plot (Figure 12.6).

```
ggdb + geom_raster(aes(fill = ghat),
          data = diabetes_grid, alpha = 0.25, interpolate = TRUE) +
    geom_point(data = as_tibble(centers), pch = "+", size = 8) +
    geom_path(aes(colour = group), data = ellipses) +
    scale_x_continuous(expand = c(0, 0)) +
    scale_y_continuous(expand = c(0, 0))
```

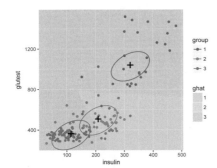

Figure 12.6: As Figure 12.5, with the classification regions from the LDA model shown. The three ellipses represent the class centers and the covariance matrix of the LDA model; note that there is only one covariance matrix, which is the same for all three classes. Therefore the sizes and orientations of the ellipses are also the same for the three classes – only their centers differ. They represent contours of equal class membership probability.

▶ Question **12.2** Why is the boundary between the prediction regions for groups 1 and 2 not perpendicular to the line between the cluster centers? ◀

▶ Solution **12.2** The boundaries would be perpendicular if the ellipses were circles. In general, a boundary is tangential to the contours of equal class probabilities, and due the elliptic shape of the contours, a boundary is in general not perpendicular to the line between centers. □

▶ Question **12.3** How confident would you be about the predictions in those areas of the 2D plane that are far from all of the cluster centers? ◀

▶ Solution **12.3** Predictions that are far from any cluster center should be assessed critically, as this amounts to an extrapolation into regions where (a) the LDA model may not be very good, and/or (b) there may be no training data nearby to support the prediction. We could use the distance to the nearest center as a measure of confidence in the prediction for any particular point, although we will see that resampling and cross-validation-based methods offer more generic and usually more reliable measures. □

▶ Question **12.4** Why is the boundary between the prediction regions for groups 2 and 3 not halfway between the centers, but shifted in favor of class 3? (Hint: have a look at the `prior` argument of `lda`.) Try again with a uniform prior. ◀

▶ Solution **12.4** The result of the following code chunk is shown in Figure 12.7. The suffix `_up` is short for "uniform prior".

```
diabetes_up = lda(group ~ insulin + glutest, data = diabetes,
  prior = with(diabetes, rep(1/nlevels(group), nlevels(group))))

diabetes_grid$ghat_up =
  predict(diabetes_up, newdata = diabetes_grid)$class

stopifnot(all.equal(diabetes_up$means, diabetes_lda$means))

ellipse_up  = unitcircle %*% solve(diabetes_up$scaling)
ellipses_up = lapply(seq_len(nrow(centers)), function(i) {
  (ellipse_up +
  matrix(centers[i, ], byrow = TRUE,
         ncol = ncol(centers), nrow = nrow(ellipse_up))) %>%
    cbind(group = i)
}) %>% do.call(rbind, .) %>% data.frame
ellipses_up$group %<>% factor

ggdb + geom_raster(aes(fill = ghat_up),
            data = diabetes_grid, alpha = 0.4, interpolate = TRUE) +
  geom_point(data = data.frame(centers), pch = "+", size = 8) +
  geom_path(aes(colour = group), data = ellipses_up) +
  scale_x_continuous(expand = c(0, 0)) +
  scale_y_continuous(expand = c(0, 0))
```

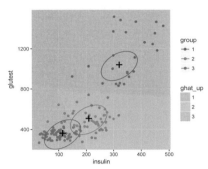

Figure 12.7: As Figure 12.6, but with uniform class priors.

The `stopifnot` line confirms that the class centers are the same, as they are independent of the prior. The joint covariance is not. □

▶ Question **12.5** Figures 12.6 and 12.7 show both the fitted LDA model (through the ellipses) and the prediction regions (through the area coloring). What part of this visualization is generic for all sorts of classification methods and what part is method specific? ◀

▶ Solution **12.5** The prediction regions can be shown for any classification method, including a "black box" method. The cluster centers and ellipses in Figures 12.6 and 12.7 are method specific. □

▶ Question **12.6** What is the difference in the prediction accuracy if we use all five variables instead of just `insulin` and `glufast`? ◀

▶ **Solution 12.6**

```
diabetes_lda5 = lda(group ~ relwt + glufast + glutest +
           steady + insulin, data = diabetes)
diabetes_lda5
## Call:
## lda(group ~ relwt + glufast + glutest + steady + insulin,
##        data = diabetes)
##
## Prior probabilities of groups:
##        1         2         3
## 0.2222222 0.2500000 0.5277778
##
## Group means:
##       relwt   glufast   glutest    steady   insulin
## 1 0.9915625 213.65625 1027.3750 108.8438 320.9375
## 2 1.0558333  99.30556  493.9444 288.0000 208.9722
## 3 0.9372368  91.18421  349.9737 172.6447 114.0000
##
## Coefficients of linear discriminants:
##                     LD1            LD2
## relwt   -1.339546e+00 -3.7950612048
## glufast  3.301944e-02  0.0373202882
## glutest -1.263978e-02 -0.0068947755
## steady   1.240248e-05 -0.0059924778
## insulin -3.895587e-03  0.0005754322
##
## Proportion of trace:
##    LD1    LD2
## 0.8784 0.1216
ghat5 = predict(diabetes_lda5)$class
table(ghat5, diabetes$group)
##
## ghat5  1  2  3
##     1 26  0  0
##     2  5 31  3
##     3  1  5 73
mean(ghat5 != diabetes$group)
## [1] 0.09722222
```

▶ **Question 12.7** Instead of approximating the prediction regions by classification from a grid of points, compute the separating lines explicitly from the linear determinant coefficients.   ◀

▶ **Solution 12.7** See Section 4.3, Equation (4.10) in Hastie et al. (2008).   □

12.3.2   Predicting embryonic cell state from gene expression

[4] Later in this chapter we will see methods that can drop this assumption and screen all available features.

Assume we already know that the four genes *FN1*, *TIMD2*, *GATA4* and *SOX7* are relevant to the classification task.[4] We want to build a classifier that predicts the developmental time (embryonic days: E3.25, E3.5, E4.5). We load the data and select four corresponding probes.

```
library("Hiiragi2013")
data("x")
probes = c("1426642_at", "1418765_at", "1418864_at", "1416564_at")
embryoCells = t(exprs(x)[probes, ]) %>% as_tibble %>%
  mutate(Embryonic.day = x$Embryonic.day) %>%
  filter(x$genotype == "WT")
```

We can use the Bioconductor annotation package associated with the microarray to verify that the probes correspond to the intended genes.

```
annotation(x)
## [1] "mouse4302"
library("mouse4302.db")
anno = AnnotationDbi::select(mouse4302.db, keys = probes,
         columns = c("SYMBOL", "GENENAME"))
anno
##        PROBEID SYMBOL
## 1 1426642_at     Fn1
## 2 1418765_at   Timd2
## 3 1418864_at   Gata4
## 4 1416564_at    Sox7
##                                                   GENENAME
## 1                                              fibronectin 1
## 2 T cell immunoglobulin and mucin domain containing 2
## 3                                    GATA binding protein 4
## 4                        SRY (sex determining region Y)-box 7
mt = match(anno$PROBEID, colnames(embryoCells))
colnames(embryoCells)[mt] = anno$SYMBOL
```

Now we are ready to visualize the data in a pairs plot (Figure 12.8).

```
library("GGally")
ggpairs(embryoCells, mapping = aes(col = Embryonic.day),
  columns = anno$SYMBOL, upper = list(continuous = "points"))
```

We can now call `lda` on these data. The linear combinations `LD1` and `LD2` that serve as discriminating variables are given in the slot `ed_lda$scaling` of the output from `lda`.

```
ec_lda = lda(Embryonic.day ~ Fn1 + Timd2 + Gata4 + Sox7,
          data = embryoCells)
round(ec_lda$scaling, 1)
##         LD1  LD2
## Fn1    -0.2 -0.4
## Timd2   0.5  0.0
## Gata4  -0.1 -0.6
## Sox7   -0.7  0.5
```

For the visualization of the learned model in Figure 12.9, we need to build the

Figure 12.8: Expression values of the discriminating genes, with the prediction target `Embryonic.day` shown by color.

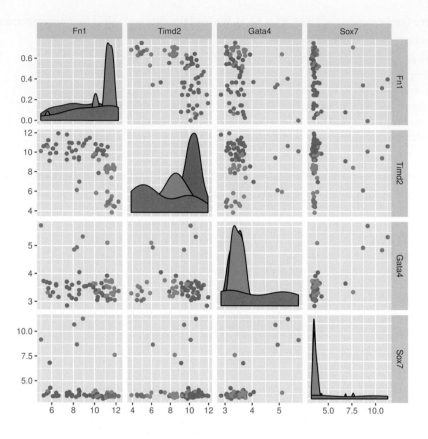

prediction regions and their boundaries by expanding the grid in the space of the two new coordinates, LD1 and LD2.

```
ec_rot = predict(ec_lda)$x %>% as_tibble %>%
            mutate(ed = embryoCells$Embryonic.day)
ec_lda2 = lda(ec_rot[, 1:2], predict(ec_lda)$class)
ec_grid = with(ec_rot, expand.grid(
  LD1 = make1Dgrid(LD1),
  LD2 = make1Dgrid(LD2)))
ec_grid$edhat = predict(ec_lda2, newdata = ec_grid)$class
ggplot() +
  geom_point(aes(x = LD1, y = LD2, colour = ed), data = ec_rot) +
  geom_raster(aes(x = LD1, y = LD2, fill = edhat),
            data = ec_grid, alpha = 0.4, interpolate = TRUE) +
  scale_x_continuous(expand = c(0, 0)) +
  scale_y_continuous(expand = c(0, 0)) +
  coord_fixed()
```

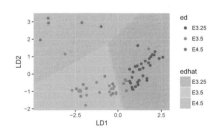

Figure 12.9: LDA classification regions for `Embryonic.day`.

▶ **Question 12.8** Repeat these analyses using *quadratic discriminant analysis* (qda). What difference do you see in the shape of the boundaries?   ◀

▶ **Solution 12.8**   See code below and Figure 12.10.

```
library("gridExtra")
```

```
ec_qda = qda(Embryonic.day ~ Fn1 + Timd2 + Gata4 + Sox7,
             data = embryoCells)

variables = colnames(ec_qda$means)
pairs = combn(variables, 2)
lapply(seq_len(ncol(pairs)), function(i) {
  grid = with(embryoCells,
    expand.grid(x = make1Dgrid(get(pairs[1, i])),
                y = make1Dgrid(get(pairs[2, i])))) %>%
    `colnames<-`(pairs[, i])

  for (v in setdiff(variables, pairs[, i]))
    grid[[v]] = median(embryoCells[[v]])

  grid$edhat = predict(ec_qda, newdata = grid)$class

  ggplot() + geom_point(
     aes_string(x = pairs[1, i], y = pairs[2, i],
     colour = "Embryonic.day"), data = embryoCells) +
  geom_raster(
     aes_string(x = pairs[1, i], y = pairs[2, i], fill = "edhat"),
     data = grid, alpha = 0.4, interpolate = TRUE) +
  scale_x_continuous(expand = c(0, 0)) +
  scale_y_continuous(expand = c(0, 0)) +
  coord_fixed() +
  if (i != ncol(pairs)) theme(legend.position = "none")
}) %>% grid.arrange(grobs = ., ncol = 2)                        □
```

▶ Question **12.9** What happens if you call `lda` or `qda` with a lot more genes, say the first 1000, in the Hiiragi dataset?   ◀

▶ Solution **12.9**

```
lda(t(exprs(x))[, 1:1000], x$Embryonic.day)

## Warning in lda.default(x, grouping, ...): variables are collinear

qda(t(exprs(x))[, 1:1000], x$Embryonic.day)

## Error in qda.default(x, grouping, ...): some group is too small for
'qda'
```

The `lda` function manages to fit a model, but complains (with the warning) about the fact that there are more variables than replicates, which means that the variables are not linearly independent, and thus are redundant with each other. The `qda` function aborts with an error, since the QDA model with so many parameters cannot be fitted from the available data.   □

12.4   Machine learning versus rote learning

Computers are really good at memorizing facts. In the worst case, a machine learning algorithm is a roundabout way of doing this.[5] The central goal in statistical learning,

[5] The not-so-roundabout way is using database technologies.

Figure 12.10: QDA for the mouse cell data. Shown are all pairwise plots of the four features; in each plot, the other two features are set to the median.

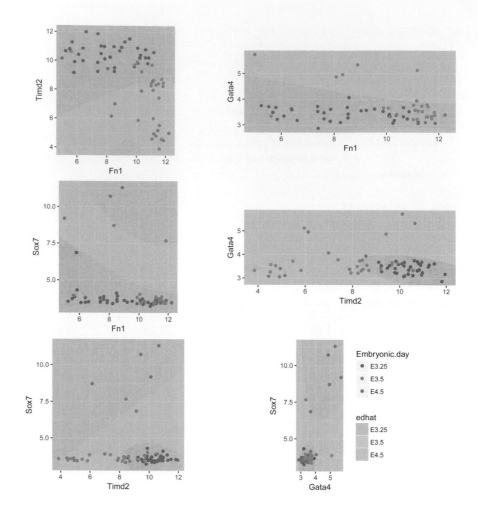

however, is **generalizability**. We want an algorithm that is able to generalize, i.e., interpolate and extrapolate from given data to make good predictions about future data.

Let's look at the following example. We generate random data (`rnorm`) for n objects, with different numbers of features (given by `p`). We train an LDA on these data and compute the **misclassification rate**, i.e., the fraction of times the prediction is wrong (`pred != resp`).

```
library("dplyr")
p = 2:21
n = 20

mcl = lapply(p, function(pp) {
  replicate(100, {
    xmat = matrix(rnorm(n * pp), nrow = n)
    resp = sample(c("apple", "orange"), n, replace = TRUE)
    fit  = lda(xmat, resp)
    pred = predict(fit)$class
    mean(pred != resp)
  }) %>% mean %>% tibble(mcl = ., p = pp)
}) %>% bind_rows
```

```
ggplot(mcl, aes(x = p, y = mcl)) + geom_line() + geom_point() +
    ylab("Misclassification rate")
```

▶ Question **12.10** What is the purpose of the `replicate` loop in the above code? What happens if you omit it (or replace the 100 with 1)?   ◀

▶ Solution **12.10** For each single replicate, the curve is a noisier version of Figure 12.11. Averaging the measured misclassifications rate over 100 replicates makes the estimate more stable. We can do this since we are working with simulated data.   □

Figure 12.11 seems to imply that we can perfectly predict random labels from random data, if we only fit a complex enough model, i.e., one with many parameters. What is wrong about this absurd conclusion? The problem with the above code is that the model performance is evaluated on the same data on which it was trained. The model looks good, but it is not predicting; it is essentially memorizing and regurgitating. How can we overcome this problem? The key idea is to assess model performance on *different* data from those on which the model was trained.

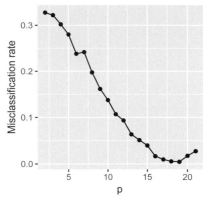

Figure 12.11: Misclassification rate of LDA applied to random data. While the number of observations n is held constant (at 20), we are increasing the number of features p starting from 2 up to 21. The misclassification rate becomes almost zero as p approaches 20. The LDA model becomes so elaborate and overparameterized that it manages to learn the random labels "by heart". (As p becomes even larger, the "performance" degrades again somewhat, apparently due to numerical properties of the lda implementation used here.)

12.4.1 Cross-validation

A naive approach would be to split the data into two halves, and use the first half for learning ("training") and the second half for assessment ("testing"). It turns out that this is needlessly variable and needlessly inefficient. It is needlessly variable because, by splitting the data only once, our results can be quite affected by where the split happens to fall. It seems better to do the splitting many times and average. Averaging will give us more stable results. It is needlessly inefficient because the performance of machine learning algorithms depends on the number of observations, and performance measured on half the data is likely to be worse than performance with all the data.[6] For this reason, it is better to use unequal sizes of training and test datasets. In the extreme case, we'll use as many as $n - 1$ observations for training, and the remaining one for testing. After we've done this likewise for all observations, we can average our performance metric. This procedure is called **leave-one-out cross-validation**. An alternative is k-**fold cross-validation**, where the samples are repeatedly split into a training set of size around $n(k - 1)/k$ and a test set of size around n/k.

Both methods of splitting have pros and cons, and there is not a universally best choice. An advantage of leave-one-out is that the amount of data used for training is close to the maximally available data; this is especially important if the sample size is limiting and "every little bit matters" for the algorithm. A drawback of leave-one-out is that the training sets are all very similar, so they may not model sufficiently well the kind of sampling changes to be expected when a new dataset comes along. For large n, leave-one-out cross-validation can be needlessly time-consuming.[7]

[6] Unless we have such an excess of data that it doesn't matter.

[7] See the chapter "Model Assessment and Selection" in the book by Hastie et al. (2008) for further discussion of these trade-offs.

```
estimate_mcl_loocv = function(x, resp) {
  vapply(seq_len(nrow(x)), function(i) {
    fit  = lda(x[-i, ], resp[-i])
    ptrn = predict(fit, newdata = x[-i,, drop = FALSE])$class
    ptst = predict(fit, newdata = x[ i,, drop = FALSE])$class
    c(train = mean(ptrn != resp[-i]), test = (ptst != resp[i]))
  }, FUN.VALUE = numeric(2)) %>% rowMeans %>% t %>% as_tibble
}

xmat = matrix(rnorm(n * last(p)), nrow = n)
resp = sample(c("apple", "orange"), n, replace = TRUE)

mcl = lapply(p, function(k) {
  estimate_mcl_loocv(xmat[, 1:k], resp)
}) %>% bind_rows %>% data.frame(p) %>% melt(id.var = "p")

ggplot(mcl, aes(x = p, y = value, col = variable)) + geom_line() +
  geom_point() + ylab("Misclassification rate")
```

The result is shown in Figure 12.12.

▶ **Question 12.11** Why are the curves in Figure 12.12 more variable ("wiggly") than in Figure 12.11? How can you overcome this? ◀

▶ **Solution 12.11** Only one dataset (`xmat`, `resp`) was used to calculate Figure 12.12, whereas for Figure 12.11 the data were generated within a `replicate` loop. You could similarly extend the above code to average the misclassification rate curves over many replicate simulated datasets. □

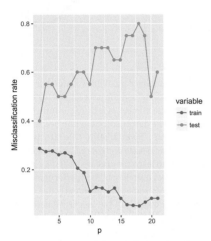

Figure 12.12: Cross-validation: the misclassification rate of LDA applied to random data, when evaluated on test data that were not used for training, hovers around 0.5, independent of `p`. The misclassification rate on the training data is also shown. It behaves similarly to what we saw in Figure 12.11.

12.4.2   The curse of dimensionality

In Section 12.4.1 we saw overfitting and cross-validation on random data, but how does it look if there is in fact a relevant class separation?

```
p   = 2:20
mcl = replicate(100, {
  xmat = matrix(rnorm(n * last(p)), nrow = n)
  resp = sample(c("apple", "orange"), n, replace = TRUE)
  xmat[, 1:6] = xmat[, 1:6] + as.integer(factor(resp))

  lapply(p, function(k) {
    estimate_mcl_loocv(xmat[, 1:k], resp)
  }) %>% bind_rows %>% cbind(p = p) %>% melt(id.var = "p")
}, simplify = FALSE) %>% bind_rows

mcl =  group_by(mcl, p, variable) %>%
  summarise(value = mean(value))

ggplot(mcl, aes(x = p, y = value, col = variable)) + geom_line() +
  geom_point() + ylab("Misclassification rate")
```

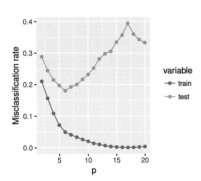

Figure 12.13: As we increase the number of features included in the model, the misclassification rate initially improves; as we start including more and more irrelevant features, it increases again, as we are fitting noise.

The result is shown in Figure 12.13. The group centers are the vectors (in $\mathbb{R}^{20}$) given by the coordinates $(1, 1, 1, 1, 1, 1, 0, 0, 0, \dots)$ (apples) and $(2, 2, 2, 2, 2, 2, 0, 0, 0, \dots)$

(oranges), and the optimal decision boundary is the hyperplane orthogonal to the line between them. For p smaller than 6, the decision rule cannot reach this hyperplane – it is biased. As a result, the misclassification rate is suboptimal, and it decreases with p. But what happens for p larger than 6? The algorithm is, in principle, able to model the optimal hyperplane, and it should not be distracted by the additional features. The problem is that it *is* distracted. The more additional features that enter the dataset, the higher the probability that one or more of them happen to fall in a way that they *look like* good discriminating features in the training data – only to mislead the classifier and degrade its performance on the test data. Shortly we'll see how to use penalization to (try to) control this problem.

The term **curse of dimensionality** was coined by Bellman (1961). It refers to the fact that high-dimensional spaces are very hard, if not impossible, to sample thoroughly: for instance, to cover a 2D square of side length 1 with grid points that are 0.1 apart, we need $10^2 = 100$ points. In 100 dimensions, we need 10^{100} – which is already more than the number of protons in the universe.[8] In genomics, we often aim to fit models to data with thousands of features. Also, our intuitions about distances between points or about the relationship between a volume and its surface break down in high-dimensional settings. We'll explore some of the weirdness of high-dimensional spaces in the next few questions.

▶ Question **12.12** Assume you have a dataset with 1 million data points in p dimensions. The data are uniformly distributed in the unit hypercube (i.e., all features lie in the interval $[0, 1]$). What's the side length of a hypercube that can be expected to contain just 10 of the points, as a function of p? ◀

▶ Solution **12.12** See Figure 12.15.

```
sideLength = function(p, pointDensity = 1e6, pointsNeeded = 10)
   (pointsNeeded / pointDensity) ^ (1 / p)
ggplot(tibble(p = 1:400, sideLength = sideLength(p)),
      aes(x = p, y = sideLength)) + geom_line(col = "red") +
  geom_hline(aes(yintercept = 1), linetype = 2)
```
□

Next, let's look at the relation between inner regions of the feature space versus its boundary regions. Generally speaking, prediction at the boundaries of a feature space is more difficult than in its interior, as it tends to involve extrapolation rather than interpolation. In the next question you'll see how this difficulty explodes with feature space dimension.

▶ Question **12.13** What fraction of a unit cube's total volume is closer than 0.01 to any of its surfaces, as a function of the dimension? ◀

▶ Solution **12.13** See code below and Figure 12.16.

```
tibble(
  p = 1:400,
  volOuterCube = 1 ^ p,
  volInnerCube = 0.98 ^ p,    # 0.98 = 1 - 2 * 0.01
  `V(shell)` = volOuterCube - volInnerCube) %>%
ggplot(aes(x = p, y = `V(shell)`)) + geom_line(col = "blue")
```
□

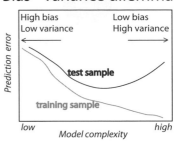

Bias - variance dilemma

Figure 12.14: Idealized version of Figure 12.13, from Hastie et al. (2008). A recurrent goal in machine learning is finding the sweet spot in the variance–bias trade-off.

[8] See *Eddington number* on Wikipedia.

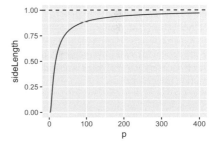

Figure 12.15: Side length of a p-dimensional hypercube expected to contain 10 out of 1 million uniformly distributed data points, as a function of p. While for $p = 1$ this length is conveniently small, namely $10/10^6 = 10^{-5}$, for larger p it approaches 1, i.e., becomes the same as the range of each the features. This means that a "local neighborhood" of 10 points encompasses almost the same data range as the whole dataset.

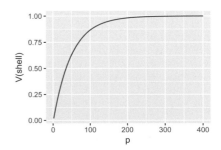

Figure 12.16: Fraction of a unit cube's total volume that is in its "shell" (here operationalized as those points that are closer than 0.01 to its surface) as a function of the dimension p.

Solution by simulation

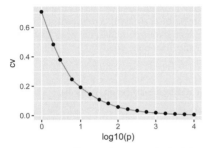

Figure 12.17: Coefficient of variation (CV) of the distance between randomly picked points in the unit hypercube as a function of the dimension. As the dimension increases, everyone is equally far away from everyone else: there is now almost no variation in the distances.

▶ **Question 12.14** What is the coefficient of variation (ratio of standard deviation over average) of the distance between two randomly picked points in the unit hypercube, as a function of the dimension? ◀

▶ **Solution 12.14** We solve this one by simulation. We generate n pairs of random points in the hypercube (x1, x2) and compute their Euclidean distances. See Figure 12.17. This result can also be predicted from the central limit theorem.

```
n = 1000
df = tibble(
  p = round(10 ^ seq(0, 4, by = 0.25)),
  cv = vapply(p, function(k) {
    x1 = matrix(runif(k * n), nrow = n)
    x2 = matrix(runif(k * n), nrow = n)
    d = sqrt(rowSums((x1 - x2)^2))
    sd(d) / mean(d)
  }, FUN.VALUE = numeric(1)))
ggplot(df, aes(x = log10(p), y = cv)) + geom_line(col = "orange") +
  geom_point()                                                    □
```

12.5   Objective functions

We've already seen the **misclassification rate** (MCR) used to assess our classification performance in Figures 12.11–12.13. Its population version is defined as

$$MCR = E\left[\mathbb{1}(\hat{y} \neq y)\right],\tag{12.1}$$

and for a finite sample

$$\widehat{MCR} = \frac{1}{n}\sum_{i=1}^{n}\mathbb{1}(\hat{y}_i \neq y_i).\tag{12.2}$$

This is not the only choice we could have made. Perhaps we care more about the misclassification of apples as oranges than vice versa; we can reflect this by introducing weights that depend on the type of error made into the sum of Equation (12.2) (or the integral of Equation (12.1)). This can get even more elaborate if we have more than two classes. Often we want to see the whole **confusion table**, which we can obtain as follows.

```
table(truth, response)
```

An important special case is binary classification with asymmetric costs – think about, say, a medical test. Here, the **sensitivity** (aka **true positive rate** or **recall**) is related to the misclassification of healthy as ill, and the **specificity** (or **true negative rate**) depends on the probability of misclassification of ill as healthy. Often, there is a single parameter (e.g., a threshold) that can be moved up and down, allowing a trade-off between sensitivity and specificity (and thus, equivalently, between the two types of misclassification). In those cases, we usually are not content to know the classifier performance at one single choice of threshold, but want to know it at many (or all) of them. This information is encapsulated in **receiver operating characteristic** (**ROC**) or **precision-recall curves**.

▶ Question **12.15** What are the exact relationships between the per-class misclassification rates and sensitivity and specificity? ◀

▶ Solution **12.15** The sensitivity or true positive rate is

$$\text{TPR} = \frac{\text{TP}}{\text{P}},$$

where TP is the number of true positives and P the number of all positives. The specificity or true negative rate is

$$\text{SPC} = \frac{\text{TN}}{\text{N}},$$

where TN is the number of true negatives and N the number of all negatives. See also the Wikipedia article on *sensitivity and specificity*. □

Another cost function can be computed from the **Jaccard index**, which we saw in Chapter 5:

$$J(A, B) = \frac{|A \cap B|}{|A \cup B|}, \tag{12.3}$$

where A is the set of observations for which the true class is 1 ($A = \{i \mid y_i = 1\}$) and B is the set of observations for which the predicted class is 1. The number J is between 0 and 1, and when J is large, it indicates high overlap of the two sets. Note that J does not depend on the number of observations for which both true and predicted classes are 0, so it is particularly suitable for measuring the performance of methods that try to find *rare events*.

We can also consider probabilistic class predictions, which come in the form $\hat{P}(Y \mid X)$. In this case, a possible risk function would be obtained by looking at distances between the true and estimated probability distributions. For two classes, the finite sample version of the log loss is

$$\text{log loss} = -\frac{1}{n} \sum_{i=1}^{n} y_i \log(\hat{p}_i) + (1 - y_i) \log(1 - \hat{p}_i), \tag{12.4}$$

The log loss will be infinite if a prediction is totally confident ($\hat{p}_i$ is exactly 0 or 1) but wrong.

where $\hat{p}_i \in [0, 1]$ is the prediction, and $y_i \in \{0, 1\}$ is the truth.

For continuous response variables (regression), a natural choice is the **mean squared error (MSE)**. It is the average squared error

$$\widehat{\text{MSE}} = \frac{1}{n} \sum_{i=1}^{n} (\hat{Y}_i - Y_i)^2. \tag{12.5}$$

The population version is defined analogously, by turning the summation into an integral as in Equations (12.1) and (12.2).

Statisticians have various names, such as **risk function**, **cost function** and **objective function**, for functions like Equations (12.1)–(12.5), depending on context and predisposition.[9]

[9] There is even an R package dedicated to evaluation of statistical learners, called *metrics*.

12.6   Variance–bias trade-off

An important fact that helps us to understand the trade-offs in picking a statistical learning model is that the MSE is the sum of two terms, and the choices we can make are often such that one of those terms goes down while the other goes up. The **bias** measures how far the average of all the different estimates is from the truth. **Variance** measures how much individual estimates might be scattered from the average value (Figure 12.18). In applications, we often get only one shot; therefore being reliably almost on target can beat being right over the long-term average but really off today. The decomposition

$$\text{MSE} = \underbrace{\text{var}(\hat{Y})}_{\text{variance}} + \underbrace{E[\hat{Y} - Y]^2}_{\text{bias}} \tag{12.6}$$

follows by straightforward algebra.

When trying to minimize the MSE, it is important to realize that sometimes we can choose to pay the price of a small bias to greatly reduce variance, and thus overall improve MSE. We encountered shrinkage estimation in Chapter 8. In classification (i.e., when we have categorical response variables), different objective functions than the MSE are used, and there is usually no such straightforward decomposition, as in Equation (12.6). The good news is that we can usually go even further than in the case of continuous responses with our tactic of trading bias for variance. This is because the discreteness of the response absorbs certain biases (Friedman, 1997), so that the cost of higher bias is almost zero, while we still get the benefit of better (smaller) variance.

12.6.1   Penalization

In high-dimensional statistics, we are constantly plagued by variance: there is just not enough data to fit all the possible parameters. One of the most fruitful ideas in high-dimensional statistics is **penalization**, a tool to actively control and exploit the variance–bias trade-off. Penalization is part of a larger class of **regularization** methods that are used to ensure stable estimates.

Although generalization of LDA to high-dimensional settings is possible (Clemmensen et al., 2011; Witten and Tibshirani, 2011), it turns out that logistic regression is a more general approach,[10] and therefore we will now switch to that, using the *glmnet* package.

Multinomial – or, for the special case of two classes, binomial – **logistic regression** models the posterior log-odds between k classes and can be written in the form[11]

$$\log \frac{P(Y = i \mid X = x)}{P(Y = k \mid X = x)} = \beta_i^0 + \beta_i x, \tag{12.7}$$

where the index $i = 1, \ldots, k - 1$ counts over the different classes. The data matrix x has dimensions $n \times p$, where n is the number of observations and p the number of features. The p-dimensional vector β_i determines how the classification odds for class i versus

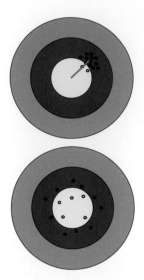

Figure 12.18: In the upper bull's-eye, the estimates are systematically off-target, but in a reproducible manner. The green segment represents the bias. In the lower bull's-eye, the estimates are not biased, as they are centered in the correct place; however, they have high variance. We can distinguish the two scenarios since we see the results from many shots. If we have only one shot and miss the bull's-eye, we cannot easily know whether that's because of bias or variance.

[10] It fits into the framework of *generalized linear models*, which we encounted in Chapter 8.

[11] See Hastie et al. (2008) for a complete presentation.

class k depend on x. The numbers β_i^0 are intercepts and depend on, among other things, the prior probabilities of the classes. Instead of the log odds (12.7), i.e., ratios of class probabilities, we can also write down an equivalent model for the class probabilities themselves, and the fact that we here used the kth class as a reference is an arbitrary choice, as the model estimates are equivariant under this choice (Hastie et al., 2008). The model is fit by maximizing the log-likelihood $\ell(\beta, \beta^0; x)$, where $\beta = (\beta_1, \dots, \beta_{k-1})$ and analogously for β^0.

Equivariant here means the estimates result in an equivalent model.

So far, so good. But as p gets larger, there is an increasing chance that some of the estimates go wildly off the mark, due to random sampling happenstances in the data (remember Figure 12.1!). This is true even if, for each individual coordinate of the vector β_i, the error distribution is bounded: the probability of there being one coordinate in the far tails increases the more coordinates there are, i.e., the larger p is.

A related problem can also occur, not in (12.7), but in other, nonlinear models, as the model dimension p increases while the sample size n remains the same: the likelihood landscape around its maximum becomes increasingly flat, and the maximum likelihood estimate of the model parameters becomes more and more variable. Eventually, the maximum is no longer a point, but something higher dimensional (a submanifold), and the maximum likelihood estimate is unidentifiable.

Both of these limitations can be overcome with a modification of the objective; instead of maximizing the bare log-likelihood, we maximize a penalized version of it:

$$\hat{\beta} = \arg\max_{\beta} \ell(\beta, \beta^0; x) + \lambda\, \text{pen}(\beta), \tag{12.8}$$

where $\lambda \geqslant 0$ is a real number, and pen is a convex function, called the **penalty function**. Popular choices are $\text{pen}(\beta) = |\beta|^2$ (**ridge regression**) and $\text{pen}(\beta) = |\beta|^1$ (**lasso**). In the **elastic net**, ridge and lasso are hybridized by using the penalty function $\text{pen}(\beta) = (1-\alpha)|\beta|^1 + \alpha|\beta|^2$ with some further parameter $\alpha \in [0, 1]$. The crux, of course, is how to choose the right λ, and we will discuss that in the following example.

Here, $|\beta|^v = \sum_i \beta_i^v$ is the L_v-norm of the vector β. Variations are possible. We could instead include in this summation only some but not all of the elements of β, or we could scale different elements differently, for instance based on some prior belief about their scale and importance.

12.6.2   Example: predicting colon cancer from stool microbiome composition

Zeller et al. (2014) studied metagenome sequencing data from fecal samples of 156 humans that included colorectal cancer patients and tumor-free controls. Their aim was to see whether they could identify biomarkers (presence or abundance of certain taxa) that could help with early tumor detection. The data are available from *Bioconductor* through its **ExperimentHub** service under the identifier EH361.

```
library("ExperimentHub")
eh = ExperimentHub()
zeller = eh[["EH361"]]
```

```
table(zeller$disease)
```

```
##
##       cancer large_adenoma          n small_adenoma
##           53            15         61            27
```

▶ **Question 12.16** Explore the `eh` object to see what other datasets there are.   ◀

▶ **Solution 12.16** Type `eh` into the R prompt and study the output.   □

For the following analysis, let's focus on the normal and cancer observations and set the adenomas aside.

```
zellerNC = zeller[, zeller$disease %in% c("n", "cancer")]
```

Before jumping into model fitting, it is, as always, a good idea to explore the data. First, let's look at the sample annotations. The following code prints the data from three randomly picked observations. (Looking only at the first ones, say with the R function `head`, is also an option, but they may not be representative of the whole dataset.)

```
pData(zellerNC)[ sample(ncol(zellerNC), 3), ]
##                      subjectID age gender bmi country disease
## CCIS07277498ST-4-0      FR-276  63   male  NA  france       n
## CCIS12656533ST-4-0      FR-654  51   male  30  france  cancer
## CCIS94417875ST-3-0      FR-110  59 female  25  france       n
##                      tnm_stage ajcc_stage localization    fobt
## CCIS07277498ST-4-0        <NA>       <NA>        <NA>    <NA>
## CCIS12656533ST-4-0       t2n1m1         iv      rectum negative
## CCIS94417875ST-3-0        <NA>       <NA>        <NA> negative
##                      wif-1_gene_methylation_test   group bodysite
## CCIS07277498ST-4-0                      negative control    stool
## CCIS12656533ST-4-0                      negative     crc    stool
## CCIS94417875ST-3-0                      negative control    stool
##                      ethnicity number_reads
## CCIS07277498ST-4-0       white     66936604
## CCIS12656533ST-4-0       white     45546920
## CCIS94417875ST-3-0       white     44052987
```

Next, let's explore the feature names.

We define the helper function `formatfn` to line-wrap these long character strings for the available space here.

```
formatfn = function(x)
  gsub("|", "| ", x, fixed = TRUE) %>% lapply(strwrap)

rownames(zellerNC)[1:4]
## [1] "k__Bacteria"
## [2] "k__Viruses"
## [3] "k__Bacteria|p__Firmicutes"
## [4] "k__Bacteria|p__Bacteroidetes"
rownames(zellerNC)[nrow(zellerNC) + (-2:0)] %>% formatfn
## [[1]]
## [1] "k__Bacteria| p__Proteobacteria| c__Deltaproteobacteria|"
## [2] "o__Desulfovibrionales| f__Desulfovibrionaceae|"
## [3] "g__Desulfovibrio| s__Desulfovibrio_termitidis"
##
## [[2]]
## [1] "k__Viruses| p__Viruses_noname| c__Viruses_noname|"
## [2] "o__Viruses_noname| f__Baculoviridae|"
## [3] "g__Alphabaculovirus|"
## [4] "s__Bombyx_mori_nucleopolyhedrovirus|"
```

```
## [5] "t__Bombyx_mori_nucleopolyhedrovirus_unclassified"
##
## [[3]]
## [1] "k__Bacteria| p__Proteobacteria| c__Deltaproteobacteria|"
## [2] "o__Desulfovibrionales| f__Desulfovibrionaceae|"
## [3] "g__Desulfovibrio| s__Desulfovibrio_termitidis|"
## [4] "t__GCF_000504305"
```

As you can see, the features are a mixture of abundance quantifications at different taxonomic levels, from **k**ingdom over **p**hylum to **s**pecies. We could select only some of these, but here we continue with all of them. Next, let's look at the distribution of some of the features. Here, we show an arbitrary choice of two, numbered 510 and 527; in practice, it is helpful to scroll through many such plots quickly to get an impression (Figure 12.19).

```
ggplot(melt(exprs(zellerNC)[c(510, 527), ]), aes(x = value)) +
    geom_histogram(bins = 25) +
    facet_wrap( ~ Var1, ncol = 1, scales = "free")
```

In the simplest case, we fit model (12.7) as follows.

```
library("glmnet")
glmfit = glmnet(x = t(exprs(zellerNC)),
                y = factor(zellerNC$disease),
                family = "binomial")
```

A remarkable feature of the `glmnet` function is that it fits (12.7) not only for one choice of λ, but for all possible λs at once. For now, let's look at the prediction performance for, say, $\lambda = 0.04$. The name of the function parameter is `s`.

```
predTrsf = predict(glmfit, newx = t(exprs(zellerNC)),
                   type = "class", s = 0.04)
table(predTrsf, zellerNC$disease)

##
## predTrsf cancer  n
##    cancer    51   0
##    n          2  61
```

Not bad – but remember that this is on the training data, without cross-validation. Let's have a closer look at `glmfit`. The *glmnet* package offers a **diagnostic plot** that is worth looking at (see Figure 12.20).

```
plot(glmfit, col = brewer.pal(12, "Set3"), lwd = sqrt(3))
```

▶ **Question 12.17** What is the *x*-axis in Figure 12.20? What are the different lines? ◀

▶ **Solution 12.17** Consult the manual page of the function `plot.glmnet` in the *glmnet* package. □

Let's get back to the question of how to choose the parameter λ. We could try many different choices – indeed, all possible choices – of λ, assess classification performance in each case using cross-validation, and then choose the best λ. We could do so by writing a loop, as we did in the `estimate_mcl_loocv` function in Section 12.4.1. It turns out

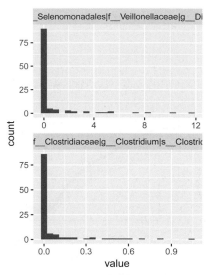

Figure 12.19: Histograms of the distributions for two randomly selected features. The distributions are highly skewed, with many zero values and a thin, long tail of non-zero values.

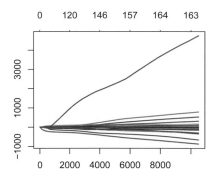

Figure 12.20: Regularization paths for `glmfit`.

You'll already realize from the description of this strategy that if we optimize λ in this way, the resulting apparent classification performance will likely be exaggerated. We need a truly independent dataset, or at least another, outer cross-validation loop to get a more realistic impression of the generalizability. We will get back to this question at the end of the chapter.

that the *glmnet* package already has built-in functionality for that with the function `cv.glmnet`, which we can use instead.

```
cvglmfit = cv.glmnet(x = t(exprs(zellerNC)),
                     y = factor(zellerNC$disease),
                     family = "binomial")
plot(cvglmfit)
```

The diagnostic plot is shown in Figure 12.21. We can access the optimal value.

```
cvglmfit$lambda.min
## [1] 0.06680157
```

As this value of λ results from finding a minimum in an estimated curve, it turns out that it is often too small, i.e., that the implied penalization is too weak. A heuristic recommended by the authors of the *glmnet* package is to use a somewhat larger value instead, namely the largest value of λ such that the performance measure is within one standard error of the minimum.

```
cvglmfit$lambda.1se
## [1] 0.1114317
```

► Question **12.18** What does the confusion table look like for λ = `lambda.1se`? ◄

► **Solution 12.18**

```
s0 = cvglmfit$lambda.1se
predict(glmfit, newx = t(exprs(zellerNC)),type = "class", s = s0) %>%
    table(zellerNC$disease)

##
## .         cancer   n
##   cancer      32   8
##   n           21  53
```

► Question **12.19** What features drive the classification? ◄

► **Solution 12.19**

```
coefs = coef(glmfit)[, which.min(abs(glmfit$lambda - s0))]
topthree = order(abs(coefs), decreasing = TRUE)[1:3]
as.vector(coefs[topthree])
## [1] -2.8132116 -0.7858018 -0.2364431
formatfn(names(coefs)[topthree])
## [[1]]
## [1] "k__Bacteria| p__Candidatus_Saccharibacteria|"
## [2] "c__Candidatus_Saccharibacteria_noname|"
## [3] "o__Candidatus_Saccharibacteria_noname|"
## [4] "f__Candidatus_Saccharibacteria_noname|"
## [5] "g__Candidatus_Saccharibacteria_noname|"
## [6] "s__candidate_division_TM7_single_cell_isolate_TM7b"
##
## [[2]]
## [1] "k__Bacteria| p__Firmicutes| c__Clostridia|"
## [2] "o__Clostridiales| f__Lachnospiraceae|"
```

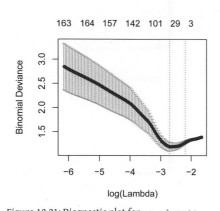

Figure 12.21: Diagnostic plot for `cv.glmnet`: shown is a measure, the deviance, as a function of λ, of cross-validated prediction performance. The dashed vertical lines show `lambda.min` and `lambda.1se`.

```
## [3] "g__Lachnospiraceae_noname|"
## [4] "s__Lachnospiraceae_bacterium_7_1_58FAA"
##
## [[3]]
## [1] "k__Bacteria| p__Firmicutes| c__Clostridia|"
## [2] "o__Clostridiales| f__Clostridiaceae| g__Clostridium|"
## [3] "s__Clostridium_symbiosum"                                          □
```

▶ Question 12.20 How do the results change if we transform the data, say, with the `asinh` transformation that we saw in Chapter 5?   ◀

▶ Solution 12.20 See Figure 12.22.

```
cv.glmnet(x = t(asinh(exprs(zellerNC))),
          y = factor(zellerNC$disease),
          family = "binomial") %>% plot                                    □
```

▶ Question 12.21 Would a good classification performance on these data mean that this assay is ready for screening and early cancer detection?   ◀

▶ Solution 12.21 No. The performance here is measured on a sample in which the cases have similar prevalence to the controls. This serves well enough to explore the biology. However, in a real-life application, the cases will be much less frequent. To be practically useful, the assay must have much higher specificity, i.e., it must rarely diagnose disease where there is none. To establish specificity, a much larger dataset with many more normal controls needs to be tested.   □

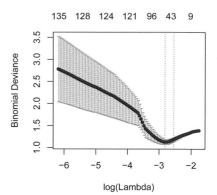

Figure 12.22: As Figure 12.21, but using an asinh transformation of the data.

12.6.3   Example: classifying mouse cells from their expression profiles

Figures 12.21 and 12.22 are textbook examples of how we expect the dependence of (cross-validated) classification *performance* versus *model complexity* (λ) to look. Now let's get back to the mouse embryo cell data. We'll try to classify the cells from embryonic day `E3.25` with respect to their genotype.

```
sx = x[, x$Embryonic.day == "E3.25"]
embryoCellsClassifier = cv.glmnet(t(exprs(sx)), sx$genotype,
               family = "binomial", type.measure = "class")
plot(embryoCellsClassifier)
```

In Figure 12.23 we see that the misclassification error is (essentially) monotonically increasing with λ, and gets smaller as $\lambda \to 0$, i.e., if we apply no penalization at all.

▶ Question 12.22 What is going on with these data?   ◀

▶ Solution 12.22 It looks as though inclusion of more, and even all, features does not harm the classification performance. In a way, these data are "too easy". Let's do a t-test for all features.

```
mouse_de = rowttests(sx, "genotype")
ggplot(mouse_de, aes(x = p.value)) +
  geom_histogram(boundary = 0, breaks = seq(0, 1, by = 0.01))
```

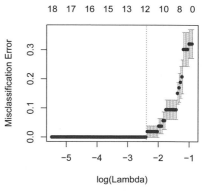

Figure 12.23: Cross-validated misclassification error versus penalty parameter for the mouse cell data.

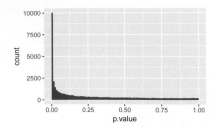

Figure 12.24: Histogram of p-values for the per-feature *t*-tests between genotypes in the E3.25 data.

The result, shown in Figure 12.24, reveals that a large number of genes are differentially expressed, and thus informative for the class distinction. We can also compute the pairwise distances between all cells, using all features.

```
dists = as.matrix(dist(scale(t(exprs(x)))))
diag(dists) = +Inf
```

Then, for each cell, determine the class of its nearest neighbor.

```
nn = sapply(seq_len(ncol(dists)), function(i) which.min(dists[, i]))
table(x$sampleGroup, x$sampleGroup[nn]) %>% `colnames<-`(NULL)
##
##                 [,1] [,2] [,3] [,4] [,5] [,6] [,7] [,8]
##   E3.25           33    0    0    0    3    0    0    0
##   E3.25 (FGF4-KO)  1   15    0    1    0    0    0    0
##   E3.5 (EPI)       2    0    3    0    6    0    0    0
##   E3.5 (FGF4-KO)   0    0    0    8    0    0    0    0
##   E3.5 (PE)        0    0    0    0   11    0    0    0
##   E4.5 (EPI)       0    0    0    0    2    2    0    0
##   E4.5 (FGF4-KO)   1    0    0    0    0    0    9    0
##   E4.5 (PE)        0    0    0    0    2    0    0    2
```

Using all features, the 1-nearest neighbor classifier is correct in almost all cases, including the E3.25 wild-type versus FGF4-KO distinction. This means that for these data, there is no apparent benefit in penalization or feature selection. Limitations of using all features might become apparent with truly new data, but that is out of reach for cross-validation. □

12.7 A large choice of methods

We have now seen three classification methods: linear discriminant analysis (`lda`), quadratic discriminant analysis (`qda`) and logistic regression using elastic net penalization (`glmnet`). In fact, there are hundreds of different learning algorithms[12] available in R and its add-on packages. You can get an overview in the *CRAN task view on machine learning & statistical learning*. Some examples are:

[12] For an introduction to the subject that uses R and provides many examples and exercises, we recommend James et al. (2013).

- Support vector machines: the function `svm` in the package *e1071*; `ksvm` in *kernlab*.
- Tree-based methods in the packages *rpart*, *tree* and *randomForest*.
- Boosting methods: the functions `glmboost` and `gamboost` in the package *mboost*.
- `PenalizedLDA` in the package *PenalizedLDA*, `dudi.discr` and `dist.pcaiv` in *ade4*.

The complexity and heterogeneity in the choice of learning strategies, tuning parameters and evaluation criteria in each of these packages can be confusing. You will already have noted differences in the interfaces of the `lda`, `qda` and `glmnet` functions, i.e., in how they expect their input data to be presented and what they return. There is even greater diversity across all the other packages and functions. At the same time, there are common tasks such as cross-validation, parameter tuning and performance assessment that are more or less the same no matter what method is used. As you have seen, e.g., in our `estimate_mcl_loocv` function, the looping and data shuffling involved led to rather verbose code.

So what to do if you want to try out and explore different learning algorithms? Fortunately, several projects provide unified interfaces to the large number of different machine learning interfaces in R, and also try to provide "best practice" implementations of common tasks such as parameter tuning and performance assessment. The two best known are the packages *caret* and *mlr*. Here we have a look at *caret*. You can get a list of supported methods through its `getModelInfo` function. There are quite a few; we show just the first eight.

```
library("caret")
caretMethods = names(getModelInfo())
head(caretMethods, 8)

## [1] "ada"       "AdaBag"     "AdaBoost.M1" "adaboost"
## [5] "amdai"     "ANFIS"      "avNNet"      "awnb"

length(caretMethods)

## [1] 238
```

We check out a neural network method, the `nnet` function from the eponymous package. The `parameter` slot informs us about the available **tuning** parameters.[13]

```
getModelInfo("nnet", regex = FALSE)[[1]]$parameter

##   parameter  class        label
## 1      size  numeric  #Hidden Units
## 2     decay  numeric  Weight Decay
```

[13] They are described in the manual of the `nnet` function.

Let's try it out.

```
trnCtrl = trainControl(
  method = "repeatedcv",
  repeats = 3,
  classProbs = TRUE)

tuneGrid = expand.grid(
  size = c(2, 4, 8),
  decay = c(0, 1e-2, 1e-1))

nnfit = train(
  Embryonic.day ~ Fn1 + Timd2 + Gata4 + Sox7,
  data = embryoCells,
  method = "nnet",
  tuneGrid  = tuneGrid,
  trControl = trnCtrl,
  metric = "Accuracy")
```

That's quite a mouthful, but the nice thing is that this syntax is standardized and applies across many different methods. All you need to do is specify the name of the method and the grid of tuning parameters that should be explored via the `tuneGrid` argument.

Now we can have a look at the output (Figure 12.25).

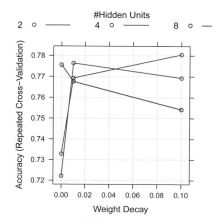

Figure 12.25: **Parameter tuning** of the neural net by cross-validation.

```
nnfit

## Neural Network
##
## 66 samples
##  4 predictor
##  3 classes: 'E3.25', 'E3.5', 'E4.5'
##
## No pre-processing
## Resampling: Cross-Validated (10 fold, repeated 3 times)
## Summary of sample sizes: 58, 58, 60, 60, 59, 60, ...
## Resampling results across tuning parameters:
##
##   size  decay  Accuracy   Kappa
##   2     0.00   0.7221825  0.4532811
##   2     0.01   0.7763492  0.6139365
##   2     0.10   0.7692857  0.5952203
##   4     0.00   0.7327778  0.5325809
##   4     0.01   0.7691667  0.6035691
##   4     0.10   0.7803968  0.6137389
##   8     0.00   0.7755556  0.6112717
##   8     0.01   0.7676190  0.5967545
##   8     0.10   0.7542063  0.5732210
##
## Accuracy was used to select the optimal model using
##  the largest value.
## The final values used for the model were size = 4 and decay
##  = 0.1.

plot(nnfit)
predict(nnfit) %>% head(10)

##  [1] E3.25 E3.25 E3.25 E3.25 E3.25 E3.25 E3.25 E3.25 E3.25 E3.25
## Levels: E3.25 E3.5 E4.5
```

▶ Question **12.23** Will the accuracy that we obtained above for the optimal tuning parameters generalize to a new dataset? What could you do to address that?   ◀

▶ Solution **12.23**   No, it is likely to be too optimistic, as we have picked the optimum. To get a somewhat more realistic estimate of prediction performance when generalized, we could formalize (into computer code) all our data preprocessing choices and the above parameter-tuning procedure, and embed this in another, outer cross-validation loop (Ambroise and McLachlan, 2002). However, this is still unlikely to be enough, as we discuss in the next section.   □

12.7.1   Method hacking

In Chapter 6 we encountered **p-value hacking**. A similar phenomenon exists in statistical learning: given a dataset, we explore various different methods of preprocessing (such as normalization, outlier detection, transformation, feature selection), try out different machine learning algorithms and tune their parameters until we are content with the result. The measured accuracy is likely to be too optimistic, i.e., will not generalize to a new dataset. Embedding as many of our methodical choices into a computational formalism and having an outer cross-validation loop (not to be confused with the inner loop that does the parameter tuning) will ameliorate the problem. But it is unlikely to address it completely, since not all our choices can be formalized.

The gold standard remains validation on truly unseen data. In addition, it is never a bad thing if the classifier is not a black box but can be interpreted in terms of domain knowledge. Finally, report not just summary statistics, such as misclassification rates, but lay open the complete computational **workflow**, so that anyone (including your future self) can convince themselves of the robustness of the result or of the influence of the preprocessing, model selection and tuning choices (Holmes, 2018).

12.8   Summary of this chapter

We have seen examples of machine learning applications; we have focused on predicting categorical variables (like diabetes type or cell class). Predicting continuous outcomes is also part of machine learning, although we have not considered it here. There are many parallels and overlaps between *machine learning* and *statistical regression* (which we studied in Chapter 8). One can regard them as two different names for pretty much the same activity, although each has its own flavors: in machine learning, the emphasis is on the prediction of the outcome variables, whereas in regression we often care at least as much about the role of the covariates – which of them have an effect on the outcome, and what is the nature of these effects? In other words, we do not only want predictions, we also want to understand them.

We saw linear and quadratic discriminant analysis, two intuitive methods for partitioning a two-dimensional data plane (or a p-dimensional space) into regions using either linear or quadratic separation lines (or hypersurfaces). We also saw logistic regression, which takes a slightly different approach but is more amenable to operating in higher dimensions and to regularization.

We encountered the main challenge of machine learning: how can we avoid overfitting? We explored why overfitting happens in the context of the so-called curse of dimensionality, and we learned how it may be overcome using penalization.

In other words, machine learning would be easy if we had infinite amounts of data representatively covering the whole space of possible inputs and outputs.[14] The challenge is to make the best of a finite amount of training data, and to generalize these to new, unseen inputs. There is a vigorous trade-off between the amount, resolution and coverage of training data and the complexity of the model. Many models have continuous parameters that enable us to "tune" their complexity or the strength of their regularization. Cross-validation can help us with such tuning, although it is not a panacea, and caveats apply, as we saw in Section 12.6.3.

[14] It would "simply" be a formidable database or data management problem.

12.9   Further reading

- An introduction to statistical learning that employs many concrete data examples and uses little mathematical formalism is given by James et al. (2013). An extension, with more mathematical background, is the textbook by Hastie et al. (2008).
- The *CRAN task view on machine learning & statistical learning* gives an overview of machine learning software in R.
- *RStudio's API for the "deep learning" platforms Keras and TensorFlow* and the associated teaching materials and demos are a good place to try out some of the recent developments in this field.

12.10   Exercises

▶ Exercise **12.1** Apply a *kernel support vector machine*, available in the *kernlab* package, to the `zeller` microbiome data. What kernel function works well?   ◀

▶ Exercise **12.2** Use `glmnet` for *prediction of a continous variable*, i.e., for regression. Use the prostate cancer data from Chapter 3 of (Hastie et al., 2008). The data are available in the CRAN package *ElemStatLearn*. Explore the effects of using a ridge versus a lasso penalty.   ◀

▶ Exercise **12.3** Consider *smoothing as a regression and model selection problem* (remember Figure 12.1). What is the equivalent quantity to the penalization parameter λ in Equation (12.8)? How do you choose it?   ◀

▶ Exercise **12.4** **Scale invariance**. Consider a rescaling of one of the features in the (generalized) linear model (12.7). For instance, denote the vth column of x by $x_{\cdot v}$, and suppose that $p \geqslant 2$ and that we rescale $x_{\cdot v} \mapsto s\,x_{\cdot v}$ with some number $s \neq 0$. What will happen to the estimate $\hat{\beta}$ from Equation (12.8) in (a) the unpenalized case ($\lambda = 0$), and (b) the penalized case ($\lambda > 0$)?   ◀

▶ Exercise **12.5** It has been quipped that all classification methods are just refinements of *two archetypal ideas*: discriminant analysis and k-nearest neighbors. In what sense might that be a useful description?   ◀

CHAPTER 13

Design of High-Throughput Experiments and Their Analyses

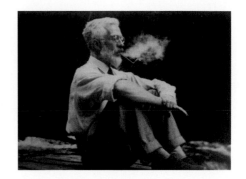

We have now seen many different biological datasets and data types, and methods for analyzing them. To conclude this book, we recapitulate some of the general lessons we learned. Three great pieces of good advice are:

How to analyze? R.A. Fisher, one of the fathers of experimental design (Fisher, 1935), is quoted as saying: *To consult the statistician after an experiment is finished is often merely to ask him to conduct a post mortem examination. He can perhaps say what the experiment died of.*[1] So it is important to design an experiment with the analysis already in mind. Do not delay thinking about how to analyze the data until after they have been acquired.

When? Dailies: start with the analysis as soon as you have acquired some data. Don't wait until everything is collected, as then it's too late to troubleshoot.

What? Start writing the paper while you're analyzing the data. Only once you're writing and trying to present your results and conclusions will you realize what you should have done to properly support them.

dailies

In the same way a film director will view daily takes to correct potential lighting or shooting issues before they affect too much footage, it is a good idea not to wait until all the runs of an experiment have been finished before looking at the data. Intermediate data analyses and visualizations will track unexpected sources of variation and enable you to adjust the protocol. Much is known about sequential design of experiments (Mead, 1990), but even in a more pragmatic setting it is important to be aware of sources of variation as they occur and adjust for them.

[1] Presidential Address to the First Indian Statistical Congress, 1938. Sankhya 4, 14-17.

13.1 Goals for this chapter

In this chapter we will:

- Develop a simple categorization of what types of experiments there are and the varying amounts of control we have with each of them.
- Recap how to distinguish the different types of variability: error, noise and bias.
- Discuss the things that we need to worry about: confounding, dependencies, batch effects. We'll ask the famous question: *how many replicates?*
- Recap the essential ideas behind mean–variance relationships and how they inform us about whether and how to transform our data.
- Computational techniques and tools are essential for getting the job done. We will discuss efficient workflow design, data representation and computation.

- Try to be aware of data summarization steps and questions of sufficiency in our analytical workflows – so that we don't throw away important information in some "upstream" step, which is then missing and making trouble downstream.

13.2   Types of experiments

The art of "good enough".   We need experimental design in order to deal with the fact that our resources are finite, our instruments are not perfect and the real world is complicated. We want to get the best possible outcome nonetheless. This invariably results in hard decisions and trade-offs. **Experimental design** aims to rationalize such decisions. Our experimental interventions and our measurement instruments have limited precision and accuracy; often we don't know these limitations at the outset and have to collect **preliminary data** to estimate them. We may only be able to observe the phenomenon of interest indirectly rather than directly. Our treatment conditions may have undesired but hard-to-avoid side effects; our measurements may be overlaid with interfering signals or "background noise". Sample sizes are limited for practical and economic reasons. There is little point in prescribing unrealistic ideals – we need to make choices that are pragmatic and feasible. A quote from Bacher and Kendziorski (2016) explains this clearly: "Generally speaking, a well-designed experiment is one that is sufficiently powered and one in which technical artifacts and biological features that may systematically affect measurements are balanced, randomized or controlled in some other way in order to minimize opportunities for multiple explanations for the effect(s) under study".

To start with, let's discuss the major different types of experiments, since each of them requires a different approach.

In a **controlled experiment**, we have control over all relevant variables: the (model) system under study, the environmental conditions, the experimental readout. For instance, we could have a well-characterized cell line growing in laboratory conditions in defined media, temperature and atmosphere, we'll administer a precise amount of a drug, and after 72 hours we measure the activity of a specific pathway reporter.

In a **study**, we have less control: important conditions that may affect the measured outcome are not under the control of the researcher, usually because of ethical concerns or logistical constraints. For instance, in an ecological field study, this could be the weather, the availabilty of nutrition resources or the activity of predators. In an **observational study**, even the variable of interest is not controlled by the researcher. For instance, in a clinical trial, this might be the assignment of the individual subjects to groups. Since there are many possibilities for confounding (see Section 13.4.1), interpreting an observational study can be difficult. Here's where the old adage "correlation is not causation" applies.

In a **randomized controlled trial**, we still have to deal with lack of control over many of the factors that impact the outcome, but we control assignment of the variable of interest (say, the type of treatment in a clinical trial); therefore, we can expect that – with large enough sample size – all the nuisance effects average out and the observed effect can really be causally assigned to the intervention. Such trials are usually **prospective**;[2] i.e., the outcome is not known at the time of the assignment of patients to groups.

A **meta-analysis** is an observational study on several previous experiments or studies. One motivation for a meta-analysis is to increase power by increasing effective sample size. Another is to overcome the limitations of individual experiments or studies, which might suffer from researcher or other bias, be underpowered, or otherwise be flawed or random. The hope is that by pooling results from many studies, such "study-level" problems average out.

[2] The antonym is retrospective; observational studies can be prospective or retrospective.

13.3   Partitioning error: bias and noise

We broadly distinguish between two types of error. The first, which we call **noise**, "averages out" if we just perform enough replicates. The second, which we call **bias**, remains; it even becomes more apparent with more replication. Recall the bull's-eye in Figure 12.18: in the lower panel, there is a lot of noise, but no bias, and the center of the cloud of points is in the right place. In the upper panel, there is much less noise, but there is bias. No amount of replication will remedy the fact that the center of the points is in the wrong place.

Bias is more difficult to deal with than noise. Noise is easily recognized just from looking at replicates, and it averages out as we analyze more and more replicates. With bias, it can be hard to even recognize that it is there, and then we need to find ways to measure it and adjust for it, usually with some quantitative model.

▶ Question **13.1** Give two examples in previous chapters where we modeled bias in high-throughput data.   ◀

▶ Solution **13.1** For instance, in Chapter 8, we modeled the sampling noise with the gamma–Poisson distribution. We estimated sequencing-depth bias with the library size factors and took it into account when testing for differential expression. We also modeled sampling bias caused by the two different protocols used (single end, paired end) by introducing a *blocking factor* into our generalized linear model.   □

Statisticians use the term **error** for any deviation of a measured value from the true value. This is different from the everyday use of the word. In statistics, error is an unavoidable aspect of life. It is not "bad", it is something to be cherished, reckoned with, tamed and controlled.

13.3.1   Error models: noise is in the eye of the beholder

The efficiency of most biochemical or physical processes involving DNA polymers depends on their sequence content. For instance, occurrences of long homopolymer stretches, palindromes, or overall or local GC content can modify the efficiency of PCR or the dynamics of how the polymer is being pulled through a nanopore. The size and nature of such effects is challenging to model. They depend in subtle ways on factors such as concentration, temperature, enzyme used, etc. So, when looking at RNA-Seq data, should we treat GC content as noise or as bias?

Remember that the noun *sample* here, by convention, refers to one column of the count matrix, e.g., one sequencing library corresponding to one replicate of one biological condition. The same term (here as the verb form *sampling*) is also used in its more general, statistical sense, as in "a sample of data from a distribution". There is no easy way around this ambiguity, so we just need to be aware of it.

▶ **Question 13.2** How does the *DESeq2* method address this issue? ◀

▶ **Solution 13.2** *DESeq2* offers both options. If size factors are used to model per-sample sampling bias, then such effects are not explicitly modeled. The assumption is then that, for each gene, any such bias would affect the counts in the same way across all samples, so that for the purpose of differential expression analysis, it cancels out. To the extent that such effects are sample specific, they are treated as noise. However, as described in its vignette, *DESeq2* also allows specifying sample- *and* gene-dependent normalization factors for a matrix, and these are intended to contain explicit estimates of such biases.

□

Formal error models can help us decompose the **variability** into noise and bias. A standard decomposition you may have encountered is called ANOVA (analysis of variance). In these types of models, variability is measured by sums of squares and apportioned according to its origin. For instance, when doing supervised classification in a linear discriminant analysis (LDA) in Chapter 12, we computed the total sum of squares C as

$$C_{\text{total}} = C_{\text{within group}} + C_{\text{between groups}}. \tag{13.1}$$

However, there are usually multiple ways of doing such a decomposition: an effect that at one stage is considered within-group variation (noise) might be considered a between-groups effect once the right (sub)groups are assigned.

Maybe this is akin to the vision of "personalized medicine": better patient stratification that converts within-group variation (including unsuccessful or unnecessary treatments) into between-groups variation (where every group of people get exactly what they need).

Determinism versus chance. Everyone thinks of the outcome of a coin toss as random, thus a perfect example of noise. But if we meticulously registered the initial conditions of the coin flip and solved the mechanical equations, we could predict which side has a higher probability of coming up (Diaconis et al., 2007b).

So, rather than asking whether a certain effect or process *is* random or deterministic, it is more fruitful to say whether *we care* to model it deterministically (as bias) or ignore the details, treat it as stochastic and use probabilistic modeling (noise). In this sense, probabilistic models are a way of quantifying our ignorance, taming our uncertainty.

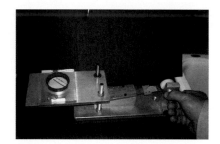

Figure 13.1: A carefully contructed coin-tossing machine can be made to provide deterministic coin flips.

Latent factors. Sometimes we explicitly know about factors that cause bias, for instance, when different reagent batches were used in different phases of the experiment. We call these **batch effects** (Leek et al., 2010). At other times, we may expect that such factors are at work but have no explicit record of them. We call these **latent factors**. We can treat them as adding to the noise, and in Chapter 4 we saw how to use mixture models to do so. But this may not be enough; with high-dimensional data, noise caused by latent factors tends to be correlated, and this can lead to faulty inference (Leek et al., 2010). The good news is that these same correlations can be exploited to estimate latent factors from the data, model them as bias and thus reduce the noise (Leek and Storey, 2007; Stegle et al., 2010).

13.3.2   Biological versus technical replicates

▶ Question **13.3** Imagine you want to test whether a weight-loss drug works. Which of the following study designs would you use?

- A person is weighed on a milligram precision scale, with 20 replicates. He follows the diet, and four weeks later, he is weighed again, with 20 replicates.
- Ten people weigh themselves once on their bathroom scale and report the number. Four weeks later, they weigh themselves and report again.

Surely the first option must be better, since it has 20 replicates on a very precise instrument rather than only 10 on an older piece of equipment?   ◄

▶ Solution **13.3** What we have here is a (placative) instance of the difference between **technical** versus **biological replicates**. The number of replicates is less important than what types of variation are allowed to affect them. The 20 replicates in the first design are wasted on remeasuring something that we already know with more than enough precision, whereas the far more important question – how does the effect generalize to different people – starts to be addressed with the second design, although in practice more people would be needed.   □

Inference or generalizations can only be made to a wider population if we have a representative randomized sample of that population in our study. In the first case, if weight loss occurs, one could infer only about that person at that time.

Analogous questions arise in biological experimentation. For example, should you do five replicates on the same cell line, or one replicate each on three different cell lines?

▶ Question **13.4** For reliable variant calling with the sequencing technology used by the 1000 Genomes Project, one needs about 30× coverage per genome. However, the average depth of the data produced was 5.1 for 1092 individuals (1000 Genomes Project Consortium, 2012). Why was that study design chosen?   ◄

The technical versus biological replicates terminology has some value, but is often too coarse. The observed effect may or may not be generalizable at many different levels: different labs, different operators within one lab, different technologies, different machines from the same technology, different variants of the protocol, different strains, litters, sexes, individual animals, and so forth. It's better to name the levels of replication more explicitly.

13.3.3   Units versus fold changes

Measurements in physics are usually reported as multiples of SI units,[3] such as meters, kilograms, seconds. A length measured in meters by a lab in Australia using one instrument is directly comparable to one measured a year later by a lab in Canada using a different instrument, or by alien scientists in a faraway galaxy. In biology, it is rarely possible or practical to make measurements that are as standardized. The situation here is more like when human body parts (feet, hands, etc.) were used for length measurements and the sizes of these body parts were different in different towns and countries, let alone different galaxies.

[3] International System of Units (French: Système International d'Unités).

Biologists often report measurements as multiples of (i.e., fold changes with regard to) some local, more or less ad hoc reference. The challenge with this practice is that fold changes and proportions are ratios. The denominator is a random variable (as it changes from lab to lab and probably from experiment to experiment), which can create high instability and very unequal variances between experiments; see the sections on transformations and sufficiency a little later in this chapter. Even when seemingly absolute values exist (e.g., TPKM values in an RNA-Seq experiment), because of experiment-specific sampling biases, they do not translate into universal units, and they often lack an indication of their precision.

13.3.4   Regular and catastrophic noise

Regular noise can be modeled by simple probability models such as independent normal distributions or Poissons, or by mixtures such as the gamma–Poisson or Laplace. We can use relatively straightforward methods to take such noise into account in our data analyses and to compute the probability of extraordinarily large or small values. In the real world, this is only part of the story: measurements can be completely off-scale (a sample swap, a contamination or a software bug), and they can go awry all at the same time (a whole microtiter plate went bad, affecting all data measured from it). Such events are hard to model or even correct for – our best chance of dealing with them is data quality assessment, outlier detection and documented removal.

13.4   Basic principles in the design of experiments

13.4.1   Confounding

▶ **Question 13.5** Consider the data shown in Figure 13.2. How can we decide whether the observed differences in the biomarker levels are due to disease versus healthy, or to the batch?   ◀

▶ **Solution 13.5** It is impossible to know from these data: the two variables are confounded.   □

Confounding need not only be between a biological and a technical variable, it can also be more subtle. For instance, the biomarker might have nothing to do with the disease directly – it might just be a marker of a lifestyle that causes the disease (as well as other things), or of an inflammation that is caused by the disease (as well as by many other things), etc.

13.4.2   Effect size and replicates

The effect size is the difference between the group centers, as shown by the red arrow in Figure 13.4. A larger sample size in each group increases the precision with which the locations of each group and the effect size are known, thus increasing our power to detect a difference (Figure 13.5). On the other hand, the performance of the biomarker as a diagnostic in individual samples for distinguishing between healthy and disease

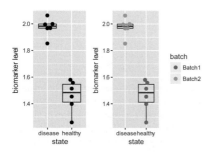

Figure 13.2: Comparison of a (hypothetical) biomarker between samples from disease and healthy states. If we are given only the information shown in the left-hand panel, we might conclude that this biomarker performs well in detecting the disease. If, in addition, we are told that the data were acquired in two separate batches (e.g., different labs, different machines, different time points) as indicated in the right-hand panel, the conclusion will be different.

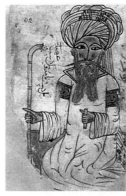

Figure 13.3: Confounding is the reason that one of the seven rules of experimental design listed by the Persian physician-scientist Abu 'Ali al-Husayn ibn Sina (Avicenna) around AD 1020 was "to study one possible cause of a disease at a time" (Stigler, 2016).

states depends on the within-group distributions (and the relative prevalences of both states), and is not improved by replication.

13.4.3 Clever combinations: Hotelling's weighting example

To get the best data out of available resources, capitalizing on cancellations and symmetries is an important tool. Here is a famous illustration of how Hotelling devised an improved weighing scheme. Suppose we are given a set of eight unknown weights $\theta = (\theta_1, \ldots, \theta_8)$. In the following code, we simulate such a set of true weights using R's random number generator.

```
theta = round((2 * sample(8, 8) + rnorm(8)), 1)
theta

## [1]  4.3 12.2  8.0 14.7 11.3  5.4  1.0 16.1
```

Method 1. Naive method, using eight weighings. Suppose we use a pharmacist's balance (Figure 13.6) that weighs each weight θ_i individually, with errors distributed normally with a standard deviation of 0.1. We compute the vector of errors `errors1` and their sum of squares as follows.

```
X = theta + rnorm(length(theta), 0, 0.1)
X

## [1]  4.303583 12.159709  8.075797 14.835033 11.105022  5.368522
## [7]  1.127750 16.018751

errors1 = X - theta
errors1

## [1]  0.003582889 -0.040291419  0.075797447  0.135033088
## [5] -0.194977866 -0.031477695  0.127749600 -0.081248674

sum(errors1^2)

## [1] 0.08754394
```

Method 2. Hotelling's method, also using eight weighings. The method is based on a Hadamard matrix (i.e., a $n \times n$ matrix H, with entries ± 1 such that $HH^\mathsf{T} = n\mathbb{I}$), which we compute here.

```
library("survey")
h8 = hadamard(6)
coef8 = 2*h8 - 1
coef8

##      [,1] [,2] [,3] [,4] [,5] [,6] [,7] [,8]
## [1,]    1    1    1    1    1    1    1    1
## [2,]    1   -1    1   -1    1   -1    1   -1
## [3,]    1    1   -1   -1    1    1   -1   -1
## [4,]    1   -1   -1    1    1   -1   -1    1
## [5,]    1    1    1    1   -1   -1   -1   -1
## [6,]    1   -1    1   -1   -1    1   -1    1
## [7,]    1    1   -1   -1   -1   -1    1    1
## [8,]    1   -1   -1    1   -1    1    1   -1
```

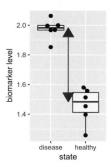

Figure 13.4: The red arrow shows the effect size, as measured by the difference between the centers of the two groups. Here we locate the centers by the medians; sometimes the mean is used.

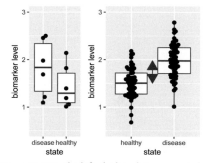

Figure 13.5: On the left, the boxplot was created with samples of size 6. On the right, the sample sizes are 60. The measurements have the same underlying error distribution in both cases.

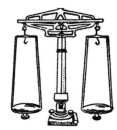

Figure 13.6: The example in this section uses the pharmacist's balance weighing analogy introduced by Yates and developed by Hotelling (1944) and Mood (1946).

We use `coef8` as the coefficients in a new weighing scheme, as follows. The first column of the matrix tells us to put all the weights on one side of the balance and to weigh that: call the result `Y[1]`. The second column tells us to place weights 1, 3, 5, 7 on one side of the balance and weights 2, 4, 6, 8 on the other. We then measure the difference and call the result `Y[2]`. And so forth, for all eight columns of `coef8`. We can express the necessary computations in matrix multiplication form.

```
Y = theta   %*% coef8 + rnorm(length(theta), 0, 0.1)
```

As in the first method, each of the eight weight measurements has a normal error with standard deviation of 0.1.

▶ Question **13.6** (a) Is `coef8` – up to an overall factor – an orthogonal matrix (i.e., $C^{T}C = \lambda \mathbb{I}$ for some $\lambda \in \mathbb{R}$)?
(b) If we multiply `theta` with `coef8` times `coef8` transposed and divide by 8, do we obtain `theta` again?   ◀

▶ Solution **13.6**

```
coef8 %*% t(coef8)

##       [,1] [,2] [,3] [,4] [,5] [,6] [,7] [,8]
## [1,]    8    0    0    0    0    0    0    0
## [2,]    0    8    0    0    0    0    0    0
## [3,]    0    0    8    0    0    0    0    0
## [4,]    0    0    0    8    0    0    0    0
## [5,]    0    0    0    0    8    0    0    0
## [6,]    0    0    0    0    0    8    0    0
## [7,]    0    0    0    0    0    0    8    0
## [8,]    0    0    0    0    0    0    0    8

theta %*% coef8 %*% t(coef8) / ncol(coef8)

##      [,1] [,2] [,3] [,4] [,5] [,6] [,7] [,8]
## [1,]  4.3 12.2    8 14.7 11.3  5.4    1 16.1
```
                                                                                              □

We combine these results to estimate `theta` using the orthogonality of `coef8`.

```
thetahat = Y %*% t(coef8) / ncol(coef8)
```

Since we know the true θ, we can compute the errors and their sum of squares.

```
errors2 = as.vector(thetahat) - theta
errors2

## [1] -0.02977399  0.09910284 -0.01224720 -0.02595442 -0.01332818
## [6] -0.01684828  0.02326719 -0.06796711

sum(errors2^2)

## [1] 0.01715389
```

We see that the sum of squares here is substantially smaller than that of the first procedure. Were we just lucky?

▶ Question **13.7** (a) Repeat the above experiment $B = 10,000$ times, each time using a different `theta`. What do the sampling distributions of sum-of-squares errors in both schemes look like?

(b) What do you think the relationship between the two variances is?   ◄

▶ **Solution 13.7**

```
B  = 10000
tc = t(coef8) / ncol(coef8)
sse = replicate(B, {
  theta = round((2 * sample(8, 8)) + rnorm(8), 1)
  X = theta + rnorm(length(theta), 0, 0.1)
  err1 = sum((X - theta)^2)
  Y = coef8 %*% theta + rnorm(length(theta), 0, 0.1)
  thetahat = tc %*% Y
  err2 = sum((thetahat - theta)^2)
  c(err1, err2)
})
rowMeans(sse)
## [1] 0.08010581 0.01001430
```

```
ggplot(tibble(lr = log2(sse[1, ] / sse[2, ])), aes(x = lr)) +
  geom_histogram(bins = 50) +
  geom_vline(xintercept = log2(8), col = "orange") +
  xlab("log2 ratio of SSE, Method 1 vs 2")
```

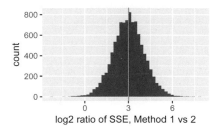

Figure 13.7: Logarithm (base 2) of the ratios of sum-of-squares error for the two methods. The vertical orange line corresponds to 8 ($3 = \log_2 8$).

The second scheme is more **efficient** than the first by a factor of eight, because the errors generated by the measurement have a sum of squares that is eight times smaller (Figure 13.7).   □

This example shows us that when several quantities are to be ascertained, there is an opportunity to increase the accuracy and reduce the cost by combining measurements in one experiment and making comparisons between similar groups.

Ibn Sina's rule that an optimal design can vary only one factor at a time was superseded in the 20th century by R.A. Fisher. He realized that one could modify the factors in combinations and still come to a conclusion – sometimes an even better conclusion, as in the weighing example – as long as the contrasts were carefully designed.

13.4.4 Blocking and pairing

Darwin suspected that corn growth is affected by the composition of the soil and the humidity in the pots. For this reason, when he wanted to compare plants grown from cross-pollinated seeds with plants grown from self-pollinated seeds, he planted one seedling of each type in each of 15 pots. Each pot in Darwin's *Zea mays* experiment is a block; only the factor of interest (pollination method), called the **treatment**, is different within each block (Figure 13.8).

> "Block what you can, randomize what you cannot."
>
> George Box, 1978

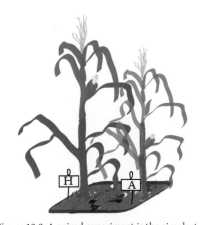

Figure 13.8: A paired experiment is the simplest case of blocking.

In fact, R.A. Fisher criticized Darwin's experiment because he systematically put the cross-pollinated plants on the same side of the pot. This could have induced confounding of a "side" effect with the cross effect, if one side of the pot received more sunlight, for instance. It would have been preferable to randomize the side of the pot, e.g., by flipping a coin.

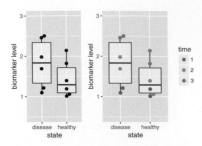

Figure 13.9: On the left, two samples each of size six are being compared. On the right, the same data are shown, but colored by the time of data collection. We note a tendency of the data to fall into blocks according to these times. Because of this, comparison between the groups is diluted. This effect can be mitigated by comparing within times, i.e., by blocking into three groups. Paired analysis, such as demonstrated in Questions 13.8–13.10, is a special case of blocking.

Comparing a paired versus an unpaired design

When comparing various possible designs, we do **power simulations** similar to what we saw in Chapter 1. Let's suppose the sample size is 15 in each group and the **effect size** is 0.2. We also need to make assumptions about the standard deviations of the measurements. Here we suppose both groups have the same standard deviation of 0.25 and simulate data.

```
n = 15
effect = 0.2
pots   = rnorm(n, 0, 1)
noiseh = rnorm(n, 0, 0.25)
noisea = rnorm(n, 0, 0.25)
hybrid = pots + effect + noiseh
autoz  = pots + noisea
```

▶ Question **13.8** Perform both a simple *t*-test and a paired *t*-test. Which is more powerful in this case?   ◀

▶ Solution **13.8**

```
t.test(hybrid, autoz, paired = FALSE)

##
##   Welch Two Sample t-test
##
## data:  hybrid and autoz
## t = 0.61871, df = 27.917, p-value = 0.5411
## alternative hypothesis: true difference in means is not equal to 0
## 95 percent confidence interval:
##   -0.5665392  1.0567862
## sample estimates:
##   mean of x  mean of y
## -0.3011246 -0.5462481

t.test(hybrid, autoz, paired = TRUE)

##
##   Paired t-test
##
## data:  hybrid and autoz
## t = 2.7153, df = 14, p-value = 0.01675
## alternative hypothesis: true difference in means is not equal to 0
## 95 percent confidence interval:
##   0.05150616 0.43874086
## sample estimates:
## mean of the differences
##                0.2451235
```
□

Were we just lucky with our simulated data here?

▶ Question **13.9** Check which method is generally more powerful. Repeat the above computations 1000 times and compute the average probability of rejection for these 1000 trials, using a false positive rate $\alpha = 0.05$.   ◀

▶ Solution 13.9

```
B     = 1000
alpha = 0.05
what  = c(FALSE, TRUE)
pvs = replicate(B, {
  pots   = rnorm(n, 0, 1)
  noiseh = rnorm(n, 0, 0.25)
  noisea = rnorm(n, 0, 0.25)
  hybrid = pots + effect + noiseh
  autoz  = pots + noisea
  vapply(what,
    function(paired)
      t.test(hybrid, autoz, paired = paired)$p.value,
    double(1)) %>% setNames(paste(what))
})
rowMeans(pvs <= alpha)

## FALSE   TRUE
## 0.001 0.497
```

We can compare the p-values obtained using both methods (Figure 13.10).

```
library("reshape2")
ggplot(melt(pvs), aes(x = value, fill = Var1)) +
  geom_histogram(binwidth = 0.01, boundary = 0, alpha = 1/3) +
  scale_fill_discrete(name = "Paired")
```  □

▶ Question 13.10 (a) Write a function that compares the power of the two types of tests for different values of the effect size, sample size, size of the pot effects (as measured by their standard deviation), noise standard deviation and sample size.

(b) Use your function to find out which of the standard deviations (pots or noise) has the largest effect on the improvement produced by pairing for $n = 15$.

(c) How big should n be to attain a power of 80% if the two standard deviations are both 0.5? ◀

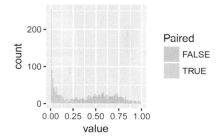

Figure 13.10: Results from the power calculation: comparing the p-value distributions from the ordinary unpaired and paired t-tests.

▶ Solution 13.10

```
powercomparison = function(effect = 0.2, n = 15, alpha = 0.05,
                 sdnoise, sdpots, B = 1000) {
  what = c(FALSE, TRUE)
  pvs = replicate(B, {
    pots   = rnorm(n, 0, sdpots)
    noiseh = rnorm(n, 0, sdnoise)
    noisea = rnorm(n, 0, sdnoise)
    hybrid = pots + effect + noiseh
    autoz  = pots + noisea
    vapply(what,
      function(paired)
        t.test(hybrid, autoz, paired = paired)$p.value,
      double(1)) %>% setNames(paste(what))
  })
  rowMeans(pvs <= alpha)
}
```

```
pwr.t.test(n = 15, d = 0.4, sig.level = 0.05, type = "paired")
##
##          Paired t-test power calculation
##
##              n = 15
##              d = 0.4
##      sig.level = 0.05
##          power = 0.3031649
##    alternative = two.sided
##
## NOTE: n is number of *pairs*
```

If we want to know what sample size would be required to detect a given effect size:

```
pwr.t.test(d = 0.4, sig.level = 0.05, type = "two.sample", power=0.8)
##
##          Two-sample t test power calculation
##
##              n = 99.08032
##              d = 0.4
##      sig.level = 0.05
##          power = 0.8
##    alternative = two.sided
##
## NOTE: n is number in *each* group

pwr.t.test(d = 0.4, sig.level = 0.05, type = "paired", power=0.8)
##
##          Paired t-test power calculation
##
##              n = 51.00945
##              d = 0.4
##      sig.level = 0.05
##          power = 0.8
##    alternative = two.sided
##
## NOTE: n is number of *pairs*
```

We see that we would need about twice as many observations for the same power when not using a paired test.

Effective sample size

A sample of independent observations is more informative than the same number of dependent observations. Suppose you want to do an opinion poll by knocking at people's doors and asking them a question. In the first scenario, you pick n people at n random places throughout the country. In the second scenario, to save travel time, you pick $n/3$ random places, and then at each of these interview three people who live next door to each other. In both cases, the number of people polled is n, but if we assume that people living in the same neighborhood are more likely to have the same opinion, the data from the second scenario are (positively) correlated. To explore this, let's do a simulation.

```
doPoll = function(n = 100, numPeoplePolled = 12) {
  opinion = sort(rnorm(n))
  i1 = sample(n, numPeoplePolled)
  i2 = sample(seq(3, n, by = 3), numPeoplePolled / 3)
  i2 = c(i2, i2 - 1, i2 - 2)
  c(independent = mean(opinion[i1]), correlated = mean(opinion[i2]))
}
responses = replicate(5000, doPoll())
ggplot(melt(responses), aes(x = value, col = Var1)) + geom_density() +
  geom_vline(xintercept = 0) + xlab("Opinion poll result")
```

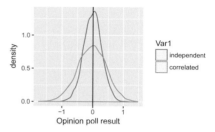

Figure 13.12: Density estimates for the polling result using the two sampling methods. The correlated method has higher spread. The truth is indicated by the vertical line.

There are 100 people in the country, of whom in the first approach (i1) we randomly sample 12. In the second approach, we sample 4 people as well as 2 neighbors for each (i2). The "opinion" in our case is a real number, normally distributed in the population with mean 0 and standard deviation 1. We model the spatio-sociological structure of the country by sorting the houses from most negative to most positive opinion in the first line of the doPoll function. The output is shown in Figure 13.12.

13.5   Mean–variance relationships and variance-stabilizing transformations

In Chapters 4 and 8 we saw examples of data transformations that compress or stretch the space of quantitative measurements in such a way that the measurements' variance is more similar throughout. Thus the variance between replicate measurements is no longer highly dependent on the mean value.

The mean–variance relationship of our data *before* transformation can, in principle, be any function, but in many cases, the following prototypic relationships are found, at least approximately:

1. Constant: the variance is independent of the mean, $v(m) = c$.
2. Poisson: the variance is proportional to the mean, $v(m) = am$.
3. Quadratic: the standard deviation is proportional to the mean; therefore the variance grows quadratically, $v(m) = bm^2$.

Here $v(m)$ is the function that describes the trend of the variance v as a function of the mean m. The real numbers $a, b, c \geqslant 0$ parameterize factors other than the mean that affect the variance.

▶ Question **13.12** Give examples of biological assays or measurement technologies whose data show these types of mean–variance relationships.   ◀

The mean–variance relationship in real data can also be a *combination* of these basic types. For instance, with DNA microarrays, the fluorescence intensities are subject to a combination of background noise that is largely independent of the signal, and multiplicative noise whose standard deviation is proportional to the signal (Rocke and

Durbin, 2001). Therefore, the mean–variance relationship is $v(m) = bm^2 + c$. For bright spots (large m), the multiplicative noise dominates (the bm^2 term), whereas for faint spots, the background term, c, does.

▶ Question **13.13** What is the point of applying a variance-stabilizing transformation? ◀

▶ Solution **13.13** Analyzing the data on the transformed scale tends to:

- Improve visualization, since the physical space on the plot is used more "fairly" throughout the range of the data. A similar argument applies to the color space in the case of a heatmap.
- Improve the outcome of ordination methods such as PCA or clustering based on correlation, as the results are not so much dominated by the signal from a few very highly expressed genes, but more uniformly from many genes throughout the dynamic range.
- Improve the estimates and inference from statistical models that are based on the assumption of identically distributed (and, hence, homoscedastic) noise.   □

13.6   Data quality assessment and quality control

We distinguish between data quality assessment (QA) – steps taken to measure and monitor data quality – and quality control (QC) – the removal of bad data. These activities pervade all phases of an analysis, from assembling the raw data over transformation, summarization, model fitting, hypothesis testing or screening for "hits" to interpretation. QA-related questions include:

- How do the marginal distributions of the variables look (histograms, ECDF plots)?
- How do their joint distributions look (scatterplots, pairs plot)?
- How well do replicates agree (as compared to different biological conditions)? Are the magnitudes of the differences between several conditions plausible?
- Is there evidence of batch effects? These could be of a categorical (stepwise) or continuous (gradual) nature, e.g., due to changes in experimental reagents, protocols or environmental factors. Factors associated with such effects may be explicitly known, or unknown and latent, and often they are somewhere in between (e.g., when a measurement apparatus slowly degrades over time, and we have recorded the times, but don't really know exactly when the degradation becomes bad).

For the last two sets of questions, heatmaps, principal component plots and other ordination plots (as we have seen in Chapters 7 and 9) are useful.

It's not easy to define **quality**, and the word is used with many meanings. The most pertinent for us is **fitness for purpose**,[4] and this contrasts with other definitions of quality that are based on normative specifications. For instance, in differential expression analysis with RNA-Seq data, our purpose may be the detection of differentially expressed genes between two biological conditions. We can check specifications such as the number of reads, read length, base calling quality and fraction of aligned reads, but

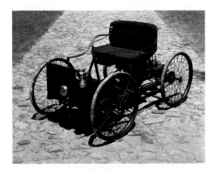

Figure 13.13: Henry Ford's (possibly apocryphal) quote, "If I had asked people what they wanted, they would have said faster horses", expresses the view of quality as *fitness for purpose*, versus adherence to specifications. Image credit: MPI/StringerGetty Images.

[4] See *quality (business)* on Wikipedia.

ultimately these measures in isolation have little bearing on our purpose. More to the point will be the identification of samples that are not behaving as expected, e.g., because of a sample swap or degradation, or genes that were not measured properly. We saw an example of this in Section 8.10.3. Useful plots include ordination plots, such as Figure 8.6, and heatmaps, such as Figure 8.7. A **quality metric** is any value that we use to measure quality, and having explicit quality metrics helps in automating QA/QC.

13.7   Longitudinal data

Longitudinal data[5] have time as a covariate. The first question is whether we are looking at a handful of time points – say, the response of a cell line measured 48h, 72h and 96h after exposure to a drug – or a long and densely sampled time series – say, patch clamp data in electrophysiology or a movie from life-cell microscopy.

In the first case, time is usually best thought of as just another discrete experimental factor. Perhaps the multiple time points were chosen because the experimenter was not sure which ones would give the most useful results. One can then try to identify the best time point and focus on that. Depending on the data, the other time points could serve for validation, as "more or less" replicates. When designing the experiment, we'll try to cover more densely those time periods when we expect the most to happen, e.g., directly after a perturbation.

In a screening context, we can ask whether there is any effect at all, whatever the time point and shape, using something like an F-test. We then just need to make sure that we account for the *dependencies* between the measurements at the different time points and determine the null distribution accordingly.

In the second case, with time series, we may want to fit dynamical models to the data. We can write $X(t)$ for the *state* of our system at time t; we have many choices, depending on whether:

- X is continuous or discrete,
- the *dynamics*[6] of X are deterministic or stochastic,
- the dynamics are smooth and/or jumpy, or
- we observe X directly or observe only some noisy and/or reduced version, $Y = g(X) + \varepsilon$, of it.[7]

We have many modeling tools at hand, including:

- Markov models: discrete state space; the dynamics are stochastic and occur by jumping between states.
- Ordinary or partial differential equations: continuous state space; the dynamics are deterministic and smooth and are described by a differential equation, possibly derived from first principles rooted in physics or chemistry.
- Master equation, Fokker–Planck equation: the dynamics are stochastic and are described by (partial) differential equations for the probability distribution of X in space and time.

[5] A related but different concept is *survival data*, where time is the outcome variable.

[6] The value of $X(t + \Delta t)$, given $X(t)$ – in other words, the temporal evolution.

[7] Here g denotes a function that loses information, e.g., by dropping some of the variables of a vector-valued X, and ε is a noise term.

- Piece-wise deterministic stochastic processes: a combination of the above. Samples from the process involve deterministic, smooth movements as well as occasional jumps.

If we don't observe X directly, but only a noisy and/or summarized version Y, then in the case of Markov models, the formalism of **hidden Markov models** (Durbin et al., 1998) makes it relatively straightforward to fit such models. For the other types of processes, analogous approaches are possible, but these are technically more demanding, and we refer to specialized literature.

Taking a more data-driven (rather than model-driven) view, methods for analyzing time series data include:

- Nonparametric smoothing followed by clustering or classification into prototypic shapes.
- Change point detection.
- Autoregressive models.
- Fourier and wavelet decomposition.

It's outside the scope of this book to go into details, and there is a huge amount of choice.[8] Many methods originated in physics, econometrics or signal processing, so it's worthwhile to scan the literature in these fields.

13.8   Data integration: use everything you (could) know

Don't pretend you are dumb.

There is an attraction to seemingly "unbiased" approaches that analyze the data at hand without reference to what is already known. Such tendencies are reinforced by the fact that statistical methods have often been developed to be generic and self-contained, for instance, to work for a general matrix without specific reference to what the rows and columns mean in an application, or what other, more or less relevant, data might be around.

Generic approaches are a good way to get started, and for analyses that are straightforward and highly powered, such an approach might work out. But often it is wasteful. Recall the example of an RNA-Seq experiment for differential expression. As we saw in Chapters 6 and 8, we could perform a hypothesis test for each recorded gene, regardless of its signal strength[9] or anything else, and then run a multiple testing method that treats all tests the same (i.e., as exchangeable). But this is inefficient: we can improve our detection power by **filtering out** or **down-weighting** hypotheses with lower power or with higher prior probability π_0 of being true.

Similarly, in the interpretation of single p-values, we don't need to ignore everything else we know and, for instance, blindly stick to an arbitrary 5% cutoff no matter what; rather, we can let prior knowledge of the test's power and of π_0 guide our interpretation (Altman and Krzywinski, 2017).

Other potential examples of misplaced objectivity include:

- Penalization or feature selection in high-dimensional regression or classification. It is easy to use schemes that treat all features the same and, for instance, standardize all of them to zero mean and unit variance. But sometimes we know that some classes of features are likely to be more, or less, informative than others (Wiel et al., 2016). We can also use graphs or networks to represent "other" data and use an approach like the group or graph lasso (Jacob et al., 2009) to structure penalties in high-dimensional modeling.
- Unsupervised clustering of our objects of interest (samples, genes or sequences) and subsequent search for overrepresented annotations. We may be better off incorporating the different uncertainties with which these were measured and their different frequencies into the clustering algorithm. We can use probabilities and similarities to check whether the members of clusters are more similar than two randomly picked objects (Callahan et al., 2016b).

When embarking on an analysis, it's important to anticipate that we'll rarely be done by applying a single method and getting a straightforward result. We need to dig out other, related datasets, look for confirmation (or otherwise) of our results, make further interpretations. An example is gene set enrichment analysis: after we've analyzed our data and found a list of genes that appear to be related to our comparison of interest, we'll overlap them with other gene lists, such as those from the *Molecular Signatures Database* (Liberzon et al., 2011), in order to explore the broader biological processes involved, or we might load up datasets to look at levels of regulation[10] upstream or downstream of ours in search of context.

[10] Genome, chromatin state, transcription, mRNA life cycle, translation, protein life cycle, localization and interactions; metabolites, …

13.9   Sharpen your tools: reproducible research

Analysis projects often begin with a simple script, perhaps to try out a few initial ideas and explore the quality of the pilot data. Then more ideas are added, more data come in, other datasets are integrated, more people become involved. Eventually the paper needs to be written, figures need to be done "properly" and the analysis needs to be saved for the scientific record and to document its integrity. Here are a few principles that can help with such a process.[11]

[11] An excellent and very readable outline of good computing practices for researchers, including data management, programming, collaborating with colleagues, organizing projects, tracking work and writing manuscripts, is given by Wilson et al. (2017).

Use an integrated development environment.   **RStudio** is a great choice. There are also other platforms, such as Emacs and Eclipse.

Use literate programming tools.   Examples are **Rmarkdown** and **Jupyter**. This makes code more readable (for yourself and for others) than burying explanations and usage instructions in comments in the source code or in separate README files. In addition, you can directly embed figures and tables in these documents. Such documents are good starting points for the supplementary material of your paper. Moreover, they're great for reporting analyses to your collaborators.

Anticipate re-engineering of data formats and software.   The first version of how you represent the data and structure the analysis workflow will rarely be capable of supporting the project as it evolves. Don't be afraid[12] to make a clean cut and redesign as soon as you notice that you are doing a lot of awkward data manipulations or repetitive steps. This is time well invested. Almost always, it also helps to unearth bugs.

[12] The professionals do it, too: "Most software at Google gets rewritten every few years" (Henderson, 2017).

Reuse existing tools.   Don't reinvent the wheel; your time is better spent on things that are actually new. Before using a self-made "heuristic" or a temporary "shortcut", spend a couple of minutes researching to see if something like this hasn't been done before. More often than not, it has, and sometimes there is a clean, scalable and already tested solution.

Use version control.   An example is *git*. This takes time to learn, but the time is well invested. In the long run, it will be infinitely better than all your self-grown attempts at managing evolving code with version numbers, switches and the like. Moreover, this is the sanest option for collaborative work on code, and it provides an extra backup of your codebase, especially if the server is distinct from your personal computer.

Use functions.   It's better than copy-pasting (or repeatedly `source`-ing) stretches of code.

Use the R package system.   Soon you'll note recurring function or variable definitions that you want to share between your different scripts. It is fine to use the R function `source` to manage them initially, but it is never too early to move them into your own package – at the latest when you find yourself starting to write emails or code comments explaining to others (or to yourself) how to use some functionality. Assembling existing code into an R package is not hard, and it offers you many goodies, including standardized ways of composing documentation, showing code usage examples, code testing, versioning and provision to others. And quite likely you'll soon appreciate the benefits of using namespaces.

Centralize the location of the raw data files and automate the derivation of intermediate data.   Store the input data on a centralized file server that is professionally backed up. Mark the files as read-only. Have a clear and linear workflow for computing the derived data (e.g., normalized, summarized, transformed, etc.) from the raw files, and store these in a separate directory. Anticipate that this workflow will need to be run several times,[13] and version it. Use the *BiocFileCache* package to mirror these files on your personal computer.[14]

[13] Always once more than the "final, final" time before the final data freeze…

[14] A more basic alternative is the *rsync* utility. A popular solution offered by some organizations is based on *ownCloud*. Commercial options are Dropbox, Google Drive and the like.

Think in terms of cooking recipes and try to automate them.   When developing downstream analysis ideas that bring together several different data types, you don't want to do the conversion from data-type-specific formats into a representation suitable for machine learning or a generic statistical method each time anew, on an ad hoc basis. Have a *recipe* script that assembles the different ingredients and cooks them up as an easily consumable[15] matrix, dataframe or Bioconductor *SummarizedExperiment*.

[15] In computer science, the term *data warehouse* is sometimes used for such a concept.

Keep a hyperlinked webpage with an index of all analyses.   This is helpful for collaborators (especially if the page and the analysis can be accessed via a web browser) and also a good starting point for the methods part of your paper. Structure it in chronological or logical order, or a combination of both.

13.10   Data representation

Getting data ready for analysis or visualization often involves a lot of shuffling until they are in the right shape and format for an analytical algorithm or a graphics routine. As we saw in Chapter 3, *ggplot2* likes its data in dataframe objects and, more specifically, in the long format. The reasons behind this choice are well explained in Hadley Wickham's paper on **tidy data** (Wickham, 2014).

13.10.1   Wide versus long table format

Recall the Hiiragi data (for space reasons we print only the first five columns of `xwdf`).

```
library("Hiiragi2013")
library("magrittr")
data("x")
xwdf = tibble(
  probe  = c("1420085_at", "1418863_at", "1425463_at", "1416967_at"),
  symbol = c(      "Fgf4",      "Gata4",      "Gata6",      "Sox2"))
xwdf %<>% bind_cols(as_tibble(exprs(x)[xwdf$probe, ]))
dim(xwdf)

## [1]    4 103

xwdf[, 1:5]

## # A tibble: 4 x 5
##    probe      symbol `1 E3.25` `2 E3.25` `3 E3.25`
##    <chr>      <chr>      <dbl>     <dbl>     <dbl>
## 1 1420085_at Fgf4        3.03      9.29      2.94
## 2 1418863_at Gata4       4.84      5.53      4.42
## 3 1425463_at Gata6       5.50      6.16      4.58
## 4 1416967_at Sox2        1.73      9.70      4.16
```

Each row of this dataframe reports 101 expression values, one for each sample. In addition, there is a column that reports the probe identifiers and one for the gene symbols. The sample identifiers, together with information on the time point when the sample was taken, are recorded in the column names. This is an example of a data table in **wide format**. Now let's call the `melt` function from the *reshape2* package.

```
xldf = melt(xwdf, id.vars = c("probe", "symbol"),
                    variable.name = "sample")
dim(xldf)
## [1] 404    4
head(xldf)
##          probe symbol   sample    value
## 1 1420085_at   Fgf4 1 E3.25 3.027715
## 2 1418863_at   Gata4 1 E3.25 4.843137
## 3 1425463_at   Gata6 1 E3.25 5.500618
## 4 1416967_at   Sox2 1 E3.25 1.731217
## 5 1420085_at   Fgf4 2 E3.25 9.293016
## 6 1418863_at   Gata4 2 E3.25 5.530016
```

In `xldf`, each row corresponds to exactly one of the 404 measured values stored in the column `value`. Then there are additional columns, `probe`, `symbol` and `sample`, which store the associated covariates. This is an instance of **long format**.

In `xwdf`, some columns refer to data from all the samples (namely, `probe` and `symbol`), whereas other columns (those with the expression measurements) contain information that is sample specific. We somehow have to "know" which is which when interpreting the dataframe. This is what Hadley Wickham calls **untidy data**.[16] In contrast, in the tidy dataframe `xldf`, each row forms exactly one observation, its value is in the column named `value`, and all other information associated with that observation is in the other colums of the same row. If we want to add additional columns, say, Ensembl gene identifiers or chromosome locations, we can simply add them, and we can be sure that we will not break existing code – in contrast to `xwdf`, where we cannot be sure how code using it differentiates between data columns (with measured values) and covariate columns.

[16] Recall the Anna Karenina principle: there are many different ways for data to be untidy.

The plotting functions in *ggplot2* and the data manipulation functions in *dplyr* are designed to work with data in the long format. Don't try using them on wide format tables – this will only lead to frustration. Rather, use the *reshape2* package and its `melt` function to reshape the data.

13.11   Tidy data – using it wisely

In tidy data (Wickham, 2014):

1. each variable forms a column,
2. each observation forms a row, and
3. each type of observational unit forms a table.

The success of the *tidyverse* attests to the power of its underlying ideas and the quality of its implementation. Much of the code for this book has adopted these ideas and uses the tidyverse.

Nevertheless, dataframes in the long format are not a panacea. Here are some things to keep in mind.

Efficiency and integrity.   Even though there are only four probe-gene symbol relationships, we repeatedly store them 404 times in the rows of `xldf`. In this instance, the extra storage cost is negligible. In other cases, it could be considerable. More important is the cost of diffuse information: when we are given an object like `xldf` and want to know all the probe-gene symbol relationships it uses, we have to gather this information back from the many copies of it in the dataframe. We cannot be sure, without further checking, that the redundant copies of the information are consistent with each other; if we want to update the information, we have to change it in many places. This speaks for workflow designs in which an object like `xldf` is not used for long-term data storage, but is assembled at a relatively late stage of analysis from more normalized[17] data containers that contain the primary data objects.

[17] Data normalization is the process of organizing a database to reduce redundancy and improve integrity; see, e.g., the Wikipedia article on *database normalization*.

Lack of contracts and standardization.   When we write a function that expects to work on an object like `xldf`, we have no guarantee that the column `probe` does indeed contain valid probe identifiers, or that such a column even exists. There is not even a proper way to express programmatically what "an object like `xldf`" means in the tidyverse. Object-oriented (OO) programming, and its incarnation S4 in R, solves such questions. For instance, the above-mentioned checks could be performed by a `validObject` method for a suitably defined class, and the class definition would formalize the notion of "an object like `xldf`". Addressing such issues is behind the object-oriented design of the data structures in Bioconductor, such as the *SummarizedExperiment* class. Other potentially useful features of OO data representations include:

- Abstraction of interface from implementation and encapsulation: the user accesses the data only through defined channels and does not need to see how the data are stored "inside" – which means the inside can be changed and optimized without breaking user-level code.
- Polymorphism: you can have different functions with the same name, such as `plot` or `filter`, for different classes of objects, and R figures out for you which to call.
- Inheritance: you can build up more complex data representations from simpler ones.
- Reflection and self-documentation: you can send programmatic queries to an object to ask for information about itself.

All of these make it easier to write high-level code that focuses on the "big picture" functionality rather than on implementation details of the building blocks – albeit at the cost of more initial investment in infrastructure and "bureaucracy".

Data provenance and metadata.   There is no obvious place in an object like `xldf` to add information about data provenance; e.g., who performed the experiment, where it was published, where the data were downloaded from, or which version of the data we're looking at (data bugs exist. . .). Neither are there any explanations of the columns, such as units and assay type. Again, the data classes in Bioconductor try to address this.

Matrix-like data.   Many datasets in biology have a natural matrix-like structure, since a number of features (e.g., genes: conventionally, the rows of the matrix) are assayed on

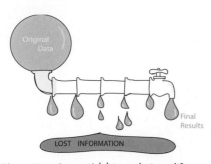

Figure 13.14: Sequential data analysis *workflows* can be leaky. If insufficient information is passed from one stage to the next, the procedure will end up being suboptimal and losing power.

[18] For instance, for the RNA-Seq differential expression analysis that we saw in Chapter 8, we needed the actual read counts, not "normalized" versions; for some analyses, gene-level summaries might suffice, for others, we'll want to look at the exon or isoform level.

[19] `http://stats.stackexchange.com/a/744`

several samples (conventionally, the columns of the matrix). Unrolling the matrix into a long form like `xldf` makes some operations (say, PCA, SVD, clustering of features or samples) more awkward.

13.12 Leaky pipelines and statistical sufficiency

Data analysis pipelines in high-throughput biology often work as "funnels" that successively summarize and compress the data. In high-throughput sequencing, we may start with individual sequencing reads, then align them to a reference, then only count the aligned reads for each position, summarize positions to genes (or other kinds of regions), then "normalize" these numbers by library size to make them comparable across libraries, etc. At each step, we lose information, yet it is important to make sure we still have enough information for the task at hand.[18] The problem is particularly acute if we build our data pipeline with a series of components from separate developers.

Statisticians have a concept for whether certain summaries enable the reconstruction of all the relevant information in the data: **sufficiency**. In a binomial random experiment with a known number n of trials, the number of successes is a sufficient statistic for estimating the probability of success p.

▶ Question **13.14** In a four-state Markov chain (A, C, G, T) such as the one we saw in Chapter 10, what are the sufficient statistics for estimating the transition probabilities?

◀

Iterative approaches akin to what we saw when we used the EM algorithm can sometimes help to avoid information loss. For instance, when analyzing *mass spectroscopy* data, a first run guesses at peaks individually for each sample. After this preliminary spectrum-spotting, another iteration allows us to borrow strength from the other samples to spot spectra that may have been overlooked (or looked like noise) before.

13.13 Efficient computing

The rapid progress in data acquisition technologies leads to ever larger datasets, and dealing with these is a challenge. It is tempting to jump right into software technologies that are designed for big data and scalability. But usually it is more helpful to first take a step back. Software engineers know the risks of **premature optimization**, or to paraphrase John Tukey:[19] "A slow and clumsy solution to the right problem is worth a good deal more than a fast and scalable solution to the wrong problem." Sometimes a good strategy is to figure out the right solution on a subset of the data before embarking on the quest for scalability and performance.

It's also good to keep in mind the value of your own time versus that of the CPU. If you can save some of your time developing code, even at the cost of longer computations, that can be a worthwhile trade-off.

Having considered all that, let's talk about performance. R has a reputation for being slow and wasteful of memory, and that perception sometimes motivates the choice of another platform. In some cases, this is justified: nobody would advocate writing a short-read aligner or the steering logic of a self-driving car in R. For statistical analyses, however, it is possible to write very efficient code using one or more of these concepts:

Vectorization. Consider the following alternatives for computing the same result.

```
a = runif(1e6)
b = runif(length(a))
system.time({
  z1 = numeric(length(a))
  for (i in seq(along = a))
    z1[i] = a[i]^2 * b[i]
})
##     user   system  elapsed
##    0.178    0.004    0.390
system.time({
  z2 = a^2 * b
})
##     user   system  elapsed
##    0.004    0.003    0.018
identical(z1, z2)
## [1] TRUE
```

The vectorized version ($z2$) is many times faster than the explicitly indexed one ($z1$) and even easier to read. Sometimes translating an algorithm that is formulated with indices is a little harder – say, if there are `if` conditions, or if the computation for index i involves results from index $i-1$. Language constructs such as vectorized conditionals with `ifelse`, shifting of vectors with functions such as `lead` and `lag` in the *dplyr* package, and generally the infrastructure of *dplyr*, which is designed to express computations on whole dataframes (rather than row by row), can help.

Parallelization. Parallelizing computations with R is easy, not least because it is a functional language in which it is natural to express computations as functions with explicit input and output, and no side effects. The landscape of R packages and functionality to support parallelized computing is fast-moving; the *CRAN task view on high-performance & parallel computing with R* and the package *BiocParallel* are good starting points.

Out-of-memory data and chunking. Some datasets are too big to load into random access memory (RAM) and manipulate all at once. Chunking means splitting the data into manageable portions ("chunks") and then sequentially loading each portion, computing on it, storing the result and removing it from memory before loading the next portion. R also offers infrastructure for working with large datasets that are stored on disk in a relational database management systems (the *DBI* package) or in *HDF5* (the *rhdf5* package). The Bioconductor project provides the class *SummarizedExperiment*, which can store big data matrices either in RAM or in an HDF5 backend in a manner that is transparent to the user of objects of this class.

Judicious use of lower level languages. The *Rcpp* package makes it easy to write portions of your code in C++ and include them seamlessly within your R code. Many convenient wrappers are provided, such as, below, the C++ class `NumericVector` that wraps the R class *numeric* vector.

```
library("Rcpp")
cppFunction("
  NumericVector myfun(NumericVector x, NumericVector y) {
    int n = x.size();
    NumericVector out(n);
    for(int i = 0; i < n; ++i) {
      out[i] = pow(x[i], 2) * y[i];
    }
    return out;
  }")
z3 = myfun(a, b)
identical(z1, z3)
## [1] TRUE
```

In practice, the above code should also contain a check on the length of `y`. Here, we provided the C++ code to *Rcpp* as an R character vector, and this is convenient for short injections. For larger functions, you can store the C++ code in an extra file. The idea is, of course, not to write a lot of code in C++, but only the most time-critical parts.

13.14   Summary of this chapter

In this final chapter, we have tried to collect, generalize and sort some of the concepts and ideas that popped up throughout the book, and that can help you to design informative experiments or studies and analyze them effectively. Some of these ideas are intuitive and natural. Others are perhaps less intuitive, such as Hotelling's weighting example in Section 13.4.3, which requires formal mathematical reasoning. Even when you cannot do an analytical computation, you might be able to do simulations or compute on similar existing data to benchmark different, non-obvious design choices.

Yet again, other ideas require discipline and foresight: for instance, the need to look at "dailies" might easily be forgotten or rationalized away in the heat of an experimental campaign, with so many other concerns competing for time and attention. You might get away with occasionally not keeping your kitchen tidy or not eating healthily – as a general approach, it is not recommended.

We have emphasized the importance of computing practices. Throughout the book, with its quantity of interwoven code and almost all "live" data visualizations, we have seen many examples of how to set up computational analyses. Nevertheless, running your own analysis on your own data is a very different experience from following the computations in a book – just like reading a cookbook is very different from preparing a banquet, or even just one dish. To equip you further, we highly recommend the resources mentioned in Section 13.15. And we wish you good cooking!

13.15 Further reading

- This chapter presented a pragmatic and brief introduction to *experimental design*. There are many book-length treatments that offer detailed advice on setting up experiments to *avoid confounding* and *optimize power*. Examples are Wu and Hamada (2011), Box et al. (1978) and Glass (2007).
- We have not even scratched the surface of more sophisticated procedures. For instance, if you have the possibility of setting up a sequence of experiments that you might stop once you can make a decision, you will need to study **sequential design** (Lai, 2001). Exploring *complex response surfaces* by choosing "good" starting points and then using successive results to choose further points can be very effective; Box et al. (1987) is an invaluable resource.
- Gentleman et al. (2004) explain the ideas behind Bioconductor data structures and software design, and Huber et al. (2015) give an update on how Bioconductor supports collaborative software development for users and developers.
- **Git and GitHub.** Jenny Bryan's website *Happy Git and GitHub for the useR* is a great introduction to using version control with R.
- Wickham (2014) explains the principles of *tidy data.*
- *Good enough practices.* Wilson et al. (2017) give a pragmatic and wise set of recommendations for how to be successful in scientific computing.
- The manual *Writing R Extensions* is the ultimate reference for R package authoring. It can be consumed in conjunction with the Bioconductor package guidelines.

13.16 Exercises

▶ Exercise **13.1** Set up a simulation experiment to decide how many subjects you need, given that you know your measurements will be affected by noise that follows a symmetric Laplace distribution (infinite mixture of normal distributions as defined in Chapter 4). You need to set up a table with different possible noise levels and effect sizes. ◀

▶ Exercise **13.2** Use the Bioconductor package *PROPER* to decide the number of samples for an RNA-Seq experiment, and compare your results to those from the *RNASeqPower* Bioconductor package. ◀

▶ Exercise **13.3** Check out R's `model.matrix` function. Read its manual page and explore the examples given there. ◀

▶ Exercise **13.4** Go back to one of your recent data analyses and assemble it into an R package. ◀

▶ Exercise **13.5** Open an account at GitHub and upload your package. Hint: follow the instructions at Jenny Bryan's *Happy Git and GitHub for the useR* site. ◀

Acknowledgements

This work would not be imaginable without the R language and environment for statistical computing, the Comprehensive R Archive Network (CRAN) and the Bioconductor project. We thank everyone who has contributed to these projects. Today virtually every statistical algorithm, every imaginable interface for data handling and visualization, and many methods from all over computer science and mathematics are readily accessible through these projects.

We thank J.J. Allaire and the RStudio team for making available such a powerful development environment and many useful R packages, which we have greatly enjoyed when writing this book.

We particularly thank the Bioconductor project, started by Robert Gentleman, led by Martin Morgan and powered by its amazing community of developers, for fostering interoperability, scalability and usability of R-based methods for genome-scale data, for making a vast range of biological data and annotation resources easy to work with in R, and for orchestrating collaborative, distributed development – all these aspects are essential for the complex biological data analysis workflows that you will see in this book.

We are grateful to the package developers we have worked with and whose packages play at center stage in the different chapters of this book, including Simon Anders, Ben Callahan, Michael Love, Joey McMurdie and Andrzej Oleś.

Trevor Martin was a student in Stats 366 at Stanford in 2012 and co-taught the class with Susan in 2013, 2014 and 2015. As a graduate student in genetics, he brought many of the examples to life and participated in earlier versions of the material we present here. We are thankful for his help and perspective. Teaching assistants for Stats 366 who have helped develop exercises and questions include Julia Fukuyama, Austen Head, Nikolaos Ignatiadis, Haben Michael, Lan Huong Nguyen and Christof Seiler. Their enthusiasm for making interesting quizzes and lab material helped nurture students from a wide range of backgrounds on the arduous journey of approaching challenging new concepts within a computational environment that has tremendous power, yet can also be overwhelming.

Many students have provided valuable feedback over the years, and we are grateful for the many questions and quizzical looks that fed our motivation to keep evolving this course. In particular, we have received extensive feedback from Jessica Grembi, Varun Gupta, Chao Jiang and Kris Sankaran.

We thank David Tranah and Diana Gillooly from Cambridge University Press for their constant effort helping us to make the book grammatically correct, aesthetically attractive and pedagogically coherent. Much potential for improvement remains, the responsibility for which stays with us.

We thank our family and supporters who have encouraged us and provided feedback on preliminary chapters: Catherine Blish, Persi Diaconis, Don Knuth, Gretchen and Barry Mazur, David Relman, Alfred Spormann, …

Susan Holmes	Wolfgang Huber
Stanford	Heidelberg

January 2018

Bibliography

1000 Genomes Project Consortium. An integrated map of genetic variation from 1,092 human genomes. *Nature*, 491(7422):56–65, 2012.

Abbott, Edwin A . *Flatland: A Romance of Many Dimensions*. Oxford University Press, 1884.

Agresti, Alan. *An Introduction to Categorical Data Analysis*. Wiley, 2007.

Altman, Naomi, and Martin Krzywinski. Points of significance: interpreting p-values. *Nature Methods*, 14(3):213–214, 2017.

Ambroise, Christophe, and Geoffrey J. McLachlan. Selection bias in gene extraction on the basis of microarray gene-expression data. *PNAS*, 99(10):6562–6566, 2002.

Anders, Simon, and Wolfgang Huber. Differential expression analysis for sequence count data. *Genome Biology*, 11:R106, 2010.

Anders, Simon, Alejandro Reyes, and Wolfgang Huber. Detecting differential usage of exons from RNA-Seq data. *Genome Research*, 22(10):2008–2017, 2012.

Anscombe, Francis J. The transformation of Poisson, binomial and negative-binomial data. *Biometrika*, 35:246–254, 1948.

Aure, Miriam Ragle, Valeria Vitelli, Sandra Jernström, Surendra Kumar, Marit Krohn, Eldri U Due, Tonje Husby Haukaas, Suvi-Katri Leivonen, Hans Kristian Moen Vollan, Torben Lüders, et al. Einar Rødland, Charles J. Vaske, Wei Zhao, Elen K. Møller, Silje Nord, Guro F. Giskeødegård, Tone Frost Bathen, Carlos Caldas, Trine Tramm, Jan Alsner, Jens Overgaard, Jürgen Geisler, Ida R.K. Bukholm, Bjørn Naume, Ellen Schlichting, Torill Sauer, Gordon B. Mills, Rolf Kåresen, Gunhild M. Mælandsmo, Ole Christian Lingjærde, Arnoldo Frigessi, Vessela N. Kristensen, Anne-Lise Børresen-Dale, Kristine K. Sahlberg. Integrative clustering reveals a novel split in the luminal A subtype of breast cancer with impact on outcome. *Breast Cancer Research*, 19(1):44, 2017.

Bacher, Rhonda, and Christina Kendziorski. Design and computational analysis of single-cell RNA-sequencing experiments. *Genome Biology*, 17(1):1, 2016.

Baddeley, Adrian J. Spatial sampling and censoring. In *Stochastic Geometry: Likelihood and Computation*, edited by O.E. Barndorff-Nielsen, W.S. Kendall, and M.N.M. van Lieshout, pages 37–78. Chapman and Hall, 1998.

Baddeley, Adrian, Jesper Moller, and Rasmus Waagepetersen. Non- and semi-parametric estimation of interaction in inhomogeneous point patterns. *Statistica Neerlandica*, 54:329–350, 2000.

Beisser, Daniela, Gunnar W. Klau, Thomas Dandekar, Tobias Müller, and Marcus T. Dittrich. BioNet: an R-package for the functional analysis of biological networks. *Bioinformatics*, 26(8):1129–1130, 2010.

Belkin, Mikhail, and Partha Niyogi. Laplacian eigenmaps for dimensionality reduction and data representation. *Neural Computation*, 15(6):1373–1396, 2003.

Bellman, Richard Ernest. *Adaptive Control Processes: A Guided Tour*. Princeton University Press, 1961.

Bendall, Sean C., Garry P. Nolan, Mario Roederer, and Pratip K. Chattopadhyay. A deep profiler's guide to cytometry. *Trends in Immunology*, 33(7):323–332, 2012.

Bengio, Yoshua, Jean-François Paiement, Pascal Vincent, Olivier Delalleau, Nicolas Le Roux, and Marie Ouimet. Out-of-sample extensions for LLE, isomap, MDS, eigenmaps, and spectral clustering. *Advances in Neural Information Processing Systems*, 16:177–184, 2004.

Benjamini, Yoav, and Marina Bogomolov. Selective inference on multiple families of hypotheses. *Journal of the Royal Statistical Society B*, 76(1):297–318, 2014.

Benjamini, Yoav, and Yosef Hochberg. Controlling the false discovery rate: a practical and powerful approach to multiple testing. *Journal of the Royal Statistical Society B*, 57:289–300, 1995.

Benjamini, Yoav, and Daniel Yekutieli. Hierarchical FDR testing of trees of hypotheses. Technical report, Department of Statistics and Operations Research, Tel Aviv University, 2003.

Bhattacharya, Bhaswar B. Power of graph-based two-sample tests. arXiv:1508.07530, 2015.

Boland, Michael V., and Robert F. Murphy. A neural network classifier capable of recognizing the patterns of all major subcellular structures in fluorescence microscope images of HeLa cells. *Bioinformatics*, 17(12):1213–1223, 2001.

Bouckaert, Remco, Joseph Heled, Denise Kühnert, Tim Vaughan, Chieh-Hsi Wu, Dong Xie, Marc A. Suchard, Andrew Rambaut, and Alexei J. Drummond. BEAST 2: a software platform for Bayesian evolutionary analysis. *PLoS Computational Biology*, 10(4):e1003537, 2014.

Bourgon, Richard, Robert Gentleman, and Wolfgang Huber. Independent filtering increases detection power for high-throughput experiments. *PNAS*, 107(21):9546–9551, 2010.

Box, George E.P., William G. Hunter, and J. Stuart Hunter. *Statistics for Experimenters: An Introduction to Design, Data Analysis, and Model Building.* John Wiley and Sons, 1978.

Box, George E.P., and Norman Richard Draper. *Empirical Model Building and Response Surfaces.* Wiley, 1987.

Brodie, Eoin L., Todd Z. DeSantis, Dominique C. Joyner, Seung M. Baek, Joern T. Larsen, Gary L. Andersen, Terry C. Hazen, Paul M. Richardson, Donald J. Herman, T.K. Tokunaga, J.M. Wan, and M.K. Firestone. Application of a high-density oligonucleotide microarray approach to study bacterial population dynamics during uranium reduction and reoxidation. *Applied and Environmental Microbiology*, 72(9):6288–6298, 2006.

Brooks, Angela N., Li Yang, Michael O. Duff, Kasper D. Hansen, Jung W. Park, Sandrine Dudoit, Steven E. Brenner, and Brenton R. Graveley. Conservation of an RNA regulatory map between *Drosophila* and mammals. *Genome Research*, 21(2):193–202, 2011.

Bulmer, Michael George. *Francis Galton: Pioneer of Heredity and Biometry.* Johns Hopkins University Press, 2003.

Callahan, Ben J., Kris Sankaran, Julia A. Fukuyama, Paul J. McMurdie, and Susan P. Holmes. Bioconductor workflow for microbiome data analysis: from raw reads to community analyses. *F1000Research*, 5, 2016a.

Callahan, Benjamin J., Paul J. McMurdie, Michael J. Rosen, Andrew W. Han, Amy J. Johnson, and Susan P. Holmes. DADA2: High resolution sample inference from amplicon data. *Nature Methods*, 1–4, 2016b.

Callahan, Benjamin J., Paul J. McMurdie, and Susan P. Holmes. Exact sequence variants should replace operational taxonomic units in marker gene data analysis. *ISME Journal*, 1–5, 2017.

Cannings, Chris, and Anthony W.F. Edwards. Natural selection and the de Finetti diagram. *Annals of Human Genetics*, 31(4):421–428, 1968.

Caporaso, J.G., J. Kuczynski, J. Stombaugh, K. Bittinger, F.D. Bushman, E.K. Costello, N. Fierer, A.G. Peña, J.K. Goodrich, J.I. Gordon, and R. Knight. QIIME allows analysis of high-throughput community sequencing data. *Nature Methods*, 7(5):335–336, 2010.

Carpenter, Anne E., Thouis R. Jones, Michael R. Lamprecht, Colin Clarke, In Han Kang, Ola Friman, David A. Guertin, Joo Han Chang, Robert A. Lindquist, and Jason Moffat. CellProfiler: image analysis software for identifying and quantifying cell phenotypes. *Genome Biology*, 7:R100, 2006.

Carr, Daniel B., Richard J. Littlefield, W.L. Nicholson, and J.S. Littlefield. Scatterplot matrix techniques for large N. *Journal of the American Statistical Association*, 82(398):424–436, 1987.

Chakerian, John, and Susan Holmes. Computational tools for evaluating phylogenetic and hierarchical clustering trees. *Journal of Computational and Graphical Statistics*, 21(3):581–599, 2012.

Chen, Min, Yang Xie, and Michael Story. An exponential-gamma convolution model for background correction of Illumina BeadArray data. *Communications in Statistics Theory and Methods*, 40(17):3055–3069, 2011.

Chessel, Daniel, Anne Dufour, and Jean Thioulouse. The ade4 package – i: One-table methods. *R News*, 4(1):5–10, 2004.

Chiu, Sung Nok, Dietrich Stoyan, Wilfrid S. Kendall, and Joseph Mecke. *Stochastic Geometry and Its Applications.* Springer, 2013.

Clemmensen, Line, Trevor Hastie, Daniela Witten, and Bjarne Ersbøll. Sparse discriminant analysis. *Technometrics*, 53:406–413, 2011.

Cleveland, William S. *The Collected Works of John W. Tukey: Graphics 1965-1985*, volume 5. CRC Press, 1988.

Cleveland, William S., Marylyn E. McGill, and Robert McGill. The shape parameter of a two-variable graph. *Journal of the American Statistical Association*, 83:289–300, 1988.

Cole, J.R., Q. Wang, E. Cardenas, J. Fish, B. Chai, R.J. Farris, A.S. Kulam-Syed-Mohideen, D.M. McGarrell, T. Marsh, G.M. Garrity, and J.M. Tiedje. The ribosomal database project: improved alignments and new tools for rrna analysis. *Nucleic Acids Research*, 37(Supplement 1):D141–D145, 2009.

Cook, R. Dennis. Detection of influential observation in linear regression. *Technometrics*, 19:15–18, 1977.

Cressie, Noel A. *Statistics for Spatial Data*. John Wiley and Sons, 1991.

de Chaumont, Fabrice, Stéphane Dallongeville, Nicolas Chenouard, Nicolas Hervé, Sorin Pop, Thomas Provoost, Vannary Meas-Yedid, Praveen Pankajakshan, Timothé Lecomte, Yoann Le Montagner, Thibault Lagache, Alexandre Dufour, and Jean-Christophe Olivo-Marin. Icy: an open bioimage informatics platform for extended reproducible research. *Nature Methods*, 9:690–696, 2012.

de Finetti, Bruno. Considerazioni matematiche sull'ereditarieta mendeliana. *Metron*, 6:3–41, 1926.

Diaconis, Persi, and David Freedman. Finite exchangeable sequences. *Annals of Probability*, 8:745–764, 1980.

Diaconis, Persi, and Susan Holmes. Gray codes for randomization procedures. *Statistics and Computing*, 4(4):287–302, 1994.

Diaconis, Persi, Sharad Goel, and Susan Holmes. Horseshoes in multidimensional scaling and kernel methods. *Annals of Applied Statistics*, 2:777–807, 2007a.

Diaconis, Persi, Susan Holmes, and Richard Montgomery. Dynamical bias in the coin toss. *SIAM Review*, 49(2):211–235, 2007b.

Diday, Edwin, and M. Paula Brito. Symbolic cluster analysis. In *Conceptual and Numerical Analysis of Data*, Otto Opitz (ed.), pp. 45–84. Springer, 1989.

Diggle, Peter J. *Statistical Analysis of Spatial and Spatio-Temporal Point Patterns*. Chapman and Hall/CRC, 2013.

DiGiulio, Daniel B., Benjamin J. Callahan, Paul J. McMurdie, Elizabeth K. Costello, Deirdre J. Lyelle, Anna Robaczewska, Christine L. Sun, Daniela S. Aliaga-Goltsman, Ronald J. Wongand, Gary M. Shaw, David K. Stevenson, Susan P. Holmes, and David A. Relman. Temporal and spatial variation of the human microbiota during pregnancy. *PNAS*, 112(35):11060-11065, 2015.

Dundar, Murat, Ferit Akova, Halid Z. Yerebakan, and Bartek Rajwa. A non-parametric Bayesian model for joint cell clustering and cluster matching: identification of anomalous sample phenotypes with random effects. *BMC Bioinformatics*, 15(1):1–15, 2014.

Durbin, Richard, Sean Eddy, Anders Krogh, and Graeme Mitchison. *Biological Sequence Analysis*. Cambridge University Press, 1998.

Efron, Bradley. *Large-Scale Inference: Empirical Bayes Methods for Estimation, Testing, and Prediction*. Cambridge University Press, 2010.

Efron, Bradley, and Robert J Tibshirani. *An Introduction to the Bootstrap*. Chapman and Hall/CRC, 1994.

Ekman, Gosta. Dimensions of color vision. *Journal of Psychology*, 38(2):467–474, 1954.

Elson, D., and E. Chargaff. On the desoxyribonucleic acid content of sea urchin gametes. *Experientia*, 8(4):143–145, 1952.

Felsenstein, Joseph. *Inferring Phylogenies*. Sinauer, 2004.

Fénelon, Jean-Pierre. *Qu'est-ce que l'analyse des données?* Lefonen Paris, 1981.

Fisher, Ronald Aylmer. *The Design of Experiments*. Oliver and Boyd, 1935.

Flury, Bernard. *A First Course in Multivariate Statistics*. Springer, 1997.

Freedman, David A. Statistical models and shoe leather. *Sociological Methodology*, 21(2):291–313, 1991.

Freedman, David, Robert Pisani, and Roger Purves. *Statistics*. W.W. Norton, 1997.

Friedman, Jerome H. On bias, variance, 0/1–loss, and the curse-of-dimensionality. *Data Mining and Knowledge Discovery*, 1: 55–77, 1997.

Friedman, Jerome H., and Lawrence C. Rafsky. Multivariate generalizations of the Wald–Wolfowitz and Smirnov two-sample tests. *Annals of Statistics*, 7:697–717, 1979.

Fukuyama, Julia, Paul J. McMurdie, Les Dethlefsen, David A. Relman, and Susan Holmes. Comparisons of distance methods for combining covariates and abundances in microbiome studies. In *Proc. Pacific Symposium on Biocomputing*, pp. 213–224, World Scientific, 2012.

Gentleman, Robert C., Vincent J. Carey, Douglas M. Bates, Ben Bolstad, Marcel Dettling, Sandrine Dudoit, Byron Ellis, Laurent Gautier, Yongchao Ge, Jeff Gentry, Kurt Hornik, Torsten Hothorn, Wolfgang Huber, Stefano Iacus, Rafael Irizarry, Friedrich Leisch, Cheng Li, Martin Maechler, Anthony J. Rossini, Gunther Sawitzki, Colin Smith, Gordon Smyth, Luke Tierney, Jean Y.H. Yang, and Jianhua Zhang. Bioconductor: open software development for computational biology and bioinformatics. *Genome Biology*, 5(10):R80, 2004.

Glass, David J. *Experimental Design for Biologists*. Cold Spring Harbor Laboratory Press, 2007.

Goslee, Sarah C., and Dean L. Urban. The ecodist package for dissimilarity-based analysis of ecological data. *Journal of Statistical Software*, 22(7):1–19, 2007.

Grantham, Richard, Christian Gautier, Manolo Gouy, M. Jacobzone, and R. Mercier. Codon catalog usage is a genome strategy modulated for gene expressivity. *Nucleic Acids Research*, 9(1):213–213, 1981.

Greenacre, Michael J. *Correspondence Analysis in Practice*. Chapman and Hall, 2007.

Grün, Bettina, Theresa Scharl, and Friedrich Leisch. Modelling time course gene expression data with finite mixtures of linear additive models. *Bioinformatics*, 28(2):222–228, 2012.

Guillot, Gilles, and François Rousset. Dismantling the mantel tests. *Methods in Ecology and Evolution*, 4(4):336–344, 2013.

Hallett, Robin M., Anna Dvorkin-Gheva, Anita Bane, and John A. Hassell. A gene signature for predicting outcome in patients with basal-like breast cancer. *Scientific Reports*, 2:227, 2012.

Hastie, Trevor, and Werner Stuetzle. Principal curves. *Journal of the American Statistical Association*, 84(406):502–516, 1989.

Hastie, Trevor, Robert Tibshirani, and Jerome Friedman. *The Elements of Statistical Learning*. Springer, 2nd edition, 2008.

Head, Megan L., Luke Holman, Rob Lanfear, Andrew T. Kahn, and Michael D. Jennions. The extent and consequences of p-hacking in science. *PLoS Biology*, 13(3):e1002106, 2015.

Held, M., M.H.A. Schmitz, B. Fischer, T. Walter, B. Neumann, M.H. Olma, M. Peter, J. Ellenberg, and D.W. Gerlich. CellCognition: time-resolved phenotype annotation in high-throughput live cell imaging. *Nature Methods*, 7:747, 2010.

Henderson, Fergus. Software engineering at Google. arXiv:1702.01715, 2017.

Hoeting, Jennifer A., David Madigan, Adrian E. Raftery, and Chris T. Volinsky. Bayesian model averaging: a tutorial. *Statistical Science*, 14:382–417, 1999.

Holmes, Susan. Phylogenetic trees: an overview. In *Statistics and Genetics*, 81–118. Springer, 1999.

Holmes, Susan. Bootstrapping phylogenetic trees: theory and methods. *Statistical Science*, 18(2):241–255, 2003a.

Holmes, Susan. Statistics for phylogenetic trees. *Theoretical Population Biology*, 63(1):17–32, 2003b.

Holmes, Susan. Multivariate analysis: The French way. In *Probability and Statistics: Essays in Honor of David A. Freedman*, D. Nolan and T.P. Speed, editors. IMS, 2006.

Holmes, Susan. Statistical proof? The problem of irreproducibility. *Bulletin of the AMS*, 55(1):31–55, 2018.

Holmes, Susan, Michael He, Tong Xu, and Peter P. Lee. Memory T cells have gene expression patterns intermediate between naive and effector. *PNAS*, 102(15):5519–5523, 2005.

Holmes, Susan, Adam Kapelner, and Peter P. Lee. An interactive Java statistical image segmentation system: GemIdent. *Journal of Statistical Software*, 30(10), 2009.

Holmes, Susan, Alexander V. Alekseyenko, Alden Timme, Tyrrell Nelson, Pankaj Jay Pasricha, and Alfred Spormann. Visualization and statistical comparisons of microbial communities using R packages on phylochip data. In *Proc. Pacific Symposium on Biocomputing*, 142–153. World Scientific, 2011.

Holmes Junca, Susan. *Outils Informatiques pour l'Évaluation de la Pertinence d'un Résultat en Analyse des Données*. PhD thesis, Université Montpellier II, France, 1985.

Hornik, Kurt. A CLUE for CLUster Ensembles. *Journal of Statistical Software*, 14(12), 2005.

Hotelling, Harold. Analysis of a complex of statistical variables into principal components. *Journal of Educational Psychology*, 24(6):417–441, 1933.

Hotelling, Harold. Some improvements in weighing and other experimental techniques. *Annals of Mathematical Statistics*, 15(3):297–306, 1944.

Huber, Peter J. Robust estimation of a location parameter. *Annals of Mathematical Statistics*, 35:73–101, 1964.

Huber, Wolfgang, Vincent J. Carey, Robert Gentleman, Simon Anders, Marc Carlson, Benilton S. Carvalho, Hector Corrada Bravo, Sean Davis, Laurent Gatto, Thomas Girke, Raphael Gottardo, Florian Hahne, Kasper D. Hansen, Rafael A. Irizarry, Michael Lawrence, Michael I. Love, James MacDonald, Valerie Obenchain, Andrzej K. Oleś, Hervé Pagès, Alejandro Reyes, Paul Shannon, Gordon K. Smyth, Dan Tenenbaum, Levi Waldron, and Martin Morgan. Orchestrating high-throughput genomic analysis with Bioconductor. *Nature Methods*, 12(2):115–121, 2015.

Hulett, Henry R., William A. Bonner, Janet Barrett, and Leonard A. Herzenberg. Cell sorting: automated separation of mammalian cells as a function of intracellular fluorescence. *Science*, 166(3906):747–749, 1969.

Ideker, Trey, Owen Ozier, Benno Schwikowski, and Andrew F. Siegel. Discovering regulatory and signalling circuits in molecular interaction networks. *Bioinformatics*, 18 (Supplement 1):S233–40, 2002.

Ignatiadis, Nikolaos, Bernd Klaus, Judith Zaugg, and Wolfgang Huber. Data-driven hypothesis weighting increases detection power in genome-scale multiple testing. *Nature Methods*, 13:577–580, 2016.

Ihaka, Ross. Color for presentation graphics. In *Proceedings of the 3rd International Workshop on Distributed Statistical Computing*, Kurt Hornik and Friedrich Leisch, editors. 2003.

Ihaka, Ross, and Robert Gentleman. R: A language for data analysis and graphics. *Journal of Computational and Graphical Statistics*, 5(3):299–314, 1996.

Irizarry, R.A., B. Hobbs, F. Collin, Y.D. Beazer-Barclay, K.J. Antonellis, U. Scherf, and T.P. Speed. Exploration, normalization, and summaries of high density oligonucleotide array probe level data. *Biostatistics*, 4(2):249–264, 2003.

Irizarry, Rafael A., Hao Wu, and Andrew P. Feinberg. A species-generalized probabilistic model-based definition of CpG islands. *Mammalian Genome*, 20(9-10):674–680, 2009.

Izenman, Alan Julian. Chapter 16 in *Nonlinear Dimensionality Reduction and Manifold Learning*, pp. 597–632. Springer, 2008.

Jacob, Laurent, Guillaume Obozinski, and Jean-Philippe Vert. Group lasso with overlap and graph lasso. In *Proceedings of the 26th Annual International Conference on Machine Learning*, pp. 433–440. ACM, 2009.

James, Gareth, Daniela Witten, Trevor Hastie, and Robert Tibshirani. *An Introduction to Statistical Learning*. Springer, 2013.

Jolicoeur, Pierre, James E. Mosimann, et al. Size and shape variation in the painted turtle. a principal component analysis. *Growth*, 24(4):339–354, 1960.

Jolliffe, Ian. *Principal Component Analysis*. Wilcy, 2002.

Jones, T., A. Carpenter, and P. Golland. Voronoi-based segmentation of cells on image manifolds. *Computer Vision for Biomedical Image Applications*, page 535, Lecture Notes in Computer Science, 3765. Springer, 2005.

Josse, Julie, and Susan Holmes. Measuring multivariate association and beyond. *Statistics Surveys*, 10:132–167, 2016.

Kahneman, Daniel. *Thinking, Fast and Slow*. Macmillan, 2011.

Kashyap, Purna C., Angela Marcobal, Luke K. Ursell, Samuel A. Smits, Erica D. Sonnenburg, Elizabeth K. Costello, Steven K. Higginbottom, Steven E. Domino, Susan P. Holmes, David A. Relman, J.I. Gordon, and J. Sonnenburg. Genetically dictated change in host mucus carbohydrate landscape exerts a diet-dependent effect on the gut microbiota. *PNAS*, 110(42):17059–17064, 2013.

Kaufman, Leonard, and Peter J. Rousseeuw. *Finding Groups in Data: An Introduction to Cluster Analysis*. Wiley, 2009.

Kendall, David. Incidence matrices, interval graphs and seriation in archeology. *Pacific Journal of Mathematics*, 28(3):565–570, 1969.

Kéry, Marc, and J. Andrew Royle. *Applied Hierarchical Modeling in Ecology: Analysis of Distribution, Abundance and Species Richness in R and BUGS. Volume 1: Prelude and Static Models*. Academic Press, 2015.

Kozich, James J., Sarah L. Westcott, Nielson T. Baxter, Sarah K. Highlander, and Patrick D. Schloss. Development of a dual-index sequencing strategy and curation pipeline for analyzing amplicon sequence data on the MiSeq Illumina sequencing platform. *Applied and Environmental Microbiology*, 79(17):5112–5120, 2013.

Kristiansson, Erik, Michael Thorsen, Markus J. Tamás, and Olle Nerman. Evolutionary forces act on promoter length: identification of enriched cis-regulatory elements. *Molecular Biology and Evolution*, 26(6):1299–1307, 2009.

Kuan, Pei Fen, Dongjun Chung, Guangjin Pan, James A. Thomson, Ron Stewart, and Sündüz Keleş. A statistical framework for the analysis of ChIP-Seq data. *Journal of the American Statistical Association*, 106(495):891–903, 2011.

Lai, Tze Leung. *Sequential Analysis*. Wiley, 2001.

Lange, Kenneth. *MM Optimization Algorithms*. SIAM, 2016.

Laufer, Christina, Bernd Fischer, Maximilian Billmann, Wolfgang Huber, and Michael Boutros. Mapping genetic interactions in human cancer cells with RNAi and multiparametric phenotyping. *Nature Methods*, 10:427–431, 2013.

Lawrence, Michael S., Petar Stojanov, Paz Polak, Gregory V. Kryukov, Kristian Cibulskis, Andrey Sivachenko, Scott L. Carter, Chip Stewart, Craig H. Mermel, Steven A. Roberts, Adam Kiezun, Peter S. Hammerman, Aaron McKenna, Yotam Drier, Lihua Zou, Alex H. Ramos, Trevor J. Pugh, Nicolas Stransky, Elena Helman, Jaegil Kim, Carrie Sougnez, Lauren Ambrogio, Elizabeth Nickerson, Erica Shefler, Maria L. Cortés, Daniel Auclair, Gordon Saksena, Douglas Voet, Michael Noble, Daniel DiCara, Pei Lin, Lee Lichtenstein, David I. Heiman, Timothy Fennell, Marcin Imielinski, Bryan Hernandez, Eran Hodis, Sylvan Baca, Austin M. Dulak, Jens Lohr, Dan-Avi Landau, Catherine J. Wu, Jorge Melendez-Zajgla, Alfredo Hidalgo-Miranda, Amnon Koren, Steven A. McCarroll, Jaume Mora, Ryan S. Lee, Brian Crompton, Robert Onofrio, Melissa Parkin, Wendy Winckler, Kristin Ardlie, Stacey B. Gabriel, Charles W. M. Roberts, Jaclyn A. Biegel, Kimberly Stegmaier, Adam J. Bass, Levi A. Garraway, Matthew Meyerson, Todd R. Golub, Dmitry A. Gordenin, Shamil Sunyaev, Eric S. Lander, and Gad Getz. Mutational heterogeneity in cancer and the search for new cancer-associated genes. *Nature*, 499(7457):214–218, 2013.

Leek, Jeffrey T., and John D. Storey. Capturing heterogeneity in gene expression studies by surrogate variable analysis. *PLoS Genetics*, 3(9):1724–1735, 2007.

Leek, Jeffrey T., Robert B. Scharpf, Héctor Corrada Bravo, David Simcha, Benjamin Langmead, W. Evan Johnson, Donald Geman, Keith Baggerly, and Rafael A. Irizarry. Tackling the widespread and critical impact of batch effects in high-throughput data. *Nature Reviews Genetics*, 11(10):733–739, 2010.

Li, Wen-Hsiung. *Molecular Evolution*. Sinauer, 1997.

Li, Wen-Hsiung, and Dan Graur. *Fundamentals of Molecular Evolution*. Sinauer, 1991.

Liberzon, Arthur, Aravind Subramanian, Reid Pinchback, Helga Thorvaldsdóttir, Pablo Tamayo, and Jill P. Mesirov. Molecular signatures database (MSigDB) 3.0. *Bioinformatics*, 27(12):1739–1740, 2011.

Love, Michael I., Wolfgang Huber, and Simon Anders. Moderated estimation of fold change and dispersion for RNA-Seq data with DESeq2. *Genome Biology*, 15(12):1–21, 2014.

Love, Michael I., Simon Anders, Vladislav Kim, and Wolfgang Huber. RNA-seq workflow: gene-level exploratory analysis and differential expression. *F1000Research*, 4(1070), 2015.

Mandal, Rakesh, Sophie St-Hilaire, John G. Kie, and DeWayne Derryberry. Spatial trends of breast and prostate cancers in the United States between 2000 and 2005. *International Journal of Health Geographics*, 8(1):53, 2009.

Mardia, Kanti, John T. Kent, and John M. Bibby. *Multivariate Analysis*. Academic Press, 1979.

Marin, Jean-Michel, and Christian Robert. *Bayesian Core: A Practical Approach to Computational Bayesian Statistics*. Springer, 2007.

McCormick Jr., William T., Paul J. Schweitzer, and Thomas W. White. Problem decomposition and data reorganization by a clustering technique. *Operations Research*, 20(5):993–1009, 1972.

McElreath, Richard. *Statistical Rethinking: A Bayesian Course with Examples in R and Stan*. Chapman and Hall/CRC, 2015.

McLachlan, Geoffrey, and Thriyambakam Krishnan. *The EM Algorithm and Extensions*. Wiley, 2007.

McLachlan, Geoffrey, and David Peel. *Finite Mixture Models*. Wiley, 2004.

McMurdie, Paul J., and Susan Holmes. Waste not, want not: why rarefying microbiome data is inadmissible. *PLoS Computational Biology*, 10(4):e1003531, 2014.

McMurdie, Paul J., and Susan Holmes. Shiny-phyloseq: web application for interactive microbiome analysis with provenance tracking. *Bioinformatics*, 31(2):282–283, 2015.

Mead, Roger. *The Design of Experiments: Statistical Principles for Practical Applications*. Cambridge University Press, 1990.

Moignard, Victoria, Steven Woodhouse, Laleh Haghverdi, Andrew J. Lilly, Yosuke Tanaka, Adam C. Wilkinson, Florian Buettner, Iain C. Macaulay, Wajid Jawaid, Evangelia Diamanti, Shin-Ichi Nishikawa, Nir Piterman, Valerie Kouskoff, Fabian J. Theis, Jasmin Fisher, and Berthold Göttgens. Decoding the regulatory network of early blood development from single-cell gene expression measurements. *Nature Biotechnology*, 33:269–276, 2015.

Mollon, John. Seeing colour. In *Colour: Art and Science*, T. Lamb and J. Bourriau, editors. Cambridge University Press, 1995.

Mood, Alexander M. On Hotelling's weighing problem. *Annals of Mathematical Statistics*, 17:432–446, 1946.

Mossel, Elchanan. On the impossibility of reconstructing ancestral data and phylogenies. *Journal of Computational Biology*, 10(5):669–676, 2003.

Mourant, A.E., Ada Kopec, and K. Domaniewska-Sobczak. *The Distribution of the Human Blood Groups*, Oxford University Press, 2nd edition, 1976.

Müllner, Daniel. Fastcluster: fast hierarchical, agglomerative clustering routines for R and Python. *Journal of Statistical Software*, 53(9):1–18, 2013.

Nacu, Serban, Rebecca Critchley-Thorne, Peter Lee, and Susan Holmes. Gene expression network analysis and applications to immunology. *Bioinformatics*, 23(7):850–8, 2007.

Nelson, Tyrell A., Susan Holmes, Alexander Alekseyenko, Masha Shenoy, Todd DeSantis, Cindy Wu, Gary Andersen, J. Winston, Justin Sonnenburg, Pankaj Jay Pasricha, and Alfred Spormann. PhyloChip microarray analysis reveals altered gastrointestinal microbial communities in a rat model of colonic hypersensitivity. *Neurogastroenterology and Motility*, 23:169–177, 2011.

Neumann, B., T. Walter, J.K. Heriche, J. Bulkescher, H. Erfle, C. Conrad, P. Rogers, I. Poser, M. Held, U. Liebel, C. Cetin, F. Sieckmann, G. Pau, R. Kabbe, A. Wunsche, V. Satagopam, M. H. Schmitz, C. Chapuis, D.W. Gerlich, R. Schneider, R. Eils, W. Huber, J.M. Peters, A.A. Hyman, R. Durbin, R. Pepperkok,

and J. Ellenberg. Phenotypic profiling of the human genome by time-lapse microscopy reveals cell division genes. *Nature*, 464(7289):721–727, 2010.

Neyman, Jerzy, and Egon S. Pearson. *Sufficient Statistics and Uniformly Most Powerful Tests of Statistical Hypotheses*. University of California Press, 1936.

Nolan, Daniel J., Michael Ginsberg, Edo Israely, Brisa Palikuqi, Michael G. Poulos, Daylon James, Bi-Sen Ding, William Schachterle, Ying Liu, Zev Rosenwaks, Jason M. Butler, Jenny Xiang, Arash Rafii, Koji Shido, Sina Y. Rabbani, Olivier Elemento, Shahin Rafii. Molecular signatures of tissue-specific microvascular endothelial cell heterogeneity in organ maintenance and regeneration. *Developmental Cell*, 26(2):204–219, 2013.

Ohnishi, Y., W. Huber, A. Tsumura, M. Kang, P. Xenopoulos, K. Kurimoto, A.K. Oles, M.J. Arauzo-Bravo, M. Saitou, A.K. Hadjantonakis, and T. Hiiragi. Cell-to-cell expression variability followed by signal reinforcement progressively segregates early mouse lineages. *Nature Cell Biology*, 16(1):27–37, 2014.

O'Neill, Kieran, Nima Aghaeepour, Josef Špidlen, and Ryan Brinkman. Flow cytometry bioinformatics. *PLoS Computational Biology*, 9(12):e1003365, 2013.

Ozsolak, Fatih, and Patrice M. Milos. RNA sequencing: advances, challenges and opportunities. *Nature Reviews Genetics*, 12:87–98, 2011.

Pagès, Jérôme. *Multiple Factor Analysis by Example Using R*. CRC Press, 2016.

Paradis, Emmanuel. *Analysis of Phylogenetics and Evolution with R*. Springer, 2011.

Pau, Grégoire, Florian Fuchs, Oleg Sklyar, Michael Boutros, and Wolfgang Huber. EBImage R package for image processing with applications to cellular phenotypes. *Bioinformatics*, 26(7):979–981, 2010.

Pearson, Karl. LIII. On lines and planes of closest fit to systems of points in space. *The London, Edinburgh, and Dublin Philosophical Magazine and Journal of Science*, 2(11):559–572, 1901.

Perraudeau, Fanny, Davide Risso, Kelly Street, Elizabeth Purdom, and Sandrine Dudoit. Bioconductor workflow for single-cell RNA sequencing: normalization, dimensionality reduction, clustering, and lineage inference. *F1000Research*, 6:1158, 2017.

Perrière, Guy, and Jean Thioulouse. Use and misuse of correspondence analysis in codon usage studies. *Nucleic Acids Research*, 30(20):4548–4555, 2002.

Pounds, Stan, and Stephan W. Morris. Estimating the occurrence of false positives and false negatives in microarray studies by approximating and partitioning the empirical distribution of p-values. *Bioinformatics*, 19(10):1236–1242, 2003.

Prentice, I.C. Non-metric ordination methods in ecology. *Journal of Ecology*, 65:85–94, 1977.

Purdom, Elizabeth. Analysis of a data matrix and a graph: metagenomic data and the phylogenetic tree. *Annals of Applied Statistics*, 5:2326–2358, 2011.

Purdom, Elizabeth, and Susan P. Holmes. Error distribution for gene expression data. *Statistical Applications in Genetics and Molecular Biology*, 4(1):16, 2005.

Rajaram, S., B. Pavie, L.F. Wu, and S.J. Altschuler. PhenoRipper: software for rapidly profiling microscopy images. *Nature Methods*, 9:635–637, 2012.

Reaven, G.M., and R.G. Miller. An attempt to define the nature of chemical diabetes using a multidimensional analysis. *Diabetologia*, 16(1):17–24, 1979.

Reyes, Alejandro, and Wolfgang Huber. Alternative start and termination sites of transcription drive most transcript isoform differences across human tissues. *Nucleic Acids Research*, 46(2):582–592, 2017.

Reyes, Alejandro, Simon Anders, Robert J. Weatheritt, Toby J. Gibson, Lars M. Steinmetz, and Wolfgang Huber. Drift and conservation of differential exon usage across tissues in primate species. *PNAS*, 110(38):15377–15382, sep 2013.

Rhee, Soo-Yon, Matthew J. Gonzales, Rami Kantor, Bradley J. Betts, Jaideep Ravela, and Robert W. Shafer. Human immunodeficiency virus reverse transcriptase and protease sequence database. *Nucleic Acids Research*, 31(1):298–303, 2003.

Rice, John. *Mathematical Statistics and Data Analysis*. Cengage Learning, 2006.

Ripley, B.D. *Statistical Inference for Spatial Processes*. Cambridge University Press, 1988.

Robert, Christian, and George Casella. *Introducing Monte Carlo Methods with R*. Springer, 2009.

Robins, Garry, Tom Snijders, Peng Wang, Mark Handcock, and Philippa Pattison. Recent developments in exponential random graph (p*) models for social networks. *Social Networks*, 29(2):192–215, 2007.

Robinson, M.D., D.J. McCarthy, and G.K. Smyth. edgeR: a Bioconductor package for differential expression analysis of digital gene expression data. *Bioinformatics*, 26(1):139–140, 2009.

Rocke, David M., and Blythe Durbin. A model for measurement error for gene expression arrays. *Journal of Computational Biology*, 8(6):557–569, 2001.

Ronquist, Fredrik, Maxim Teslenko, Paul van der Mark, Daniel L. Ayres, Aaron Darling, Sebastian Höhna, Bret Larget, Liang Liu, Marc A. Suchard, and John P. Huelsenbeck. Mrbayes 3.2: efficient bayesian phylogenetic inference and model choice across a large model space. *Systematic Biology*, 61(3):539–542, 2012.

Rosen, Michael J., Benjamin J. Callahan, Daniel S. Fisher, and Susan P. Holmes. Denoising PCR-amplified metagenome data. *BMC Bioinformatics*, 13(1):283, 2012.

Rousseeuw, Peter J. Silhouettes: a graphical aid to the interpretation and validation of cluster analysis. *Journal of Computational and Applied Mathematics*, 20:53–65, 1987.

Rousseeuw, Peter J., and Annick M. Leroy. *Robust Regression and Outlier Detection*. Wiley, 1987.

Roweis, Sam T., and Lawrence K. Saul. Nonlinear dimensionality reduction by locally linear embedding. *Science*, 290(5500):2323–2326, 2000.

Russ, John C., and F. Brent Neal. *The Image Processing Handbook*. CRC Press, 7th edition, 2015.

Sankaran, Kris, and Susan Holmes. structssi: simultaneous and selective inference for grouped or hierarchically structured data. *Journal of Statistical Software*, 59(1):1–21, 2014.

Schilling, Mark F. Multivariate two-sample tests based on nearest neighbors. *Journal of the American Statistical Association*, 81(395):799–806, 1986.

Schindelin, Johannes, Ignacio Arganda-Carreras, Erwin Frise, Verena Kaynig, Mark Longair, Tobias Pietzsch, Stephan Preibisch, Curtis Rueden, Stephan Saalfeld, Benjamin Schmid, Jean-Yves Tinevez, Daniel James White, Volker Hartenstein, Kevin Eliceiri, Pavel Tomancak, and Albert Cardona. Fiji: an open-source platform for biological-image analysis. *Nature Methods*, 9:676–682, 2012.

Schloss, P.D., S.L. Westcott, T. Ryabin, J.R. Hall, M. Hartmann, E.B. Hollister, R.A. Lesniewski, B.B. Oakley, D.H. Parks, C.J. Robinson, J.W. Sahl, B. Stres, G.G. Thallinger, D.J. Van Horn, and C.F. Weber. Introducing mothur: open-source, platform-independent, community-supported software for describing and comparing microbial communities. *Applied and Environmental Microbiology*, 75(23):7537–7541, 2009.

Schloss, P.D., A.M. Schuber, J.P. Zackular, K.D. Iverson, Young V.B., and Petrosino J.F. Stabilization of the murine gut microbiome following weaning. *Gut Microbes*, 3(4):383–393, 2012.

Schölkopf, Bernhard, Koji Tsuda, and Jean-Philippe Vert. *Kernel Methods in Computational Biology*. MIT Press, 2004.

Senn, Stephen. Controversies concerning randomization and additivity in clinical trials. *Statistics in Medicine*, 23:3729–3753, 2004.

Serra, Jean. *Image Analysis and Mathematical Morphology*. Academic Press, 1983.

Setiadi, A. Francesca, Nelson C. Ray, Holbrook E. Kohrt, Adam Kapelner, Valeria Carcamo-Cavazos, Edina B. Levic, Sina Yadegarynia, Chris M. Van Der Loos, Erich J. Schwartz, Susan Holmes, and P.P. Lee. Quantitative, architectural analysis of immune cell subsets in tumor-draining lymph nodes from breast cancer patients and healthy lymph nodes. *PLoS One*, 5(8):e12420, 2010.

Shalizi, Cosma. *Advanced Data Analysis from an Elementary Point of View*. Cambridge University Press, 2019.

Slonim, Noam, Gurinder Singh Atwal, Gašper Tkačik, and William Bialek. Information-based clustering. *PNAS*, 102(51):18297–18302, 2005.

Stegle, O., L. Parts, R. Durbin, and J. Winn. A Bayesian framework to account for complex non-genetic factors in gene expression levels greatly increases power in eQTL studies. *PLoS Computational Biology*, 6(5):e1000770, 2010.

Steijger, T., J.F. Abril, P.G. Engstrom, F. Kokocinski, T.J. Hubbard, R. Guigo, J. Harrow, P. Bertone, J.F. Abril, M. Akerman, T. Alioto, G. Ambrosini, S.E. Antonarakis, J. Behr, P. Bertone, R. Bohnert, P. Bucher, N. Cloonan, T. Derrien, S. Djebali, J. Du, S. Dudoit, P. Engstrom, M. Gerstein, T.R. Gingeras, D. Gonzalez, S.M. Grimmond, R. Guigo, L. Habegger, J. Harrow, T.J. Hubbard, C. Iseli, G. Jean, A. Kahles, F. Kokocinski, J. Lagarde,

J. Leng, G. Lefebvre, S. Lewis, A. Mortazavi, P. Niermann, G. Ratsch, A. Reymond, P. Ribeca, H. Richard, J. Rougemont, J. Rozowsky, M. Sammeth, A. Sboner, M.H. Schulz, S.M. Searle, N.D. Solorzano, V. Solovyev, M. Stanke, T. Steijger, B.J. Stevenson, H. Stockinger, A. Valsesia, D. Weese, S. White, B.J. Wold, J. Wu, T.D. Wu, G. Zeller, D. Zerbino, and M.Q. Zhang. Assessment of transcript reconstruction methods for RNA-seq. *Nature Methods*, 10(12):1177–1184, 2013.

Stigler, Stephen M. *The Seven Pillars of Statistical Wisdom*. Harvard University Press, 2016.

Strang, Gilbert. *Introduction to Linear Algebra*. Wellesley-Cambridge Press, 4th edition, 2009.

Tenenbaum, Joshua B., Vin De Silva, and John C. Langford. A global geometric framework for nonlinear dimensionality reduction. *Science*, 290(5500):2319–2323, 2000.

ter Braak, Cajo J.F. Correspondence analysis of incidence and abundance data: properties in terms of a unimodal response. *Biometrics*, 41:859–873, 1985.

Tibshirani, Robert. Regression shrinkage and selection via the lasso. *Journal of the Royal Statistical Society. Series B (Methodological)*, 58(1):267–288, 1996.

Tibshirani, Robert, Guenther Walther, and Trevor Hastie. Estimating the number of clusters in a data set via the gap statistic. *Journal of the Royal Statistical Society. Series B (Methodological)*, 63(2):411–423, 2001.

Trosset, Michael W., and Carey E. Priebe. The out-of-sample problem for classical multidimensional scaling. *Computational Statistics and Data Analysis*, 52(10):4635–4642, 2008.

Tseng, George C., and Wing H. Wong. Tight clustering: a resampling-based approach for identifying stable and tight patterns in data. *Biometrics*, 61(1):10–16, 2005.

Tukey, John W. *Exploratory Data Analysis*. Addison-Wesley, 1977.

Tversky, Amos, and Daniel Kahneman. Heuristics and biases: judgement under uncertainty. *Science*, 185:1124–1130, 1974.

Tversky, Amos, and Daniel Kahneman. Judgment under uncertainty: heuristics and biases. In *Utility, Probability, and Human Decision Making*, pp. 141–162. Springer, 1975.

Verhulst, Pierre-François. Recherches mathématiques sur la loi d'accroissement de la population. *Nouveaux Mémoires de l'Académie Royale des Sciences et Belles-Lettres de Bruxelles*, 18:1–42, 1845.

Vetterli, Martin, Jelena Kovačević, and Vivek Goyal. *Foundations of Signal Processing*. Cambridge University Press, 2014.

von Helmholtz, H. *Handbuch der Physiologischen Optik*. Leopold Voss, 1867.

Wang, Q., G.M. Garrity, J.M. Tiedje, and J.R. Cole. Naive Bayesian classifier for rapid assignment of RRNA sequences into the new bacterial taxonomy. *Applied and Environmental Microbiology*, 73(16):5261, 2007.

Wasserstein, Ronald L., and Nicole A. Lazar. The ASA's statement on p-values: context, process, and purpose. *The American Statistician*, 70:129–133, 2016.

Wertheim, Joel O., and Michael Worobey. Dating the age of the SIV lineages that gave rise to HIV-1 and HIV-2. *PLoS Computational Biology*, 5(5):e1000377, 2009.

Wickham, Hadley. A layered grammar of graphics. *Journal of Computational and Graphical Statistics*, 19(1):3–28, 2010.

Wickham, Hadley. Tidy data. *Journal of Statistical Software*, 59(10), 2014.

Wickham, Hadley. *ggplot2: Elegant Graphics for Data Analysis*. Springer, 2nd edition, 2016.

Wiel, Mark A., Tonje G. Lien, Wina Verlaat, Wessel N. Wieringen, and Saskia M. Wilting. Better prediction by use of co-data: adaptive group-regularized ridge regression. *Statistics in Medicine*, 35(3):368–381, 2016.

Wilkinson, Leland. Dot plots. *The American Statistician*, 53(3):276–281, 1999.

Wilkinson, Leland. *The Grammar of Graphics*. Springer, 2005.

Wills, Quin F., Kenneth J. Livak, Alex J. Tipping, Tariq Enver, Andrew J. Goldson, Darren W. Sexton, and Chris Holmes. Single-cell gene expression analysis reveals genetic associations masked in whole-tissue experiments. *Nature Biotechnology*, 31(8):748–752, 2013.

Wilson, Greg, Jennifer Bryan, Karen Cranston, Justin Kitzes, Lex Nederbragt, and Tracy K. Teal. Good enough practices in scientific computing. *PLOS Computational Biology*, 13(6):e1005510, 2017.

Witten, Daniela M., and Robert Tibshirani. Penalized classification using Fisher's linear discriminant. *Journal of the Royal Statistical Society. Series B (Methodological)*, 73(5):753–772, 2011.

Witten, Daniela M., Robert Tibshirani, and Trevor Hastie. A penalized matrix decomposition, with applications to sparse principal components and canonical correlation analysis. *Biostatistics*, 10(3): 515–534, 2009.

Wright, Erik S. DECIPHER: harnessing local sequence context to improve protein multiple sequence alignment. *BMC Bioinformatics*, 16(1):322, 2015.

Wu, C.F. Jeff, and Michael S. Hamada. *Experiments: Planning, Analysis, and Optimization*. Wiley, 2011.

Yu, Hongxiang, Diana L. Simons, Ilana Segall, Valeria Carcamo-Cavazos, Erich J. Schwartz, Ning Yan, Neta S. Zuckerman, Frederick M. Dirbas, Denise L. Johnson, Susan P. Holmes, and Peter P. Lee. PRC2/EED-EZH2 complex is up-regulated in breast cancer lymph node metastasis compared to primary tumor and correlates with tumor proliferation *in situ*. *PLOS One*, 7(12):e51239, 2012.

Zeileis, Achim, Christian Kleiber, and Simon Jackman. Regression models for count data in R. *Journal of Statistical Software*, 27(8), 2008.

Zeller, Georg, Julien Tap, Anita Y. Voigt, Shinichi Sunagawa, Jens Roat Kultima, Paul I. Costea, Aurélien Amiot, Jürgen Böhm, Francesco Brunetti, Nina Habermann, Rajna Hercog, Moritz Koch, Alain Luciani, Daniel R. Mende, Martin A. Schneider, Petra Schrotz-King, Christophe Tournigand, Jeanne Tran Van Nhieu, Takuji Yamada, Jürgen Zimmermann, Vladimir Benes, Matthias Kloor, Cornelia M. Ulrich, Magnus von Knebel Doeberitz, Iradj Sobhani, and Peer Bork. Potential of fecal microbiota for early-stage detection of colorectal cancer. *Molecular Systems Biology*, 10(11):766, 2014.

Zou, Hui, Trevor Hastie, and Robert Tibshirani. Sparse principal component analysis. *Journal of Computational and Graphical Statistics*, 15(2):265–286, 2006.

Statistical Concordance

Where are the statistical methods covered?

As a supplement to the index, we provide a list of statistical concepts and procedures and the chapters in which they are covered.

Method	Chapter	Method	Chapter
Analysis of variance	8	Markov chains	2, 10
Bayesian statistics	2	Maximum likelihood	2
Bootstrap	4, 5	Multidimensional scaling (MDS)	9
Chi-squared test	2	Multiple hypothesis testing	6
Classification	12	Multivariate regression	8, 9, 12
Clustering	4, 5	Nonlinear methods	9
Correspondence analysis	9	Ordination and gradient detection	9
Data transformations	4, 8	p-value	1, 2, 6
Differential expression analysis	8	Permutation tests	10
Distances	4, 9	Phylogenetics	10
Exploratory data analysis (EDA)	3	Power calculations	13
Fisher's exact test	10	Principal components (PCA)	7
False discovery rate (FDR)	6	Principal coordinates analysis (PCoA)	9
Goodness of fit	2	Regression	7, 8
Generalized linear models	8	RNA-Seq	8
Grammar of graphics	3	Robust methods	8
Hypergeometric test	10	Spatial statistics	11
Hypothesis testing	1, 6	Supervised learning	12

Index